Neurology

A Clinician's Approach

Neurology

A Clinician's Approach

Andrew Tarulli
Instructor in Neurology, Harvard Medical School, and Associate Residency Program Director,
Beth Israel Deaconess Medical Center, Boston, MA, USA

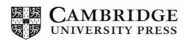

CAMBRIDGE UNIVERSITY PRESS
Cambridge, New York, Melbourne, Madrid, Cape Town, Singapore,
São Paulo, Delhi, Dubai, Tokyo, Mexico City

Cambridge University Press
The Edinburgh Building, Cambridge CB2 8RU, UK

Published in the United States of America by Cambridge University Press, New York

www.cambridge.org
Information on this title: www.cambridge.org/9780521722223

© Cambridge University Press 2011

First published 2011

Printed in the United Kingdom at the University Press, Cambridge

A catalog record for this publication is available from the British Library

Library of Congress Cataloging in Publication data
Tarulli, Andrew.
Neurology : a clinician's approach / Andrew Tarulli.
p. ; cm.
Includes bibliographical references and index.
ISBN 978-0-521-72222-3 (pbk.)
1. Nervous system–Diseases–Diagnosis.   2. Neurology.   I. Title.
[DNLM: 1. Nervous System Diseases–diagnosis.   2. Physical Examination–methods. WL 141]
RC346.T27 2011
616.8–dc22   2010034893

ISBN 978-0-521-72222-3 Paperback

For my parents, Marianne and Joe Tarulli, and my brother, Matt.

Contents

Foreword

Although there are many good textbooks of neurology – some of them extremely comprehensive and multi-volume in type, some of them presented as tabulated texts – none of them presents a basic clinical approach to the individual patient. When faced with an individual patient and an individual complaint, one must use deductive reasoning to come to a diagnosis. An accurate history leads the way and will more often than not provide the likely diagnosis. The history allows for a hypothesis, which must be tested by the clinical exam.

Dr. Tarulli has blazed a pathway from history through examination to diagnosis based on clinical acumen rather than on "blind" imaging searching for a possible diagnosis. Each chapter is in itself a pearl of information designed to teach the reader how to get from "chief complaint" to final diagnosis and then to consider further investigation when appropriate. Too often nowadays, there is a tendency to jump to technology without clearly thinking through a clinical problem, to the detriment of patient care and overutilization of expensive and sometimes unnecessary studies.

The book is written for advanced medical students and residents early in training and is a practical guide to patient care. It follows in the footsteps of classical clinical neurology and should prove invaluable to neurologists in training. These young doctors need a practical, symptom-based approach to patient care. This is the place to find it.

Michael Ronthal, MB BCh
Professor of Neurology
Harvard Medical School

Beth Israel Deaconess Medical Center
Boston, MA, USA
June 16, 2010

Preface

Does the world need another introductory neurology textbook? My initial answer was "no," but after considerable and considerate prodding by my publishers, I relented and decided to write *Neurology: A Clinician's Approach* for two reasons.

First, I wrote it because it is the book that I sought as a senior medical student and junior neurology resident. Although there were many great books that organized neurology by specific disease processes, I wanted to learn how a neurologist approached a problem. The question for me was: how does a neurologist start with a patient who comes into their office with falls and end by making a diagnosis of progressive supranuclear palsy? The answer is that they know how to ask the right questions, interpret the patient's answers, and perform a focused neurological examination that will lead them to the gold. This diagnostic process requires *basic* knowledge of anatomy and physiology, but *immeasurably more* experience with patients and recognition of both common and uncommon patterns of disease. The textbooks that I found sufficed on the anatomy and physiology fronts, but I needed the wisdom of my professors and some time to acquire the experience that would make me into a neurologist. My problem was that I was impatient and, try as I might, I could not find the wisdom I was looking for in any of the textbooks in the Countway Library of Medicine.

Secondly, it is derived from the series of case conferences that I lead on a twice-weekly basis with third-year Harvard medical students at Beth Israel Deaconess Medical Center. A student presents a case, and we begin, from the first sentence of their presentation, on a diagnostic journey that involves defining the problem, generating a list of possible anatomic localizations, discussing the utility of different tests, and considering treatments and their likely outcomes. These conferences are the highlights of my week: it gives me immense pleasure to help the students to connect the dots and put their universally impressive factual knowledge into clinical practice. My students have encouraged me to put my approach into writing, and the basic text of *Neurology: A Clinician's Approach* reflects our case conference format.

Each of the problems that face a neurologist requires a different approach. In general, however, the technique of *Neurology: A Clinician's Approach* is to start by defining the chief complaint, move to techniques concerning how to take the history and how to conduct a neurological examination relevant to the particular question, figure out which diagnostic tests to order, and then conclude with common disease processes and their management. Unlike introductory books, there is no single chapter dedicated to the neurological examination. Rather, I try to teach the examination as a tool to be used intelligently in order to reach a diagnosis. I have tried to limit redundancy through cross-referencing, but there is inevitably some overlap among the chief complaints. I have also tried to use the evidence as much as possible, but I am by no means a slave to it. Finally, I have addressed topics that are frequently ignored in other introductory neurology texts. There are discussions of fibromyalgia, Raynaud's phenomenon, and conversion disorders, for example, which are common in clinical practice but often exist outside of the vacuum of neurological diseases presented to the newcomer to the field.

I hope that many readers will find this book helpful. It is intended, as I noted, for upper-level medical students and beginning residents. The ideal target is a preliminary medicine intern who cannot wait to begin their neurology residency in July. There are others who I think may find this book valuable. Senior residents who have less exposure to outpatient neurological disease may find several sections useful. I also think that neurologists who have just finished their fellowships and face the daunting task of entering practice after a year in which they only saw neuromuscular diseases or movement disorders may enjoy it. This book may also be a good "insider's guide" for internists and psychiatrists. Regardless of your level of training, I hope that *Neurology: A Clinician's Approach* will leave you with a greater confidence (and excitement!) in approaching patients with neurological problems.

Andrew Tarulli
Boston, MA
May 16, 2010

Acknowledgments

Writing *Neurology: A Clinician's Approach* would not have been possible without my family, friends, mentors, colleagues, and students. Because I may never write another set of acknowledgments, I want to name as many of these people as possible.

I would like to thank my parents, Marianne and Joe Tarulli, and my best friend and brother, Matt Tarulli, for a lifetime of love and support.

I am fortunate to have so many great friends. Of course, this list must start with Pops and Pops, Greg Evangelista and Sal Savatta …

… and must continue with Thomas Kreibich, Patrick Huggins, Jimmy Yoo, Greg Piazza (Peter Poindexter), and Praveen Akuthota (Tall Walter Lomax). The many friends I have met during the course of my training include: Juan Acosta, Michael Benatar (for showing me that I could get something like this done while still young), Greg Esper, John Croom, Dan Cohen, Daniel Mattson (a fellow fan of S. Weir Mitchell and future brother-in-Langë), Sean Savitz, Judy Liu, Shiv Sohur, Jen Langsdorf, Ricardo Isaacson, Anh thu Nguyen, Ludy Shih, Jay Bhatt, Amy Amick, Laura Miller, Elayna Rubens, Nick Silvestri, Julie V. Roth, Marcus Yountz, and Ranee Niles.

My list of mentors must begin with Orrin Devinsky who started me on the road of academic neurology. This book would not have been possible without the guidance and attention I received as a resident at Beth Israel Deaconess Medical Center. I would like to acknowledge the entire faculty and my senior residents – sometimes I heard your voices dictating the very sentences of this book. In particular, I am indebted to Clif Saper for being the most supportive chairman I could imagine, for constantly challenging me to expand my knowledge and skill as a neurologist, and for seeing my calling before even I could; Mike Ronthal, the "generator of a generation," for being the consummate clinician whose style inspired this book and, I'm sure, many others; Frank Drislane who has been a constant source of wisdom, common sense, and humor; and Penny Greenstein for helping craft me into a neurologist through high standards and kind words.

Thanks to my colleagues in the neuromuscular division at Beth Israel Deaconess Medical Center for supporting me and understanding my need to go missing on a few Tuesdays in order to complete this project: Seward Rutkove, Beth Raynor, Pushpa Narayanaswami, Rachel Nardin, Rich Castonguay, Carrie Jarvie, Rebekah Hill, Cindy Aiello, and Maggie Fermental.

Of course, I could not forget my team at Cambridge University Press whose patience and encouragement made this project a reality: Beth Barry, Nisha Doshi, Nick Dunton, Chris Miller, and Jane Hoyle.

Thanks to all those who inspired me through this journey and life in general: James, Kirk, Dave, Marty, Jeff, Kerry, Bobby, D. D., Darrell, Eddie, Dan Gable, and of course, number 1, William Hayward Wilson.

Special thanks to those who helped me with EEG images (Julie Roth), error checking (Nick Silvestri), and pictures (Rebekah Hill, Maggie Fermental, Jed Barash, Sabra Abbott, Scott Boruchow, and Michelle Walk).

And finally, a heartfelt thanks to my students at Beth Israel Deaconess Medical Center and Harvard Medical School: opening your minds to this discipline of neurology is my passion, and it is my privilege to serve you.

Andrew Tarulli
Boston, MA
May 16, 2010

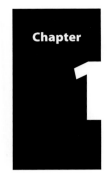

Chapter

1

Confusion

History

Confusion is a cognitive disorder characterized by loss of the normal coherent stream of thought or action.[1] Up to 50% of older hospitalized patients will develop an acute confusional state, and those who become confused are at greater risk for prolonged hospitalization and death.[2] Unfortunately, the confused patient cannot provide a reasonable account of the problem, and detailed narrative histories from family members, nurses, and primary physicians are often similarly unhelpful. The history may consist only of a single phrase such as "He's agitated," "He's not waking up," or "He's confused." Sometimes the history is comprised of examples of abnormal behavior. In many cases, especially when the physician requesting the consult does not know the patient very well, the history is summarized as nothing more than the ambiguous catch-all term "change in mental status."

The three variations of confusion are agitated delirium, somnolence, and incoherence. Despite their strikingly different phenotypes, these three states are all caused by a fundamental disturbance in the attentional matrix and a group of responsible medical conditions.

Agitated delirium

Agitated delirium is characterized by hyperactivity and aggressiveness, and is the most disruptive form of confusion. Patients with agitated delirium scream, yell, rip out intravenous catheters, and sometimes assault hospital staff or even other patients. They are often physically and chemically restrained or undergoing psychiatric evaluation by the time a neurologist is consulted.

Somnolence

Somnolent patients are sleepy and difficult to arouse. While this variant is less disruptive to the hospital staff than agitated delirium, somnolence is often serious, sometimes heralding the onset of coma. These patients,

therefore, require immediate medical and neurological attention.

Incoherence

Incoherence lies between agitated delirium and somnolent confusion on the arousal spectrum. These patients are neither aggressive nor sleepy, but lack the ability to think, speak, or act in a lucid, goal-directed manner.[1] Incoherent patients misidentify people and misinterpret situations, especially the circumstances of their hospitalization. They are easily distracted by novel but trivial stimuli and are inattentive to important ones.

Examination

Inattention

The signature mental status abnormality of the confused patient is inattention. This may become quite obvious with simple observation or when listening to the patient attempt to relate their history. Several bedside tests may help to establish inattention for patients with more subtle deficits:

Months of the year backwards

This is perhaps the best test of attention, as it allows both description and quantification of deficits. Normal people should be able to recite the months of the year backwards in 10–15 seconds. When asked to recite the months of the year backwards, the confused patient may respond in one of several ways. Agitated patients may erupt in anger at the request to perform such a silly task. Somnolent patients will give no response and quickly fall asleep. Incoherent patients may begin by starting with December, reciting November and October in the correct sequence, and then lose track of the task. Some may stop completely, while others may resume by reciting the months in calendar order. Still others may start with December, and when they reach November, start to talk about the fall or Thanksgiving.

Patients with only subtle inattention may make no mistake other than transposing the months in the May–April–March transition.

Reverse digit span

Digit span is another useful, quantifiable test of attention. To perform this test, first recite a list of random numbers at a rate of one digit per second, and then ask the patient to repeat the list to you *in sequence*. After establishing the forward digit span, ask the patient to recite a different number sequence backwards. Most people have digit spans of at least seven forwards and five backwards.

Serial sevens

Test serial sevens by asking the patient to subtract seven from 100 and then seven from that result and so on until they can subtract no more. This test of attention is somewhat dependent on the patient's mathematical abilities and education level, and is therefore less useful or quantifiable than testing the months of the year backwards or the reverse digit span.

Spelling "world" backwards

Spelling "world" backwards is generally not very useful, as the only common mistake is transposing the letters "l" and the "r," an error that is due to chance as often as it is to inattention.

Other changes in mental status

In addition to the primary disturbance in attention, confused patients often demonstrate a variety of other mental status examination abnormalities including problems with language, memory, and praxis (Chapters 3 and 4). Careful testing, however, shows that the main problem is inattention.

Asterixis

Asterixis accompanies most metabolic and some structural encephalopathies, and is not, as many believe, pathognomonic for hepatic encephalopathy. To test for asterixis, ask the patient to elevate their pronated arms and extend their wrists in front of them as if they are making stop signs. After a latent period of up to 30 seconds, both hands will drop forward slightly and then jerk backwards several times, quickly and asynchronously.[3] These movements are accompanied by tiny oscillations of the fingers. After

several jerks, the movements disappear, only to reappear a few seconds later.

Differential diagnosis

The four conditions that are most often "confused with confusion" are aphasia, neglect, transient global amnesia, and psychosis.

Aphasia

Aphasia is an acquired disorder of language resulting from brain damage (Chapter 3). It may be difficult to distinguish some patients with aphasia, particularly those with fluent varieties, from patients with acute confusional states. A patient with Wernicke's aphasia, for example, may appear confused because they produce a copious verbal output that makes little sense and because they do not appear to understand simple instructions. Confusion is best distinguished from aphasia by a more widespread pattern of cognitive dysfunction.

Neglect and the right hemispheric syndrome

Neglect[4] is a multidomain disorder of focused rather than global attention. This syndrome is seen most often in patients with right middle cerebral artery infarction, and when fully formed is almost always accompanied by left hemiparesis or hemiplegia. Many of the behaviors of a patient with neglect described here are quite unusual, and it is easy to see why a physician unfamiliar with the condition would mislabel the patient as being confused.

Visual neglect

Visual neglect is usually the most striking behavioral feature of the right hemispheric syndrome. The patient with severe neglect looks exclusively to the right side of space and may not respond to the examiner if approached from the left. Specific testing may be required to elicit neglect in patients with more subtle deficits. For example, the patient with neglect will describe fewer details of a complex visual scene. They will also have difficulty with line bisection. To perform this test, place an 8 ½″ × 11″ piece of blank paper in

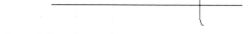

Figure 1.1 Line bisection test in a patient with neglect. Note that the line is bisected well to the right of the midline.

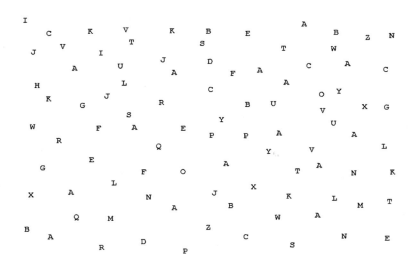

Figure 1.2 Template for the "A" cancellation task. The patient is instructed to circle the target letter "A." Patients with neglect will begin on the right side of the page and may completely ignore the left side.

landscape orientation before the patient. Draw a line across the page from left to right and instruct the patient to bisect the line. Normal subjects will come within a few millimeters of the center of the line, but the patient with neglect will bisect it to the right of the midline, sometimes within a few centimeters of the line's right side (Figure 1.1). Target cancellation is another useful test of hemineglect. Write the letter "A" in a random distribution approximately 15–20 times on a blank sheet of paper in landscape orientation (Figure 1.2). Make sure to distribute the target letter evenly on the left, right, center, top, and bottom. Next, surround the target with randomly chosen letters of the alphabet and instruct the patient to circle only the letter "A." The patient with neglect will circle the targets predominantly or even exclusively on the right side of the page.

Somatosensory neglect

To test for somatosensory neglect, first make sure that gross touch perception is preserved on both the left and right sides of the body, as somatosensory neglect cannot be diagnosed if basic sensation is impaired. Instruct the patient to close their eyes and gently stroke the dorsal surfaces of both hands. Patients with neglect will acknowledge only the sensation of being touched on the right hand, a phenomenon known as double simultaneous extinction.

Other elements of the right hemispheric syndrome

Patients with the right hemispheric syndrome are usually not aware of their deficits or deny them

explicitly, a phenomenon known as anosognosia. When asked why they are in the hospital, a patient with the right hemispheric syndrome may tell you that they should not be there because they feel well. They may tell you that they are at home rather than in the hospital. Even when confronted with incontrovertible evidence that they are sick and in the hospital, the patient may continue to deny their illness or express a lack of concern about the problem (anosodiaphoria). Because prosody, the rhythmic and melodic elements of speech, is largely a function of the right hemisphere, patients with the right hemisphere syndrome tend to speak in monotone.

Transient global amnesia

Transient global amnesia (TGA) is a sudden-onset, temporary disorder of memory encoding that often prompts consultation for confusion. Without warning, the patient starts to ask questions such as, "How did I get here?", "What happened?", and "Where am I?" After being provided with an apparently satisfactory explanation, the patient repeats the same questions a few minutes later. The typical patient is otherwise attentive and comports himself normally. They are capable of the entire spectrum of complex behaviors, including the ability to drive themselves home during an episode. Transient global amnesia typically lasts for several hours and then resolves. The precise etiology of TGA is unclear, with seizure, migraine, and stroke being implicated as possible etiologies.[5] Because TGA resolves on its own, it requires no specific treatment other than reassurance.

Psychosis

Psychosis may closely resemble an acute confusional state. Factors that help to differentiate between psychosis and confusion include the better organization and greater consistency of psychotic hallucinations and delusions, and the overall preserved level of consciousness and orientation in psychosis.[6] A normal electroencephalogram helps to exclude encephalopathy in cases that are difficult to distinguish on clinical grounds alone. Formal psychiatric assessment may help to differentiate between the two if any doubt remains.

Diagnostic testing

A complete medical history, medication list review, and chart review often disclose the source of confusion. Table 1.1 contains a basic guide to testing for some of the more common disorders that produce confusion. Many of these tests are ordered routinely in all hospitalized patients, and there are just a few additions specifically for the confused patient. EEG may help to confirm that a patient is encephalopathic (see Figures 1.3 and 1.4) if any doubt remains after the history and physical examination. EEG is also useful for determining whether a patient is in nonconvulsive status epilepticus. Almost all confused patients should undergo a neuroimaging study, generally a noncontrast head CT to exclude the possibility of a structural lesion, particularly subdural hematoma. MRI may be needed when acute stroke or inflammatory lesions are suspected. Finally, a lumbar puncture may be indicated when an infectious, inflammatory, or neoplastic process is suspected.

Etiologies

Toxic and metabolic encephalopathies

Medical diseases and intoxications are the most common causes of the acute confusional state. While essentially any medical disturbance may lead to confusion, commonly identified precipitants include pneumonia, urinary tract infections, hyponatremia, uremia, hepatic dysfunction, hypoxia, and hypercarbia (Table 1.1). In many elderly patients, subtle rather than overt metabolic derangements are often responsible for the problem. Among the medications that lead to confusion, the most common culprits are opioids, benzodiazepines, sleeping aids, and anticonvulsants. Intoxication with drugs of abuse

Table 1.1 Diagnostic testing for confusion

Test	Diagnosis
Complete blood count	Infection
Basic metabolic panel	Hyponatremia Hyperglycemia Hypoglycemia Hypercalcemia
Liver function tests, including ammonia	Hepatic encephalopathy
Arterial blood gas analysis	Hypoxia Hypercarbia
Thyroid function tests	Hyperthyroidism Hypothyroidism
Urinalysis	Urinary tract infection
Serum and urine toxicology screen	Intoxication with alcohol, cocaine, opioids, barbiturates
Chest X-ray	Pneumonia
Noncontrast head CT	Subdural hematoma Intracranial hemorrhage Space-occupying lesion
Head MRI	Acute ischemic stroke Encephalomyelitis Posterior reversible encephalopathy syndrome
Electroencephalogram	Nonconvulsive status epilepticus
Lumbar puncture	Bacterial meningitis Viral meningitis and encephalitis Subarachnoid hemorrhage Neoplastic meningitis Fungal meningitis

is another important cause of confusion. While the various toxic and metabolic encephalopathies are quite similar in their presentations, those related to ethanol consumption and hepatic failure present in distinctly different fashions and I will therefore discuss them in more detail here.

Ethanol and confusion

Ethanol intoxication

The signs of ethanol intoxication are easily identifiable and include slurred speech, incoherence, and ataxia. If there is any doubt about the diagnosis, it may be confirmed by finding an elevated serum ethanol level.

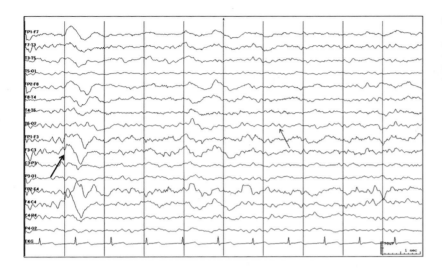

Figure 1.3 EEG in patient with moderate encephalopathy. The posterior dominant rhythm (thin arrow) is slow at approximately 5–6 Hz. There is also superimposed generalized slowing (thick arrow). Image courtesy of Dr. Julie Roth.

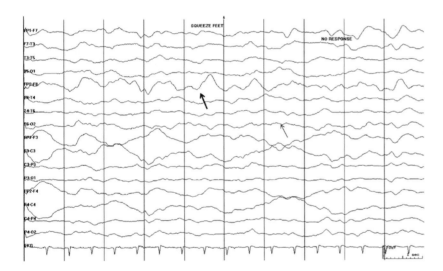

Figure 1.4 EEG in a patient with severe encephalopathy. Posterior dominant rhythm (thin arrow) is approximately 2–3 Hz. Additional slowing is noted throughout the record (thick arrow). There is no reactivity of the EEG to a request for movement. Image courtesy of Dr. Julie Roth.

Ethanol withdrawal

Withdrawal symptoms may develop as early as 6 hours after stopping heavy alcohol intake. The most common manifestation of ethanol withdrawal is tremulousness. When ethanol withdrawal causes a confusional state, it most frequently takes the form of agitated delirium, including auditory and visual hallucinations. These typically peak between 24 and 36 hours of ethanol withdrawal.[7] Delirium tremens is characterized by autonomic instability including diaphoresis, hypertension, and tachycardia, and develops between 2 and 4 days after ethanol discontinuation. If not treated properly, delirium tremens may be fatal. Benzodiazepines,

administered on a standing basis or as needed for signs of severe withdrawal (Table 1.2) are the agents of choice in reducing morbidity from ethanol withdrawal.[8]

Wernicke's encephalopathy

Chronic alcoholism and malnutrition may lead to thiamine deficiency and the clinical syndrome of Wernicke's encephalopathy. The classic clinical triad of Wernicke's encephalopathy is confusion, ophthalmoplegia, and ataxia. Because the triad is complete in only a minority of patients with Wernicke's encephalopathy, it is good practice to administer thiamine 100 mg intravenously for 5 days unless another source of confusion

Table 1.2 Benzodiazepine regimens for ethanol withdrawal

	Standing regimen	Prn regimen
Lorazepam	2 mg q6h × 24 hours followed by 1 mg q6h × 48 hours	2–4 mg q1h prn agitation or autonomic instability
Diazepam	10 mg q6h × 24 hours followed by 5 mg q6h × 24 hours	10–20 mg q1h prn agitation or autonomic instability
Chlordiazepoxide	50 mg q6h × 24 hours followed by 25 mg q6h × 48 hours	50–100 mg q1h prn agitation or autonomic instability

is identified.[9] Thiamine is a benign intervention, and if Wernicke's encephalopathy is not treated quickly, it may be irreversible. Intravenous thiamine leads to improvement in ocular symptoms in hours to days and ataxia and confusion in days to weeks.[7]

Hepatic encephalopathy

Both acute and chronic liver failure produce neurological dysfunction. In its mildest form, hepatic encephalopathy is characterized by inattention and psychomotor slowing. Deficits may not be detected at this stage unless they are sought specifically. Moderate hepatic encephalopathy produces more prominent inattention and somnolence. Asterixis, the most well-known sign of hepatic encephalopathy, is usually present at this stage. Other features of moderate hepatic encephalopathy include pyramidal and extrapyramidal signs including dysarthria, tremor, rigidity, and bradykinesia. EEG recordings may show triphasic waves, although this finding is not pathognomonic for hepatic encephalopathy. Advanced hepatic encephalopathy is characterized by seizures and more severe cognitive dysfunction, which may progress to coma and death. While a high serum ammonia level may suggest the diagnosis of hepatic encephalopathy, the substantial overlap between venous ammonia levels and the degree of hepatic encephalopathy makes following ammonia levels unhelpful for monitoring disease progression.[10] Treatment of hepatic encephalopathy includes reducing enteric bacterial ammonia production with the nonabsorbable disaccharide lactulose (30–60 mg tid) and short-term treatment with the antibiotics rifaximin (400 mg tid) or neomycin (1000–3000 mg qid). Although symptoms may be temporarily reversible, hepatic encephalopathy has a poor long-term prognosis.

Spinal fluid pleocytosis

Abnormal cells in the spinal fluid, whether they are neutrophils in bacterial meningitis, lymphocytes in viral meningitis, tumor cells in neoplastic meningitis, or red blood cells in subarachnoid hemorrhage (Chapter 19), may produce an acute confusional state.

Bacterial meningitis

The typical presentation of bacterial meningitis is fever, headache, and stiff neck. It is often accompanied by a confusional state that is otherwise indistinguishable from other toxic or metabolic encephalopathies. If you do not have a high index of suspicion for bacterial meningitis from the outset, you will miss the diagnosis, potentially leading to irreversible neurological damage and even death. Several findings may assist in making the diagnosis. Nuchal rigidity may be present in approximately 30% of patients with meningitis.[11] Kernig's sign is elicited by instructing the patient to lie flat with the hip flexed to 90° and looking for resistance or pain with attempted knee extension. Brudzinski's sign is elicited in a supine patient by observing spontaneous hip flexion when the neck is flexed. Unfortunately, Kernig's and Brudzinski's signs are unreliable, as they accompany meningitis in only 5% of cases.[11] If you suspect bacterial meningitis, then you must perform a lumbar puncture. The technique and safety of lumbar punctures is discussed in Box 1.1. The most important findings in the cerebrospinal fluid of a patient with bacterial meningitis are neutrophilic pleocytosis, elevated protein, and low glucose. Even if all three of these parameters are normal, however, until the Gram stain and cultures return, treat patients with suspected bacterial meningitis empirically with antibiotics covering the commonly responsible pathogens *Streptococcus pneumoniae*, *Neisseria meningitidis*, *Haemophilus influenzae*, and *Listeria monocytogenes*:[12,13]

- ceftriaxone 2 g IV q12h (substitute cefepime 2 g q8h in immunocompromised patients)
- vancomycin 1 g IV q12h
- ampicillin 2 g IV q4h
- dexamethasone 10 mg q6h for the first 2–4 days

Continue treatment until bacterial cultures are negative for 48 hours or a specific organism is isolated. Further tailoring and duration of antibiotic therapy depends on the organism cultured and its antibiotic sensitivity, and should be determined in consultation with an infectious disease specialist.

Box 1.1 Lumbar puncture

Many of the causes of confusion require CSF analysis. Although time is of the essence in performing a lumbar puncture, it is first necessary to exclude space-occupying intracranial lesions, as such lesions increase the risk of cerebral herniation. Not every patient, however, requires a CT scan before lumbar puncture. Risk factors for space-occupying lesions, and therefore indications for performing a head CT prior to lumbar puncture include age > 60 years, an immunocompromised state, a history of seizures within 1 week prior to presentation, papilledema, or an abnormal neurological examination.[14] In addition to cerebral herniation, the risks of the procedure include headache (30%), bleeding at the site of the puncture, and infection.

The main reason that a lumbar puncture is unsuccessful is that the patient is positioned improperly. Almost all textbooks instruct that the lumbar puncture should be performed in the lateral decubitus position. This position is ideal to obtain an accurate measurement of the cerebrospinal fluid pressure, but is also associated with a greater failure rate due to spine rotation and incomplete opening of the intervertebral space. The subarachnoid space is easier to access if the patient sits up and leans forward (Figure 1.7).

Identify the L2–3 or L3–4 interspace by drawing an imaginary line between the iliac crests as a marker of the L4 interspace. Next, sterilize the area with iodine or other sterilizing agent and place a drape over the planned lumbar puncture site. Infiltrate the target interspace with a small amount of lidocaine. Place the lumbar puncture needle into the space and advance slightly until you feel a slight decrease in resistance or "pop." Opening pressure may be measured by rotating the patient into the lateral decubitus position, withdrawing the stylet, and connecting the manometer. Be sure to collect enough spinal fluid to perform all necessary studies and to use an appropriate fixative solution when performing cytological examination to look for neoplastic cells. After all of the fluid is collected, replace the stylet and withdraw the needle. I instruct the patient to remain flat for 1 hour after the procedure to decrease the risk for headache.

Viral meningitis and encephalitis

Because they present so similarly, it may be difficult to distinguish between bacterial and viral meningitis on clinical grounds alone. Lumbar puncture is also often unhelpful in the acute setting, as viral meningitis may also cause a neutrophilic pleocytosis in the first 24 hours of infection. While waiting to repeat lumbar puncture in 24–48 hours (by which time the shift to lymphocytic pleocytosis should have occurred), check the Gram stain and bacterial cultures, and treat patients with empiric therapy for bacterial meningitis.

Viral encephalitis is characterized by viral invasion of the brain parenchyma, and therefore a greater likelihood of confusion, seizures, and serious neurological morbidity than viral meningitis. The most important causes of viral meningitis and encephalitis are:

- Enteroviruses. Most viral meningitis is due to enteroviral (e.g. coxsackievirus and echovirus) infection and does not require treatment beyond supportive care.
- Herpes simplex virus type 1 (HSV-1). HSV-1 produces encephalitis that preferentially (but not exclusively) affects the temporal lobes. The only way to make the diagnosis is by finding a positive HSV polymerase chain reaction (PCR) result in the cerebrospinal fluid. The classic findings of HSV encephalitis including T2-weighted MRI hyperintensities in the temporal lobes (Figure 1.5), periodic lateralizing epileptiform discharges on EEG, and red blood cells in the CSF are not universal, especially in the early stages. Because the HSV PCR usually requires several days to process during which time neurological deterioration may occur, treat all patients with suspected HSV encephalitis with acyclovir 10 mg/kg tid until the HSV PCR results return. Monitor kidney function while treating with acyclovir. Continue treatment for confirmed HSV infection with acyclovir for 21 days.
- Herpes simplex virus type 2 (HSV-2). Most patients with HSV-2 meningitis have genital herpes at the time of presentation. In the absence of herpetic lesions, the diagnosis is made by finding a positive HSV PCR in the CSF. Treat patients with HSV-2 meningitis with intravenous acyclovir, as described for patients with HSV-1 encephalitis.
- Human immunodeficiency virus (HIV). It may be difficult to distinguish HIV seroconversion from other causes of viral meningitis. While patients with a meningitic presentation of HIV seroconversion usually improve with little more than supportive care, it is important to recognize the pathogen for counseling purposes and for planning further treatment.

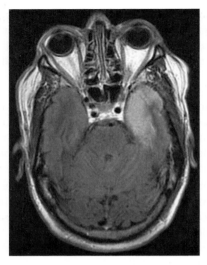

Figure 1.5 Fluid attenuation inversion recovery (FLAIR) MRI of a patient with hyperintensity in the left temporal lobe.

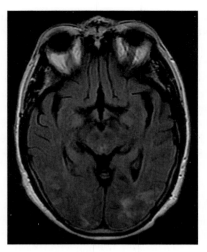

Figure 1.6 Fluid attenuation inversion recovery (FLAIR) MRI of a patient with posterior reversible encephalopathy syndrome showing the characteristic occipital lobe hyperintensities.

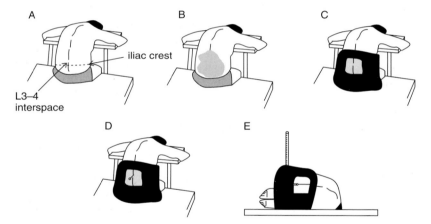

Figure 1.7 Technique for performing lumbar puncture. Identify the L3–4 interspace as the interspace superior to a line connecting the iliac crests (A). Prepare the area with iodine or another sterilizing agent (B) and a sterile drape (C). After anesthetizing the area with lidocaine or another anesthetic, place the lumbar puncture needle into the L2–3 or L3–4 interspace, advancing slowly until a sudden decrease in resistance or "pop" is heard (D). If an opening pressure needs to be measured, then rotate the patient into the lateral decubitus position, withdraw the stylet and attach the manometer (E). Collect the fluid and send to the laboratory for studies.

Neoplastic meningitis

Tumor cells that invade the CSF and leptomeninges have the potential to cause multifocal dysfunction of the CNS, cranial nerves, and nerve roots. The constellation of symptoms may include encephalopathy, headaches, seizures, increased intracranial pressure, diplopia, dysarthria, radicular pain, and weakness. The most common tumors that produce neoplastic meningitis are primary CNS tumors, carcinomas of the lung and breast, melanoma, lymphoma, and leukemia.[15] Although neoplastic meningitis usually accompanies advanced cancer, it may be the first sign of disease in some cases. Routine CSF examination shows a high cell count with lymphocytic predominance and a high protein level. A positive cytological examination of

the CSF establishes the diagnosis. Malignant cells are found after a single lumbar puncture in approximately 55% and after a second lumbar puncture in 85%.[16] Three or more lumbar punctures should therefore be performed before declaring the evaluation negative. Contrast-enhanced MRI serves an adjunctive role in diagnosis, showing leptomeningeal enhancement and focal nodular tumor deposits in about half of high-risk patients with initially normal cytological examinations.[17] If possible, perform MRI prior to lumbar puncture, as lumbar puncture itself may lead to artifactual leptomeningeal enhancement. Neoplastic meningitis is a poor prognostic sign, associated with a median survival of ≤6 months.[15] In most cases, therapy is supportive. Steroids, local radiation, and intrathecal or systemic methotrexate or cytarabine may be used for palliative purposes.[15]

Lyme meningitis

Infection with the tick-borne spirochete *Borrelia burgdorferi* produces Lyme disease, a disorder with protean neurological and systemic manifestations. Symptoms of early disseminated Lyme disease occur several weeks to months after tick bite and may include radiculopathy, Bell's palsy, or lymphocytic meningitis. There is often no history of the classical erythema chronicum migrans rash. The diagnosis is established by finding *Borrelia* antibodies in the CSF. In many patients, however, antibodies are not present and the diagnosis is made only from the relevant clinical and exposure history. Treat Lyme meningitis with ceftriaxone (2 g IV qd for 28 days).

Tuberculous meningitis

Tuberculous meningitis produces a monocytic pleocytosis with high protein and very low glucose levels. The diagnosis is made by finding acid-fast bacilli (AFB) in the CSF. This test is of low diagnostic yield, and multiple lumbar punctures may be required before finding a positive AFB stain. Treat tuberculous meningitis with a four-drug regimen (most regimens include a combination of isoniazid, pyrazinamide, rifampin, and either ethambutol or streptomycin) in consultation with an infectious disease specialist.

Fungal meningitis

Coccidioides immitis produces a lymphocytic meningitis endemic to the American Southwest. The diagnosis is made by culturing the organisms or by finding coccidioidal antibodies in the CSF. Treat patients with coccidioidal meningitis with oral fluconazole (400 mg qd).

Cryptococcus neoformans may produce a life-threatening meningitis that is mostly seen in immunocompromised patients. The CSF shows a monocytic pleocytosis, which is often modest in patients who cannot mount a robust immune response. Cryptocci stain positively with India ink. Treat cryptococcal meningitis with a combination of amphotericin B IV 0.7 mg/kg qd and flucytosine PO 25 mg/kg qid for 2 weeks followed by fluconazole 400 mg PO qd for 8 weeks.[18] Additional treatment should be determined in conjunction with an infectious disease specialist.

Drug-induced meningitis   NSAID , TMP/Smx , IUIg

The most common causes of drug-induced meningitis are nonsteroidal anti-inflammatory drugs, trimethoprim-sulfamethoxazole, and intravenous immunoglobulin. These agents usually produce a neutrophilic pleocytosis in the acute setting. Drug-induced meningitis resolves when the offending agent is withdrawn.

Limbic encephalitis

Limbic encephalitis is an immune-mediated neurological syndrome characterized by confusion, memory loss, and seizures. It generally occurs in patients with cancer (sometimes as the first sign), but in others, it is secondary to a nonneoplastic, autoimmune process. Common antibodies associated with limbic encephalitis include:

- anti-Hu (ANNA-1) associated with small-cell lung cancer[19]
- anti-Ma2 associated with testicular cancer in young men[19]
- anti-CV2/CRMP5 associated with small-cell lung cancer[20]
- voltage-gated potassium channel antibodies[20]
- *N*-methyl-D-aspartate (NMDA) receptor antibodies associated with ovarian teratoma[20,21]

Limbic encephalitis may improve with successful treatment of the underlying cancer. Intravenous immunoglobulin is often a useful adjunctive treatment.

Nonconvulsive status epilepticus

Nonconvulsive status epilepticus (NCSE) is defined as uninterrupted complex partial or absence seizures that last for at least 30 minutes. The behavior of a patient in NCSE differs little from that of a patient with any of the more common toxic or metabolic sources of confusion. Because of its obvious treatability, maintaining a high index of suspicion for NCSE when evaluating any confused patient is important. The best way to confirm the diagnosis is by finding ongoing seizures on EEG. There are many times, however, when EEG is not readily available, in which case empiric treatment with 2 mg of intravenous lorazepam may disrupt NCSE and improve the confusional state. Unlike convulsive status epilepticus, NCSE may not necessarily pose a substantial risk for brain damage or death. It is not clear, therefore, how aggressively NCSE should be treated. While small doses of benzodiazepines and initiating or augmenting maintenance doses of anticonvulsants are obviously warranted, it is less clear whether patients in NCSE require drastic measures such as propofol, midazolam, or pentobarbital infusions. The decision to proceed with aggressive pharmacological treatment of NCSE should be decided on a case-by-case basis, bearing in mind that the ultimate prognosis of NCSE is related to the process responsible for the seizures and not to the seizures themselves.

Structural lesions responsible for confusion

Because of their rarity, it is easy to become cavalier and dismiss the possibility of focal structural lesions as a source of confusion. Subdural hematoma is the diagnosis that is most often missed. Usually caused by traumatic tearing of the bridging subdural veins, subdural hematoma may result in a wide variety of neurological presentations including hemiparesis, seizures, headaches, and confusion. The head trauma that produces a subdural hematoma is often trivial and sometimes not remembered by the patient. Thus, it is almost mandatory to obtain a noncontrast head CT in every confused patient (see Chapter 21, Figure 23.3). Most subdural hematomas reabsorb without intervention, but progressive neurological deficits or radiographic evidence of hematoma expansion require surgical intervention. Although stroke is not a common cause of confusion, left posterior cerebral[22] and right middle cerebral artery[23] infarctions may rarely produce a confusional state.

Posterior reversible encephalopathy syndrome

Posterior reversible encephalopathy syndrome (PRES) is a severe encephalopathy produced by vasogenic edema.[24] The clinical syndrome may be quite variable, but usually takes the form of a rapidly developing encephalopathy accompanied by visual disturbances and sometimes by seizures. The most commonly identified precipitants are hypertensive emergency, eclampsia, and calcineurin inhibitors used as immunosuppressants after organ transplantation (most commonly tacrolimus and cyclosporine). Characteristic imaging findings of PRES are T2 hyperintensities (best visualized using fluid-attenuated inversion recovery sequences) with a predilection for the subcortical white matter of the parietal and occipital lobes (Figure 1.6). Despite its name, PRES is not necessarily restricted to the posterior part of the brain and may not be reversible: the frontal lobes, thalamus, and basal ganglia may be involved, and PRES may be associated with poor neurological outcome and death. Blood pressure correction (most commonly with a regimen including verapamil or other calcium-channel blockers), delivery of the baby for women with eclampsia, and discontinuation of calcineurin inhibitors may lead to resolution of PRES.

General approach to treatment

Most acute confusional states have an identifiable and often a reversible cause. It is essential to ensure that no more harm comes to the patient while the responsible abnormality is being corrected. This is best accomplished by providing the patient with a room of their own, soft lighting, and the company of a family member or friend. Many patients, particularly elderly ones, will require chemical or physical restraints, which must be administered judiciously. Quetiapine (25 mg prn) is the most popular agent for sedating combative patients. Haloperidol (0.5–1 mg IV) may be used for patients who refuse or cannot take oral medications. Security sitters and physical restraints may be necessary in extreme cases.

References

1. Ronthal M. Confusional states and metabolic encephalopathy. In: Samuels MA, Feske SK, eds. *Office Practice of Neurology*, 2nd edn. Philadelphia: Churchill Livingstone; 2003:886–890.
2. Inouye SK. Delirium in hospitalized older patients. *Clin Geriatr Med* 1998;**14**:745–764.
3. Leavitt S, Tyler HR. Studies in asterixis. *Arch Neurol* 1964;**10**:360–368.
4. Mesulam M. Attentional networks, confusional states, and neglect syndromes. In: Mesulam M, ed. *Principles of Behavioral and Cognitive Neurology*. Oxford: Oxford University Press; 2000:174–256.
5. Hodges JR, Warlow CP. The aetiology of transient global amnesia. *Brain* 1990;**113**:639–657.
6. Kaplan HI, Sadock BJ. *Kaplan and Sadock's Synopsis of Psychiatry*. Baltimore: Williams & Wilkins; 1998.
7. Charness ME, Simon RP, Greenberg DA. Ethanol and the nervous system. *N Engl J Med* 1989;**321**:442–454.
8. Mayo-Smith MF. Pharmacological management of alcohol withdrawal. A meta-analysis and evidence-based practice guideline. *JAMA* 1997;**278**:144–151.
9. Harper CG, Giles M, Finlay-Jones R. Clinical signs in the Wernicke–Korsakoff complex: a retrospective analysis of 131 cases diagnosed at necropsy. *J Neurol Neurosurg Psychiatry* 1986;**49**:341–345.

10. Ong JP, Aggarwal A, Krieger D, et al. Correlation between ammonia levels and the severity of hepatic encephalopathy. *Am J Med* 2003;**114**:188–193.

11. Thomas KE, Hasbun R, Jekel J, Quagliarello VJ. The diagnostic accuracy of Kernig's sign, Brudzkinski's sign, and nuchal rigidity in adults with suspected meningitis. *Clin Infect Dis* 2002;**35**:46–52.

12. van de Beek D, de Gans J, Spanjaard L, et al. Clinical features and prognostic factors in adults with bacterial meningitis. *N Engl J Med* 2004;**351**:1849–1859.

13. Tunkel AR, Hartman BJ, Kaplan SL, et al. Practice guidelines for the management of bacterial meningitis. *Clin Infect Dis* 2004;**39**:1267–1284.

14. Hasbun R, Abrahams J, Jekel J, Quagliarello VJ. Computed tomography of the head before lumbar puncture in adults with suspected meningitis. *N Engl J Med* 2001;**345**:1727–1733.

15. Herrlinger U, Forschler H, Kuker W, et al. Leptomeningeal metastasis: survival and prognostic factors in 155 patients. *J Neurol Sci* 2004;**223**:167–178.

16. Wasserstrom WR, Glass JP, Posner JB. Diagnosis and treatment of leptomeningeal metastases from solid tumors: experience with 90 patients. *Cancer* 1982;**49**:759–772.

17. Gomori JM, Heching N, Siegal T. Leptomeningeal metastases: evaluation by gadolinium enhanced spinal magnetic resonance imaging. *J Neurooncol* 1998;**36**:55–60.

18. van der Horst CM, Saag MS, Cloud GA, et al. Treatment of cryptococcal meningitis associated with the acquired immunodeficiency syndrome. *N Engl J Med* 1997;**337**:15–21.

19. Gultekin SH, Rosenfeld MR, Voltz R, et al. Paraneoplastic limbic encephalitis: neurological symptoms, immunological findings and tumour association in 50 patients. *Brain* 2000;**123**: 1481–1494.

20. Graus F, Saiz A, Lai M, et al. Neuronal surface antigen antibodies in limbic encephalitis: clinical–immunologic associations. *Neurology* 2008;**71**: 930–936.

21. Thieben MJ, Lennon VA, Boeve BF, et al. Potentially reversible autoimmune limbic encephalitis with neuronal potassium channel antibody. *Neurology* 2004;**62**:1177–1182.

22. Devinsky O, Bear D, Volpe BT. Confusional states following posterior cerebral artery infarction. *Arch Neurol* 1988;**45**:160–163.

23. Mesulam M, Waxman SG, Geschwind N, Sabin TD. Acute confusional states with right middle cerebral artery infarctions. *J Neurol Neurosurg Psychiatry* 1976;**39**:84–89.

24. Lee VH, Wijdicks EFM, Manno EM, Rabinstein AA. Clinical spectrum of reversible posterior leukoencephalopathy syndrome. *Arch Neurol* 2008;**65**:205–210.

History

Coma is a state of eyes-closed unresponsiveness in which even the most vigorous stimulation fails to arouse the patient.[1] Because comatose patients cannot communicate, the history must be assembled from family members, emergency service records, and hospital notes. Clues to the etiology of coma obtained from the history include the presence of trauma, evidence of intoxication, and history of cardiac, pulmonary, hepatic, and renal disease. The tempo of coma onset may also be helpful: sudden onset in the absence of trauma favors a cardiogenic source or intracranial hemorrhage, whereas gradual onset is more consistent with a metabolic cause or a slowly expanding mass lesion. In many cases, the history contains few details beyond the patient being "found down," and the evaluation of the comatose patient quickly shifts to physical examination and diagnostic testing.

Examination

Mental status examination

The purpose of the mental status examination of the comatose patient is to verify that they are actually comatose rather than just encephalopathic. Before beginning the examination, make sure that any short-acting sedatives such as midazolam or propofol are discontinued. By definition, a comatose patient's eyes should be closed and they should appear as if they are sleeping. If gently calling out their name does not produce any response, yell out their name or gently squeeze their hand. Attempt to awaken them with increasingly noxious stimuli: severely encephalopathic patients may respond to painful maneuvers such as rubbing the sternum, applying nailbed pressure, or pinching the areola. Comatose patients will not. Document the reaction to each stimulus and also note what happens when it is withdrawn.

Pupillary reactions

Abnormal pupillary reactions may provide insight into structural causes of coma involving the thalamus and brainstem. A quick rule of thumb (with several important exceptions) is that symmetric pupils, even if abnormal in size and unreactive, are more likely due to toxic or metabolic lesions, while asymmetric pupils are more likely due to structural lesions. Before assigning too much weight to an abnormal pupillary examination, exclude preexisting pupillary irregularities, such as those that might be due to prior cataract surgery. Chapter 7 contains a more detailed discussion of pupillary neuroanatomy and function. The following patterns of pupillary reactions are the most important ones in comatose patients:

1. Normal-sized pupils with normal reactions (Figure 2.1A). This pattern argues against a structural source of coma and is more suggestive of a toxic or metabolic disturbance.
2. Small, reactive pupils (Figure 2.1B). Although thalamic lesions may produce this pattern, patients with small, reactive pupils are more likely to have toxic or metabolic disturbances.
3. Unreactive midsized pupils (Figure 2.1C). Midbrain lesions may produce unreactive midsized pupils. More commonly, however, this pattern is the result of toxic or metabolic disturbances.
4. Unreactive pinpoint pupils (Figure 2.1D). Pontine lesions classically produce pinpoint pupils. It is more common, however, for patients with unreactive pinpoint pupils to have a toxic or metabolic disturbance, particularly opioid intoxication.
5. Asymmetric pupils, abnormal pupil is dilated (Figure 2.1E). The most common causes of this pattern in comatose patients are uncal herniation and ruptured posterior communicating artery aneurysm. Both conditions are true neurological

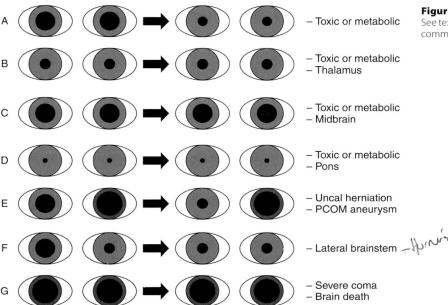

Figure 2.1 Pupillary reactions in coma. See text for details. PCOM, posterior communicating artery.

A — Toxic or metabolic

B — Toxic or metabolic
— Thalamus

C — Toxic or metabolic
— Midbrain

D — Toxic or metabolic
— Pons

E — Uncal herniation
— PCOM aneurysm

F — Lateral brainstem *Horners*

G — Severe coma
— Brain death

emergencies that require rapid evaluation and treatment.

6. Asymmetric pupils, abnormal pupil is constricted (Figure 2.1F). Coma accompanied by Horner's syndrome points to lateral brainstem damage.
7. Fixed and dilated pupils (Figure 2.1G). This pattern suggests severe coma or brain death.

Blink reflexes

The sensory nerve fibers responsible for the blink reflex originate in the cornea and travel in the ophthalmic branch of the trigeminal nerve (Figure 2.2). These trigeminal nerve fibers synapse in the ipsilateral principal sensory nucleus of the trigeminal nerve and the nucleus of the spinal trigeminal tract in the pons and medulla. Neurons originating from these trigeminal nuclei send axons to both the ipsilateral and contralateral facial nuclei. The facial nucleus gives rise to the facial nerve, which innervates the ipsilateral orbicularis oculi, contraction of which produces blinking.

To assess the corneal reflex, peel both eyelids open and gently stroke the sclera and cornea with a wisp of cotton or sterile gauze. Both eyes should blink in response to this stimulus. Test the blink reflex in each eye in sequence. The following are the important blink reflex patterns found in comatose patients (Figure 2.3):

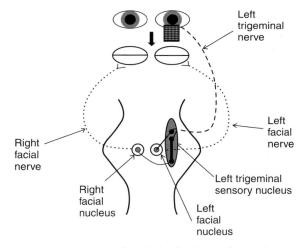

Figure 2.2 Schematic of the blink reflex. See text for details.

1. Normal responses in both eyes point to preserved integrity of the blink reflex pathways in the pons and medulla (Figure 2.3A).
2. Stimulation of the right eye produces no blink in either eye, while stimulation of the left eye produces normal blink responses in both eyes (Figure 2.3B). This pattern points to dysfunction of the right trigeminal nerve or nuclei in the pons and medulla.
3. Stimulation of either eye fails to produce a blink response in the right eye (Figure 2.3C). The lesion in this case is in the right facial nucleus or nerve.

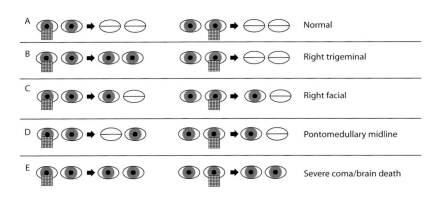

A Normal
B Right trigeminal
C Right facial
D Pontomedullary midline
E Severe coma/brain death

Figure 2.3 Common patterns on blink reflex testing in patients in coma. See text for details.

4. Stimulation of either eye produces a blink in the ipsilateral eye, but not in the contralateral eye (Figure 2.3D). This pattern suggests dysfunction of the pathways connecting the trigeminal nuclei to the contralateral facial nucleus in the pons and medulla.
5. Bilaterally absent blink responses point to severe brainstem dysfunction, which may be due to either structural or metabolic processes (Figure 2.3E). Bear in mind that patients who wear contact lenses may also lose their blink responses.

Eye position

Horizontal eye position

The frontal eye fields (FEF) in the frontal lobes are the most important structures in the supranuclear control of horizontal eye movements. Projections from the FEF synapse with the contralateral abducens nucleus. Thus, activation of the FEF or inhibition of the abducens nucleus produces contralateral eye deviation, while inhibition of the FEF or activation of the abducens nucleus leads to ipsilateral eye deviation. Supranuclear, nuclear, and infranuclear lesions may lead to abnormal eye positions, which can help to localize the process responsible for coma. In all cases, it is helpful to interpret eye deviation in the context of any associated hemiparesis (Figure 2.4):
1. Destructive right frontal lesions such as strokes or tumors produce rightward deviation of the eyes accompanied by left hemiparesis (Figure 2.4A).
2. Irritative right frontal lesions such as seizures produce leftward deviation of the eyes. There may or may not be a left hemiparesis (Figure 2.4B).
3. Right thalamic lesions produce "wrong-way eyes" that are deviated to the left and are accompanied by left hemiparesis (Figure 2.4C).[2]

4. Right pontine lesions produce leftward eye deviation. Left hemiparesis may or may not be present (Figure 2.4D).

In addition, horizontal dysconjugate gaze abnormalities (the eyes look in different directions) are often helpful in localizing coma. Common patterns include:
1. Exodeviation of both eyes. This is the pattern seen in many patients with coma, and usually does not have localizing value.
2. Hypo- and exodeviation of one eye ("down and out") secondary to ipsilateral third-nerve palsy.
3. Esodeviation of one eye secondary to sixth-nerve palsy.

Vertical eye position

The supranuclear control of vertical eye movements is more complex, and involves the bilateral frontal lobes and structures within the brainstem including the vestibular nuclei and interstitial nucleus of Cajal in the midbrain. The important abnormalities of vertical ocular eye position in coma include:
1. Downward deviation of the eyes, which suggests a severe dorsal midbrain lesion.[3]
2. Vertical ocular misalignment pointing to skew deviation from a brainstem lesion on to fourth-nerve palsy.
3. Hypo- and exodeviation of one eye ("down and out") secondary to ipsilateral third-nerve palsy.

Spontaneous eye movements

The spontaneous eye movements of comatose patients are usually slow and roving or absent altogether. Absent eye movements suggest a greater depth of coma, and possibly brain death, but do not have particular localizing value. Ocular bobbing is characterized by quick

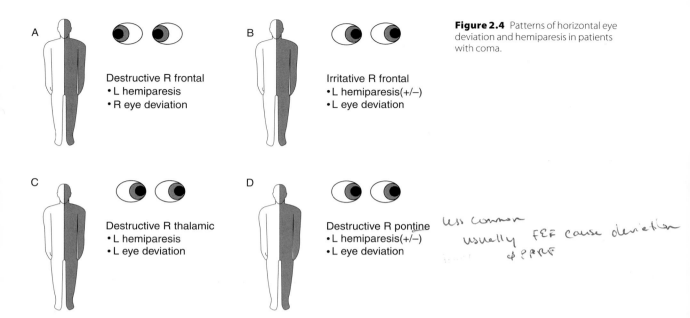

Figure 2.4 Patterns of horizontal eye deviation and hemiparesis in patients with coma.

A Destructive R frontal
• L hemiparesis
• R eye deviation

B Irritative R frontal
• L hemiparesis(+/−)
• L eye deviation

C Destructive R thalamic
• L hemiparesis
• L eye deviation

D Destructive R pontine
• L hemiparesis(+/−)
• L eye deviation

less common usually FEF cause deviation of PPRF

downward eye movements, which are followed by a slower return back to the primary position, and classically reflect pontine damage.[4] Dipping refers to slow downward eye movements with a quicker upward return: this finding has less localizing value than bobbing. Bobbing and dipping may also have inverse forms, in which the first movement is upwards rather than downwards.

Oculocephalic responses

The oculocephalic response may be assessed by the head thrust maneuver or by cold caloric testing. To test the oculocephalic response via the head thrust maneuver, grasp the head by the forehead and chin. Hold the eyes open and turn the head briskly to one side. In comatose patients with intact brainstem function, the eyes should turn in the direction opposite to head rotation. Patients with structural brainstem lesions may demonstrate dysconjugate eye movements. Those who are deeply comatose or brain dead have no eye movements at all. Do not use the head thrust maneuver in patients with possible cervical spine instability, as neck manipulation may worsen motor deficits and even lead to paralysis.

Because the head thrust maneuver is only a weak stimulus to eye movement, most comatose patients require cold caloric testing to properly assess the oculocephalic response. To test cold caloric responses, place the head of the bed at 30° above the horizontal, thereby

aligning the horizontal semicircular canal parallel to the ground. Examine the auditory canal to ensure that excessive cerumen accumulation will not interfere with the test, and disimpact the ears as necessary. Fill a 60 ml syringe with ice water and attach the syringe to a short piece of intravenous tubing. Place the tubing into the ear and infuse the ice water slowly over 5 minutes. If brainstem function is intact, then the eyes should deviate towards the side of ice water infusion. After performing the test on one ear, wait approximately 5 minutes for the vestibular system to reset and then test the opposite ear. Important patterns of oculocephalic response testing are shown in Figure 2.5:

1. Cold water placed in either ear produces ipsilateral eye deviation (Figure 2.5A). This is the expected response in a patient with a metabolic encephalopathy.
2. Cold water placed in the right ear produces no response (Figure 2.5B). Cold water placed in the left ear produces tonic ipsilateral eye deviation. This is the pattern seen in patients with right vestibular nerve or right lateral pontine damage.
3. Cold water placed in the right ear produces rightward eye deviation of the right eye only (Figure 2.5C). Cold water placed in the left ear produces leftward eye deviation of the left eye only. This is consistent with a midline lesion of the midbrain and pons producing bilateral internuclear ophthalmoplegia (Chapter 6).

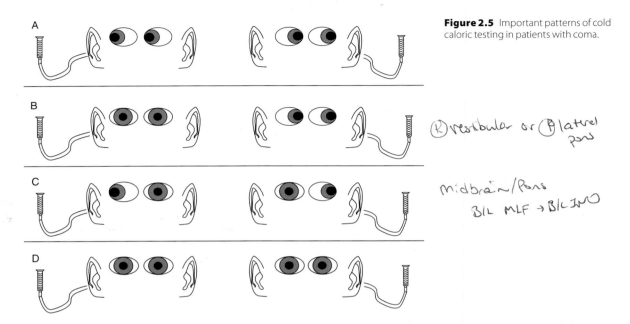

Figure 2.5 Important patterns of cold caloric testing in patients with coma.

[handwritten annotation:] ℞ vestibular or Ⓑ lateral pons

[handwritten annotation:] midbrain/pons BIL MLF → BIL INO

4. Cold water placed in either ear produces no response (Figure 2.5D). This occurs with severe coma or brain death.

Motor examination

The motor examination helps to determine the presence and severity of coma and in some cases localizes the responsible lesion. Movements may be divided into the following four categories.

Spontaneous and purposeful

Spontaneous, purposeful movements indicate that the patient is not comatose, and should prompt evaluation for encephalopathy as discussed in Chapter 1.

Spontaneous but nonpurposeful

For comatose patients, the most important spontaneous, nonpurposeful movement is polymyoclonus caused by anoxic brain injury. These movements are characterized by brief muscle jerks of the arms, legs, and face, followed by relaxation of the involved muscles. Sometimes they may take the form of violent jaw closure and result in tongue laceration or even severing of a mechanical airway (Chapter 14).

Reflexive

Comatose patients may demonstrate one of several reflex movements. In most patients, these are limited, local, nonpurposeful movements. They may be differentiated from normal movements by their lack

of habituation to repeatedly applied, painful stimuli. The most widely known reflex movements in coma are decorticate and decerebrate posturing. In decorticate posturing, a painful stimulus causes flexion at the elbows, wrists, and fingers, and adduction of the arms. In decerebrate posturing, a painful stimulus causes internal rotation of the arms with extension at the elbows and flexion–pronation at the wrists. In both decorticate and decerebrate posturing, there is extension at the hips, extension at the knees, and plantarflexion at the ankles. The anatomical basis of decorticate and decerebrate posturing is less well defined in humans than in laboratory animals, and both may result from nonstructural, metabolic processes or from brainstem pathology. Both forms of posturing are associated with a poor outcome, with decerebrate posturing portending a worse prognosis.

Absent

If the patient does not move spontaneously or in response to verbal command, compress the fingernail or toenail bed with the handle of a reflex hammer. Severely encephalopathic patients but not those in coma may purposefully move the hand or foot away from such a stimulus. In some patients, a painful stimulus may produce only a facial grimace or heart rate elevation with no visible motor response in the limbs. This lack of a motor response in the presence of a preserved autonomic response is due either to severe brain damage or to neuromuscular dysfunction (Chapter 12).

Cheyne–Stokes – Bl Frontal lobes
Hyperventilation
– Pontine
Ataxic – lower pons or upper medulla
c̄ contrast

Absent movements with no change in heart rate suggest brain death.

Respiratory patterns

Abnormal respiratory patterns may suggest specific anatomic localizations of coma.[1] The classic patterns are often not observed while the patient is intubated, sedated, and paralyzed, but may become obvious if mechanical ventilation is discontinued temporarily. Cheyne–Stokes breathing is characterized by hyperpneic phases that build to a crescendo and then taper to apneic periods lasting for 10–20 seconds. This pattern usually implies bilateral frontal lobe pathology, and is common in metabolic encephalopathies. Hyperventilation is another pattern associated with toxic and metabolic encephalopathies, generally those that produce metabolic acidosis. Central neurogenic hyperventilation is rare, and is usually seen in the context of brainstem glioma or lymphoma.[5] Apneustic breathing is characterized by 2- or 3-second pauses that occur at the end of inspiration and expiration, and reflects pontine damage. Ataxic breathing has an irregular, gasping quality, and is secondary to lower pontine or upper medullary dysfunction.

Investigation of impaired consciousness and coma

Approximately two-thirds of the causes of coma are due to medical conditions, such as metabolic abnormalities and toxins, while the remaining one-third are due to structural causes such as trauma, brain hemorrhage, and tumor.[1] Because the number of potential causes of coma is quite large, I find it helpful to divide the investigation into three phases based on the frequency of the responsible causes and the ease of obtaining diagnostic testing:

Phase 1: history, examination, and basic studies

By the time a neurologist is consulted, a basic metabolic workup and CT scan of the brain is usually available. Combined with a careful history and physical examination, these data help to establish one of the following coma diagnoses:

- Trauma. Patients with head trauma sufficient to cause coma almost always have abnormal head CT scans. In addition to skull fractures, abnormalities following trauma include epidural,

subdural, intraparenchymal, and subarachnoid hemorrhages. Some patients have no clear evidence of fracture or hemorrhage, but the CT scan (or, more likely, an MRI) shows evidence of diffuse axonal injury.
- Intracranial mass lesion. Bilateral frontal or brainstem lesions including tumors, abscesses, and intracranial hemorrhages may all lead to coma.
- Subarachnoid hemorrhage. Aneurysmal rupture leading to subarachnoid hemorrhage is an important cause of coma that may be detected with a CT scan (Chapter 19).
- Hypoxic–ischemic injury. Whether due to anoxia following cardiac arrest or to severe hypoxia secondary to pulmonary disease, irreversible brain damage occurs after just minutes of global ischemia and is among the most serious causes of coma.
- Toxic or metabolic disturbances with normal imaging studies. Comatose patients with normal CT scans usually have a toxic or metabolic disturbance, often more than one. Routine laboratory testing is generally sensitive to the conditions listed in Table 2.1, many of which are reversible.

Phase 2: MRI, electroencephalography, and lumbar puncture

Although the history, CT scan, and basic laboratory studies often disclose the etiology of coma, further evaluation is necessary should these initial investigations fail to identify the responsible process.

MRI serves several purposes in patients with coma of unclear etiology. Diffusion-weighted MRI identifies hypoxic–ischemic changes several days before they are noted on a routine head CT. MRI may also disclose two specific infarctions that may be poorly visualized by CT. The first is infarction of the intralaminar nuclei of the thalamus and rostral midbrain[6] (supplied by the paramedian thalamic artery; Figure 2.6). The second is infarction of the base of the pons leading to the locked-in state. Other causes of coma that may be missed by CT but detected by MRI include occult encephalitis or posterior reversible encephalopathy syndrome (PRES) (Chapter 1).

EEG helps to establish the presence of severe encephalopathy or brain death in unclear cases of coma. The real value of EEG in comatose patients, however, actually lies in its ability to detect nonconvulsive

Table 2.1 Medical causes of coma

Hepatic failure
Hypercalcemia
Hypoglycemia
Hyperglycemia
Hypernatremia
Hyponatremia
Hyperthyroidism
Hypothyroidism
Intoxication with:
Acetaminophen
Alcohol
Amphetamines
Barbiturates
Benzodiazepines
Cocaine
Opioids
Renal failure
Systemic infection

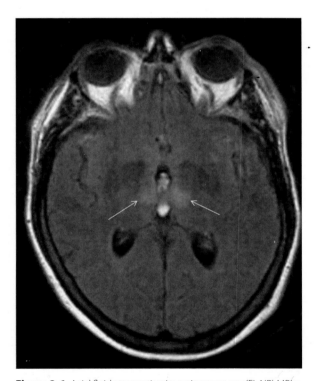

Figure 2.6 Axial fluid attenuation inversion recovery (FLAIR) MRI in a patient with paramedian thalamic artery infarction. This is an uncommon cause of coma, but it is important to recognize because it is easy to overlook. The bilateral thalamic hyperintensities are quite symmetric, and it is easy to misdiagnose this finding as an artifact.

status epilepticus (NCSE), a potentially reversible condition that often eludes clinical diagnosis (Chapters 1 and 20). Continuous rather than routine EEG should be employed if NCSE is suspected, as the first electroencephalographic evidence of seizures may appear only after more than 24 hours of monitoring in 20% of patients.[7]

Lumbar puncture should be performed to evaluate for CNS infections, particularly bacterial meningitis and herpes encephalitis (Chapter 1).

Phase 3: uncommon etiologies and coma mimics

If the diagnosis remains unclear after an initial panel of investigations, MRI, EEG, and lumbar puncture, then consider less common toxins, neuromuscular mimics of coma, and psychogenic unresponsiveness.

Some toxins that may not be detected by routine toxicology screens are listed in Table 2.2. Consultation with a toxicologist is often helpful when considering these less common agents.

Severe neuromuscular disorders may lead to a state of profound weakness that mimics coma. Conditions such as Guillain–Barré syndrome, myasthenia gravis, and botulism are usually diagnosed before weakness reaches this severity, but on some occasions, motor function declines so precipitously that the initial phase of weakness may go unrecognized. Rapidly progressive weakness and difficulty weaning from the ventilator due to neuromuscular disease acquired in the intensive care unit are discussed further in Chapter 12.

Psychogenic unresponsiveness secondary to conversion disorder, malingering, or catatonia may be profound to the point that it mimics a comatose state. Obviously, exhaustive medical evaluation must be conducted before these possibilities are even considered. For patients with conversion disorders or malingering, cold caloric testing may clinch the diagnosis and cure the coma by inciting violent nausea and vomiting. Although patients with psychiatric disorders do not have an organic explanation for coma, they require attention and life support that is just as careful as that provided to patients with organic neurological disorders.

Prognostication in coma

The ability to accurately predict the outcome of a comatose patient is essential, as it provides families with reasonable expectations about the potential for

Table 2.2 Less common toxins that lead to coma

Anticholinergics
Anticonvulsants
Antidepressants
Ethylene glycol
Ketamine
Methanol
Phencyclidine
Rohypnol

recovery and advisability of continuing life support. Prognostication is based on the proximate cause of coma, the neurological examination, and, in some instances, diagnostic test results. In general, patients with reversible causes of coma such as hypoglycemia or uremia have better prognoses than those with severe head trauma or hypoxic–ischemic injury.

The largest body of data concerning coma prognostication comes from patients with coma after cardiac arrest. Often, the goal in this patient population is to define which group of patients has a zero chance of a good neurological outcome. If any reasonable chance of a good outcome remains, aggressive supportive care must be continued. The following examination and laboratory results predict grave prognosis after cardiac arrest, and *should be applied only to patients with this specific etiology*: [8,9]

- absent brainstem reflexes
- myoclonic status epilepticus at day 1 (24 hours after cardiac arrest)
- evoked potentials showing absent N20 responses at days 1–3
- serum neuron-specific enolase >33 µg/l at days 1–3
- absent pupil or corneal response at day 3
- no motor response or extensor (decerebrate) posturing at day 3 *I.E. Wait 3 days*

This list suggests that, using the clinical examination alone, it is unwise to deliver an authoritative statement about coma prognosis until at least 72 hours after cardiac arrest. Unless supplemental tests are available, be cautious in providing too much information before this time. Keep several additional caveats in mind when using this list. First, confounders such as hypothermia, sedatives, and other toxins must be excluded, as responsible for the comatose state. Secondly, N20 evoked potentials may be difficult to measure in the intensive care unit due to electrical noise. Thirdly, the

turnaround time for neuron-specific enolase results is usually several weeks and almost always prevents it from being used in a timely fashion. Finally, the now commonplace practice of inducing mild-to-moderate hypothermia after cardiac arrest improves long-term neurological outcome, and it is not clear how this will change prognostication.[10,11]

The persistent vegetative state

After several days to a few weeks of deep coma, patients may appear to awaken and enter a vegetative state, which is given the name persistent vegetative state (PVS) if it lasts for at least 1 month.[12] This state is characterized by roving or tracking eye movements and what appears to be an irregular sleep–wake cycle. However, these patients do not interact with their environment in a meaningful way. They may grunt or moan, but they do not speak or comprehend. A PVS is the result of bilateral cortical damage with relatively preserved diencephalic and brainstem function. Although it may seem that PVS is a more favorable state than coma, its ultimate prognosis is still quite poor: of patients with nontraumatic PVS, only 1% have a good outcome at 1 year, while for patients with traumatic PVS, only 7% will have a good outcome at 1 year.[13] A PVS should be considered permanent if it persists for 3 months in patients with nontraumatic conditions and 12 months in patients with traumatic brain injuries.[14] News stories of patients recovering after years of coma or PVS are exceptional and should not be used to give family members false hope.

Brain death

Brain death is defined as the complete loss of brain function despite preserved cardiac function. It is particularly important to recognize brain death in order to allow decisions about withdrawing aggressive medical support and to plan for organ procurement. Before a patient is diagnosed with brain death, all potentially reversible causes of coma must be corrected. Sedatives such as midazolam and propofol must be discontinued and the patient's core temperature should be raised to at least 97°F. Next, the patient must be carefully examined, often using an institution-specific brain death protocol. The patient must be unarousable to any stimulus, lack pupillary and corneal reflexes, have no cold caloric responses, and not gag or cough when suctioned. Deep tendon reflexes may be (and often are) preserved. Many institutions require that the examination be confirmed several hours or a day after the initial assessment.

The apnea test is used to confirm brain death. Hypercarbia is a profound stimulus to breathe, and when it fails to produce a respiratory effort, it indicates severe brain damage incompatible with life. Before performing the apnea test, obtain a baseline arterial blood gas sample and note the partial pressure of carbon dioxide (P_{CO_2}). Next, preoxygenate the patient with 100% oxygen for at least 10 minutes. Following preoxygenation, discontinue mechanical ventilation while continuing to provide oxygen via a face mask. The apnea test is positive (i.e. consistent with brain death) if no respiratory efforts are visible after 10 minutes of ventilator discontinuation. Before reconnecting the patient to the ventilator, draw a repeat arterial blood gas sample to confirm the adequacy of hypercarbia: the P_{CO_2} level must be at least 60 mmHg or 20 mmHg greater than the baseline level.

In some patients, difficulties with interpreting the neurological examination or minor metabolic abnormalities prevent airtight confirmation of brain death. In such cases, several supplementary diagnostic tests establish brain death by showing the absence of cerebral electrical activity or cerebral blood flow. These include:

- EEG showing electrocerebral silence
- somatosensory evoked potentials showing absent N20 responses
- absent cerebral blood flow as determined by:
- transcranial Doppler ultrasound
- cerebral angiography
- nuclear scintigraphy

Increased intracranial pressure

Expansion of the intracranial contents is limited by the rigid confines of the skull. Blood, tumor, abscess, and edema are tolerated to a limit extent before symptoms and signs of increased intracranial pressure develop. In its earliest stage, increased intracranial pressure causes nonspecific headaches and visual blurring. Recognition of increased intracranial pressure at this stage may allow the responsible process to be diagnosed and reversed, thereby preventing additional neurological deterioration. Further increases in intracranial pressure lead to encephalopathy, seizures, and a variety of focal neurological findings. The most devastating consequences of increased intracranial pressure are the herniation syndromes in which brain tissue is displaced from its normal location, compressing or damaging otherwise healthy structures. The most important of these syndromes are uncal and transtentorial herniation.

Uncal herniation

A hemispheric mass or edema may cause expansion of one cerebral hemisphere relative to the other, leading to herniation of the uncus of the temporal lobe medially and inferiorly into the tentorial notch.[1] The earliest signs of uncal herniation are ipsilateral pupillary dilation produced by stretching or compression of the third nerve and a decrease in consciousness, which results from compression of the upper brainstem. Pupillary dilation in the presence of preserved consciousness, however, is essentially never due to uncal herniation.[1] As uncal herniation progresses, hemiparesis develops *ipsilateral* to the herniating mass as the *contralateral* cerebral peduncle is compressed, the so-called Kernohan's notch phenomenon. Less commonly, the ipsilateral cerebral peduncle is compressed leading to a contralateral hemiparesis. Thus, pupillary dilation is more reliable than hemiparesis in lateralizing uncal herniation. Shearing or compression of the posterior cerebral arteries in the tentorial notch may lead to cortical blindness. Because uncal herniation may progress rapidly to a state of irreversible neurological compromise or death, it must be identified as quickly as possible to allow the responsible source to be treated.

Transtentorial herniation

An expanding midline lesion may cause herniation downwards through the tentorium, compressing the thalamus and brainstem.[1] In early transtentorial herniation, the patient appears to be sleepy with small, minimally reactive pupils. It is very easy to misdiagnose the patient with a metabolic encephalopathy, and a high index of suspicion must be maintained in order to make the diagnosis at this stage, as further progression leads to a poor outcome. As herniation continues, the midbrain is compressed, leading to paresis of upgaze, unresponsiveness, and decorticate posturing. Continued downward herniation compromises the pons, resulting in loss of lateral eye movements and motor unresponsiveness or decerebrate posturing. In the final stage of transtentorial herniation, medullary compression produces irregular breathing, flaccidity, and eventually death.

Management of increased intracranial pressure

The first step in managing increased intracranial pressure is to improve cerebral venous drainage by placing the head of the patient's bed at a 45° angle. Next, intubate the patient and hyperventilate them to a P_{CO2} of 25 mmHg. This decrease in P_{CO2} produces cerebral vasoconstriction and increases the volume available for the brain parenchyma to occupy. Next, administer the osmotic diuretic mannitol (1–1.5 g/kg IV bolus and then 0.25–0.5 g/kg IV boluses q6h as needed). Measure the serum osmolality with each dose of mannitol, and discontinue the mannitol if the osmolality exceeds 315 mOsm. Consider intracranial pressure monitoring in comatose patients in whom the neurological examination cannot be monitored reliably. Other treatments including barbiturates, corticosteroids, and therapeutic hypothermia probably do not improve outcome in patients with increased intracranial pressure and should be avoided. The definitive treatment of increased intracranial pressure is removing the proximate cause, whether it is a hemorrhage, edema, tumor, or abscess. In patients in whom the relevant source cannot be addressed, consider craniotomy and temporal lobectomy to reduce rapidly increasing intracranial pressure. Because most patients who reach the stage at which this intervention is considered have a poor prognosis, decisions about neurosurgical intervention should be made very carefully.

References

1. Posner JB, Saper CB, Schiff ND, Plum, F. *Plum and Posner's Diagnosis of Stupor and Coma*. Oxford: Oxford University Press; 2007.

2. Fisher CM. Some neuro-ophthalmological observations. *J Neurol Neurosurg Psychiatry* 1967;**30**:383–392.

3. Baloh RW, Furman JM, Yee RD. Dorsal midbrain syndrome: clinical and oculographic findings. *Neurology* 1985;**35**:54–60.

4. Fisher CM. Ocular bobbing. *Arch Neurol* 1964;**11**:543–546.

5. Tarulli AW, Lim C, Bui JD, Saper CB, Alexander MP. Central neurogenic hyperventilation: a case report and discussion of pathophysiology. *Arch Neurol* 2005;**62**:1632–1634.

6. Barth A, Bogousslavsky J, Caplan LR. Thalamic infarcts and hemorrhages. In: Bogousslavsky J, Caplan LR, eds. *Stroke Syndromes*. Cambridge: Cambridge University Press; 2001; 461–468.

7. Claassen J, Mayer SA, Kowalski RG, Emerson RG, Hirsch LJ. Detection of electrographic seizures with continuous EEG monitoring in critically ill patients. *Neurology* 2004;**62**:1743–1748.

8. Levy DE, Bates D, Caronna JJ, et al. Prognosis in nontraumatic coma. *Ann Intern Med* 1981;**94**:293–301.

9. Wijdicks EF, Hijdra A, Young GB, et al. Practice parameter: prediction of outcome in comatose survivors after cardiopulmonary resuscitation (an evidence-based review). *Neurology* 2006;**67**:203–210.

10. Bernard SA, Gray TW, Buist MD, et al. Treatment of comatose survivors of out-of-hospital cardiac arrest with induced hypothermia. *N Engl J Med* 2002;**346**:557–563.

11. The Hypothermia After Cardiac Arrest Study Group. Mild therapeutic hypothermia to improve the neurologic outcome after cardiac arrest. *N Engl J Med* 2002;**346**:549–556.

12. Jennett B, Plum F. Persistent vegetative state after brain damage: a syndrome in search of a name. *Lancet* 1972;**1**:734–737.

13. The Multi-Society Task Force on PVS. Medical aspects of the persistent vegetative state – second of two parts. *N Engl J Med* 1994;**330**:1572–1579.

14. Giacino JT. The vegetative and minimally conscious states: consensus-based criteria for establishing diagnosis and prognosis. *Neurorehabilitation* 2004;**19**:293–298.

Aphasia

Introduction

Aphasia is an acquired disorder of language resulting from brain damage. Understanding the history, controversies, and neuropsychology of aphasia are requirements for every neurologist in training, and there are several excellent reviews available that discuss these topics in greater detail.[1-3] For bedside purposes, however, a simpler, clinically focused approach consisting of the following three steps is necessary:

1. Determine if the problem is aphasia or a mimic.
2. Classify the type of aphasia based on bedside examination.
3. Determine the etiology and attempt to treat it if possible.

Mimics of aphasia

The first step in evaluating a patient with a possible acute language disturbance is to determine whether they are actually aphasic. The two problems that are most often misidentified as aphasia are dysarthria and confusion.

Dysarthria is an abnormality in the mechanical production of speech (Chapter 8). It is most easily distinguished from aphasia by the absence of word-finding or comprehension difficulties. In most cases, dysarthria is secondary to intoxication with drugs (both prescription and illicit) or alcohol, or to a metabolic disturbance such as hyponatremia or hypoglycemia. In rare instances, acute-onset *isolated* dysarthria may be secondary to stroke.[4]

Differentiating confusion from aphasia is often challenging, but doing so is very important because the metabolic derangements that produce confusion are quite distinct from the vascular lesions that are most commonly responsible for aphasia. Although confusion is principally a disorder of attention, any cognitive domain, including language, may be affected (Chapter 1). Language examination in the confused patient will often show normal fluency, poor comprehension, and normal repetition, potentially leading to the erroneous impression that the patient has a transcortical sensory aphasia. Confused patients are most reliably distinguished from aphasic ones by the presence of widespread behavioral abnormalities outside the language domain.

Bedside examination of the aphasic patient

Because the most common acute cause of aphasia is ischemic stroke, it is important to evaluate the patient rapidly in order to determine their eligibility for intravenous thrombolysis. Once the patient is stabilized and any possible treatment for acute stroke is administered, you can assess language in greater detail. More than an academic exercise, the classification of aphasia helps to define the patient's language capabilities and to predict the recovery and evolution of their language. Correct classification of aphasia also allows succinct communication with other health-care providers including speech pathologists and rehabilitation experts. For a neurologist's purposes, assessment of aphasia requires evaluation of:

1. Spontaneous speech
2. Comprehension ability
3. Repetition
4. Confrontation naming
5. Reading, both aloud and for comprehension
6. Writing

Spontaneous speech

Careful listening to spontaneous speech while taking the history often provides most of the essential details about a patient's language dysfunction.

Fluent speech is characterized by a normal or increased rate of word production with normal phrase lengths, while nonfluent speech is characterized by a paucity of verbal output and short phrase lengths. Fluent aphasics use excessive numbers of "filler" words such as prepositions, conjunctions, and adjectives. Despite the excessive number of words, content is lacking. Nonfluent aphasics generally use a preponderance of content-rich words such as nouns and verbs. While their utterances are short and agrammatic, they often convey a great deal of meaning. As a general rule, fluent aphasias are caused by lesions posterior to the central sulcus, while nonfluent aphasias are caused by lesions anterior to the central sulcus.

Paraphasic errors are word substitutions, and may be classified broadly into semantic and phonemic errors. Semantic paraphasic errors are those in which the word produced is related in meaning to the target word. Examples of common semantic paraphasic errors include simplifications (e.g. *finger* for *thumb*), substitutions of one item for another of the same class (e.g. *toe* for *thumb*), and substitutions of the whole for the part (e.g. *hand* for *thumb*). Phonemic paraphasic errors are those in which individual phonemes (segments of sound) are substituted (e.g. *tadle* for *table*), omitted (e.g. *tale* for *table*), or added (e.g. *tadable* for *table*) incorrectly.

Articulatory errors are apparent word substitutions produced by patients with dysarthria. These are not technically paraphasias, but in some cases may resemble phonemic errors.

Neologisms are new words that are formed from appropriate phonemes but which do not resemble an identifiable target word. These are particularly characteristic of posterior aphasias such as Wernicke's aphasia.

Circumlocution is a circling in on the target word in which the patient uses descriptors of the word rather than the word itself (e.g. *thing you eat with* for *fork*). It is a characteristic feature of conduction aphasia.

Comprehension

While it is generally true that nonfluent aphasics comprehend spoken language better than fluent aphasics do, all aphasic patients have some degree of comprehension impairment. Conversely, the comprehension abilities of fluent aphasics (in whom comprehension is traditionally described as being poor) are often preserved to some degree. When assessing comprehension, it is important to establish a floor and a ceiling of performance. In sequence, ask the patient to do the following:

- Follow commands that involve the midline of the body, such as opening and closing the eyes and sticking out the tongue. The ability to follow these commands is preserved in patients with all but the most severe comprehension deficits.
- Answer simple yes/no questions that require only head nodding. Be sure to alternate questions that elicit both yes and no responses, as many patients may continue to nod "yes" without actually understanding the questions.
- Perform simple limb movements such as raising the left or right hand or pointing to objects around the room. Keep in mind that right arm weakness and apraxia (Chapter 4) may accompany aphasia, thus limiting the ability to perform and interpret this type of test.
- Follow sequential commands such as "point to the door, then the light, then the window."
- Follow out-of-sequence commands such as "after pointing to the door, but before pointing to the light, point to the window." These are more difficult, especially for nonfluent aphasics in whom understanding complex syntactic structures is impaired.
- Answer listening comprehension questions such as, "The wolf was chased and eaten by the sheep. Who died?" Questions such as these in which both the traditional subject–verb–object syntax and the expected logic of the sentence are altered are often helpful in detecting subtle deficits in nonfluent aphasic patients with apparently preserved comprehension.

Repetition

While the ability to repeat is seldom applied to everyday life situations, testing repetition is useful in distinguishing among the different aphasia syndromes. The general rule is that repetition is poor in aphasias derived from lesions adjacent to the Sylvian fissure, whereas repetition is relatively preserved in extrasylvian aphasias. To test repetition, start with common, single-syllable words such as "cat" and "dog." The ability to repeat these words is preserved in all but those with the most severe difficulties. Next, test the ability to repeat simple subject–verb–object sentences such as, "The boy threw the ball." Finally, ask the patient to repeat complex sequences such as, "After coming home from work, they ate breakfast in the living room." Note specific problems with repetition in each case. Patients with nonfluent aphasias tend to omit prepositions and conjunctions but repeat content-rich words correctly. Inattentive patients might be able to repeat only the first few (or last few) words of a complex phrase correctly. All repetition impairments should be judged in terms of their relative severity compared with other language deficits. For example, patients with transcortical motor aphasia may make mild errors when repeating, but compared with a near absence of spontaneous speech, any deficits in repetition are relatively minor.

Confrontation naming

Some patients with aphasia have few deficits beyond problems with confrontation naming. A commonly used bedside method to test confrontation naming is to ask the patient to name your hand, finger, thumb, knuckle, and cuticle in sequence. This is a rough screen for anomia for high-, medium-, and low-frequency items. Standardized materials such as the Boston Naming Test allow better analysis of naming deficits. Be cautious not to assign too much weight to mild anomia, as it is common in people who are older or less educated.

Reading

Reading deficits generally mirror spoken language deficits. Test for the ability to read individual words, short sentences, and brief passages of 100–200 words aloud. Look for both the ability to pronounce the words correctly and for an understanding of content.

Writing

Like reading, writing performance usually mirrors spoken language. Patients with nonfluent aphasias write short, agrammatic sentences full of content words, while those with fluent aphasias write long, often incomprehensible sentences with many paraphasic errors.

Aphasia syndromes

While the following descriptions of the classic aphasia syndromes are clinically useful, they have several important limitations. First, they are largely a cluster of language deficits associated with specific ischemic strokes. Impairments from aphasia secondary to trauma, tumor, or hemorrhage do not conform to these patterns. Secondly, there are numerous exceptions to even the most basic rules such as left-sided lesions cause aphasia in right-handed people, posterior lesions produce fluent aphasias, and extrasylvian aphasias do not affect repetition. Finally, aphasia may undergo a

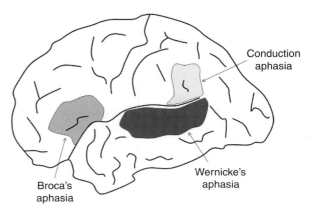

Figure 3.1 Left lateral view of the brain demonstrating the rough localizations of the classical cortical aphasias.

semiological transformation over time, resembling global aphasia at initial presentation and changing to Wernicke's aphasia several days later, for example.

Broca's aphasia

Broca's aphasia is characterized by nonfluent speech, relatively preserved comprehension, and impaired repetition. In its classical form, spontaneous output is limited to content-rich phrases of one or two words, which are produced with great effort and poor melodic intonation. While patients understand simple sentences and can follow commands, longer, syntactically complex sentences reveal important comprehension limitations. Patients may be able to repeat single words but longer phrases prove more challenging. Accompanying deficits include contralateral arm and face weakness. Broca's aphasia is traditionally due to infarction of the frontal operculum and adjacent subcortical white matter (Figure 3.1), although many patients with lesions isolated to these areas have fractional syndromes rather than full-blown Broca's aphasia.[5]

Wernicke's aphasia

Patients with Wernicke's aphasia have fluent speech, often with an increase in the rate and quantity of verbal output to the point where it can be labeled as pressured. While the quantity of output is great, the content is sparse, consisting of excessive semantic and phonemic paraphasic errors, adverbs, adjectives, and grammatical connectors. The prosody, or rhythm and inflection of verbal output, is normal. Comprehension of both spoken and written language is poor. Patients with Wernicke's aphasia are unable to repeat in a reliable manner, and in many cases are not even able to understand the request to repeat. Patients with Wernicke's aphasia may be completely unaware of or unconcerned by their deficits. Additional neurological deficits include contralateral hemibody sensory abnormalities and right-sided visual field cuts. The lesion associated with Wernicke's aphasia is in the left superior temporal gyrus (Figure 3.1) and is often produced by an embolus to the inferior division of the left middle cerebral artery.

Global aphasia

Global aphasia is most often caused by a large left middle cerebral artery infarction. Output is nonfluent and agrammatical, and in some cases the patient may be mute. Both comprehension and repetition are poor. Global aphasia is usually accompanied by a severe right hemiparesis and often by forced leftward eye deviation.

Transcortical motor aphasia

The most obvious feature of transcortical motor aphasia is poor initiation of speech, with phrases that may be only one or two words in length. Comprehension is relatively preserved. The difference between spontaneous speech and repetition is quite striking. Some patients with transcortical motor aphasia may be able to repeat long sentences almost verbatim. Others have very little spontaneous speech, but are able to repeat the examiner's questions (echolalia). The most common lesion location is in the frontal subcortical white matter anterolateral to the left lateral ventricle.[6] Transcortical motor aphasia may be due to left anterior cerebral artery infarction, in which case it is accompanied by right foot weakness.

Conduction aphasia

The most obvious feature of spontaneous speech in conduction aphasia is the excessive number of paraphasic errors, most often phonemic ones. Circumlocution is also quite striking and may take the form of *conduit d'approche* in which the patient makes successive paraphasic errors that more closely approximate the desired word before finally arriving at the target. Fluency is generally preserved, although it may be slightly reduced as the patient attempts to correct their paraphasic errors or search for the appropriate word. Comprehension is relatively normal, but repetition is very poor. Conduction aphasia may be associated with

contralateral homonymous hemianopsia or inferior quadrantanopsia. Conduction aphasia is usually due to lesions of the left supramarginal gyrus, insula, or the underlying white matter (Figure 3.1).

Transcortical sensory aphasia and mixed transcortical aphasia

These aphasias are uncommon in the acute setting. Transcortical sensory aphasia is characterized by fluent output of nonspecific words such as "that" or "things," poor comprehension, and relatively spared repetition. It is most common in Alzheimer's disease and semantic dementia (Chapter 4). Patients with mixed transcortical aphasia show poor fluency and comprehension, with relatively preserved repetition. It is uncommon, and is most often due to large frontal or anterior thalamic lesions.[1]

Subcortical aphasias

Subcortical lesions may result in a wide variety of aphasias, which I will not discuss in great detail. Deficits may resemble one of the classical aphasias or may be somewhat nonspecific, or may be restricted to anomia. The most commonly described locations for subcortical aphasia are the thalamus and the striatum.[7]

Anomic aphasia

Essentially any left hemispheric lesion may produce anomia without other language abnormalities. Anomia may be the only deficit in acute aphasia, or it may be the long-term remnant of a resolving aphasia.

Aphemia

Aphemia is characterized by severe articulatory planning deficits that may mimic nonfluent aphasia.[8] In most cases, patients are mute at presentation, and fluency improves over several days. Unlike patients with nonfluent aphasias, comprehension and written language are preserved in aphemia. The capacity to write lengthy, well-constructed sentences that contrast markedly with the sparse spontaneous verbal output is often astounding. Aphemia is caused by any number of left hemispheric lesions, including those involving Broca's area, the premotor cortex, the motor strip, and the insula. It is usually accompanied by right hemiparesis. As acute mutism resolves, speech is initially slow, effortful, and poorly articulated. Complete recovery may occur over several days to a few weeks. It is important to recognize aphemia, as it usually has a better prognosis than the nonfluent aphasia syndromes with which it is confused.

Determining the cause and treatment of aphasia

Acute aphasia is most commonly due to ischemic or hemorrhage stroke. Other sources of acute aphasia include head trauma, intracranial masses, seizures, and the postictal state. In the acute setting, a comprehensive evaluation of language must assume a secondary priority, as the pathologies that produce acute aphasia are potentially devastating and sometimes reversible. Until proven otherwise, assume that all patients who present with acute-onset aphasia have an ischemic stroke that requires immediate evaluation and treatment (Chapter 21).

Recovery and rehabilitation of acute aphasia

Most recovery from aphasia takes place within the first 3–6 months after symptom onset.[9] The traditional notion that recovery beyond 1 year is rare may not necessarily be true.[10] Predictors of better prognosis include smaller lesions, younger patient age, and left-handedness. Patients with traumatic lesions tend to have better outcomes than those with ischemic or hemorrhagic ones. Recovery is mediated by the cortex adjacent to the lesion, subcortical structures, and the right hemisphere.[11] Both formal (with a speech therapist) and informal (reintegrating the patient back into everyday communication with family, friends, and coworkers) rehabilitation programs are beneficial and should be initiated as soon as possible.[12]

References

1. Alexander MP. Aphasia: clinical and anatomical aspects. In: Feinberg TE, Farah MJ, eds. *Behavioral Neurology and Neuropsychology*. New York: McGraw Hill; 1997; 133–150.

2. Hillis AE. Aphasia: progress in the last quarter of a century. *Neurology* 2007;**69**:200–213.

3. Benson DF, Ardila A. *Aphasia: a Clinical Perspective*. Oxford: Oxford University Press; 1996.

4. Kim JS. Pure dysarthria, isolated facial paresis, or dysarthria-facial paresis syndrome. *Stroke* 1999;**25**:1994–1998.

5. Mohr J, Pessin M, Finkelstein S, et al. Broca aphasia: pathological and clinical. *Neurology* 1978;**28**:311–324.

6. Freedman M, Alexander MP, Naeser MA. Anatomic basis of transcortical motor aphasia. *Neurology* 1984;**34**:409–417.

7. Nadeau SE, Crosson B. Subcortical aphasia. *Brain Lang* 1997;**58**:355–402.

8. Ottomeyer C, Reuter B, Jager T, et al. Aphemia: an isolated disorder of speech associated with an ischemic lesion of the left precentral gyrus. *J Neurol* 2009;**256**:1166–1168.

9. Kertesz A, McCabe P. Recovery patterns and prognosis in aphasia. *Brain* 1977;**100**:1–18.

10. Moss A, Nicholas M. Language rehabilitation in chronic aphasia and time postonset: a review of single-subject data. *Stroke* 2006;**37**:3043–3051.

11. Saur D, Lange R, Baumgaertner A, et al. Dynamics of language reorganization after stroke. *Brain* 2006;**129**:1371–1384.

12. Robey RR. The efficacy of treatment for aphasic persons: a meta-analysis. *Brain Lang* 1994;**47**: 582–608.

Dementia

History

Dementia is the chronic and progressive (at least 6 months in duration) loss of memory and at least one other cognitive function (language, praxis, object knowledge, or executive function) that interferes with a person's ability to perform the activities of daily living.[1] Although the history is the most important means of establishing the diagnosis, most patients with dementia provide only a vague account of their cognitive deficits, often stating that nothing is wrong or focusing on a minor respiratory, gastrointestinal, or orthopedic complaint. The patient frequently lacks awareness of their deficits, and collateral history must be obtained from a family member or friend. Because this narrative history may also be vague and unhelpful, directed questioning about specific deficits is often the only effective strategy to establish the exact nature of the problem.

Memory

The first memory problem that families report is often that the patient repeats himself or asks the same question in the space of a few minutes. A demented patient misplaces their keys, eyeglasses, or wallet more frequently than would be expected of someone who was simply absentminded. Other memory problems include forgetting to purchase items from the grocery store, missing appointments, and getting lost. Memory problems may lead to difficulty with the finances, as the patient often forgets charges or receipts when balancing their checkbook or preparing their taxes. Although all dementias include at least a component of memory problems, these are particularly important in Alzheimer's disease (AD).

Language

Word-finding difficulties are an early deficit in many dementias, especially AD and primary progressive aphasia (PPA). The patient seems to search for the proper word for an excessive amount of time or has a tendency to substitute less specific words such as "thing," "that," or "the place" for more precise ones. Intermittent episodes in which speech appears to be slurred or garbled are a feature of dementia with Lewy bodies (DLB).

Praxis

Praxis is the ability to perform skilled movements, and deficits in praxis (apraxia) are an important feature of many dementias, especially corticobasal ganglionic degeneration and AD. Early evidence of apraxia includes difficulty with operating computers, DVD players, and other relatively newer technologies. Other patients have problems with planning and preparing meals. As dementia progresses, simpler tasks such as brushing the hair or teeth or eating become difficult.

Visuospatial function

Visuospatial deficits include problems with getting lost, applying makeup, and driving or parking. These problems are especially common in patients with DLB, but may be features of any of the dementias. Patients with more advanced dementia may have difficulties dressing properly.

Behavioral abnormalities

Behavioral abnormalities occur as early symptoms in frontotemporal dementia (FTD). Socially inappropriate behaviors including lewd comments, aggression, and excessive risk-taking are features of FTD, as are abulia in which the patient seems unmotivated, spending most of their time in bed or watching television. Personal hygiene also suffers in many demented patients. Hallucinations, particularly visual ones, are a core feature of DLB. Be cautious when asking about hallucinations, as the patient may be hesitant to admit to things that might lead to psychiatric hospitalization. To ease into inquiries about hallucinations, ask first about vivid dreams and then about seeing unusual things, and, if the patient does not endorse either of these, ask them specifically about hallucinations. Finally, ask about features of rapid eye movement (REM) sleep behavioral disorder such as punching, kicking, or screaming out in the middle of sleep, which may predate other symptoms of DLB by many years.

Gait difficulties

Although gait difficulties are common and somewhat nonspecific in the elderly (Chapter 18), they may point to specific causes of dementia including normal pressure hydrocephalus (NPH), vascular dementia, and progressive supranuclear palsy.

Relevant medical history

Obtain a complete medical history in all patients who present with suspected dementia. A history of human immunodeficiency virus (HIV) infection, cardiac surgery, renal or hepatic failure, or hypothyroidism may point to explanations for cognitive decline other than one of the degenerative dementias. It is also helpful to screen briefly for sleep disorders, disabling pain, and depression. These medical problems often mimic dementia and, because they are reversible, it is important to identify and treat them as soon as possible. Medications, especially narcotics, benzodiazepines, and anticonvulsants, may also produce reversible cognitive dysfunction.

Age of onset, tempo, and fluctuations

Noting the age of onset is often helpful in generating a differential diagnosis for dementia: while most demented patients are older than 65, FTD and early-onset AD may begin in patients in their 40s or 50s. Deficits in most dementias are acquired in a gradual fashion, but some are characterized by a subacutely progressive onset over a few weeks to months (Creutzfeldt–Jakob disease or Hashimoto's encephalopathy), or a sudden stepwise onset (vascular dementia). Fluctuation of deficits is a key feature of DLB. Examples of fluctuation include daytime drowsiness and lethargy, daytime naps lasting at least 2 hours, staring into space for long periods, and episodes of disorganized speech.[2]

Examination

Mental status examination

The mental status examination begins informally as the history is being obtained. Make note of any word-

finding difficulties, repetition of details, or vague answers. Patients with moderate-to-severe dementia may not be able to provide any relevant history whatsoever. Observe for bizarre comments or general sluggishness as might be expected in FTD, or bradykinesia or bradyphrenia, which may reflect DLB.

Keep in mind that poor performance on components of the mental status examination may represent the patient's cognitive baseline rather than an acquired cognitive problem. Before judging any deficiencies, inquire about the length of the patient's formal education, occupation, and level of intellectual activity prior to the onset of cognitive decline.

Mental status testing is often time-consuming. In some cases, thorough cognitive assessment may require more detail than a single office visit allows, particularly in the early stages of dementia when the problems may be subtle or when the patient has a high premorbid level of function. The mini mental status examination is a good brief screening examination, but is generally not good at diagnosing or classifying dementia or milder deficits.[3] The brief mental status examination summarized in Table 4.1 and described in detail in this chapter may be performed in 10 minutes and provides both a general picture of a patient's cognitive abilities and details about problems in specific cognitive domains.

Attention

A variety of bedside tests is available to assess attention (Chapter 1). After establishing basic orientation to person, place, and time, ask the patient to recite the months of the year backwards to determine whether they are sufficiently attentive to complete the remainder of the mental status examination. Attention is relatively preserved until the advanced stages of AD, while it may be affected earlier in the course of FTD or DLB.

Language

Chapter 3 provides more detailed instructions for the assessment of language. Perhaps the most important components of language evaluation in a patient with suspected dementia are tests of semantic and phonemic fluency.

Semantic fluency

To test semantic fluency, ask the patient to name as many animals as they can in 1 minute. More specific normative values stratified by age and educational level are available, but a normal older person will be able to

Table 4.1 Summary of mental status examination

Orientation to person, place, and time
Months of the year backwards
Language testing for fluency, comprehension, and repetition
Semantic fluency
Phonemic fluency
Recall of four words at 5 minutes
Target cancellation (Chapter 1)
Praxis testing
Draw a house
Place the numbers of a clock on a circle
Luria test
Stroop test
Frontal release signs

name roughly 12 different animals in a minute.[4] Early loss of semantic fluency compared with phonemic fluency suggests the possibility of AD or semantic dementia.[5] These patients may be able to name only four or five animals in 1 minute, often repeating more familiar animals several times during the course of the test.

Phonemic fluency

To test phonemic fluency, ask the patient to generate a list of words, exclusive of proper nouns, beginning with the letter "S." It may be helpful to perform this test several minutes after testing semantic fluency: many patients who perform the tests consecutively will restrict their responses to animals that begin with the letter "S." Again, there are normative values stratified by age and educational level. A healthy older person should be able to name roughly ten "S" words in 1 minute.[4] Although there is some variability in the literature, patients with DLB and FTD generally show loss of phonemic fluency that is greater than or at least equal to semantic fluency, which is distinct from patients with AD in whom phonemic fluency is relatively preserved compared with semantic fluency.[5]

Memory

Asking the patient to tell you about a few current events or sports stories is a good screening test for memory problems. If they cannot tell you anything spontaneously, try to trigger their memory by providing hints about an item in the news. If they still draw a blank, ask the patient to name the president, governor, or best player on the local baseball or football team. If they are not capable of doing even this last task, ask them if they know the date or season.

Verbal recall of a four-word list is a good test of episodic memory. Begin by telling the patient that you will ask them to recall four words in 5 minutes. When selecting target words, use both words that have physical manifestations such as "apple" and also conceptual ones to which visual tags cannot be so readily assigned, such as "wisdom." Present the word list at least three times and instruct the patient to repeat it back to you after each presentation. A patient who cannot repeat the word list has attentional problems that will prevent accurate assessment of their recall abilities. Complete the remainder of the mental status examination, and ask the patient to recall the four words after 5 minutes have elapsed. Older patients are generally able to recall three or four of the words, and usually can select the fourth word from a multiple-choice list or recall it if you give them a hint about the category to which the item belongs. Patients with AD have problems not only with recalling the words but also with recognizing them from a list or guessing them from a category. In the very early stages of memory problems, a four-item list may not be sensitive enough to detect memory deficits, and a more detailed neuropsychological evaluation may be required.

Praxis

Apraxia is defined as the inability to perform a learned movement in response to the stimulus that normally produces it. In order for the label of apraxia to be appropriate, all elemental neurological functions such as strength, sensation, language, and attention must be preserved. Apraxia was originally described by Liepman, and his division of apraxia into ideomotor, ideational, and limb-kinetic forms largely persists to this day, despite substantial controversies. Interested readers are referred to Ochipa and Gonzalez Rothi's review on the topic, as I will discuss only one type, ideomotor apraxia, in a limited format here.[6]

Ideomotor apraxia is characterized by errors in positioning, orientation, sequencing, and timing of limb movements. The manifestations and localizations of ideomotor apraxia may roughly be understood with a simplified connectionist model (Figure 4.1).[6] Verbal, visual, or somatosensory inputs synapse with movement representations in the left inferior parietal lobule. These, in turn, activate motor programs in the supplementary motor area of the left frontal lobe. These

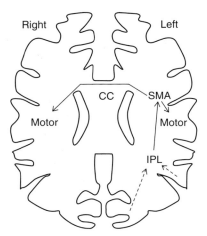

Figure 4.1 Axial section of the brain showing simplified schematic of ideomotor apraxia. Multimodal sensory information is processed by the left inferior lobule (IPL). This in turn activates motor programs in the left supplemental motor area (SMA), which projects to the left motor cortex and, via the corpus callosum (CC), to the right motor cortex.

motor programs activate movement of the right side of the body via synapses with the motor cortex of the left hemisphere. They also cross to the motor cortex of the right hemisphere via the corpus callosum, thereby activating movements of the left side of the body. Thus, lesions of the left inferior parietal lobule or supplementary motor area might be expected to produce ideomotor apraxia of both sides of the body while lesions of the corpus callosum might lead to apraxia of only the left side of the body.

A variety of tests is available to investigate for apraxia. Commonly used bedside tests include asking the patient to perform the following actions to command:

1. Wave goodbye.
2. Blow a kiss.
3. Pretend that they have a toothbrush in their hand and ask them to use it to brush their teeth.
4. Pretend that they have a hammer, and use it to put a nail into a board.
5. Pretend that they have a brush, and use it to brush their hair.

Look for errors in positioning, orientation, sequencing, and timing. If they cannot perform these actions to command, they should try to imitate them. It is also important to watch the patient use actual tools. For hospitalized patients, readily available tools include pencils, forks, remote controls, and flashlights.

Apraxia may be due to vascular, traumatic, neoplastic, or degenerative disorders involving the left frontal or parietal lobes. It is particularly common in patients with AD and corticobasal degeneration. The two most important applications of praxis testing are in patients with suspected corticobasal degeneration in whom apraxia is a prominent early finding and in patients with callosal lesions in whom isolated left limb apraxia reflects disconnection between the left supplementary motor cortex and the right motor cortex.

Construction

Common tests of construction include drawing a house and drawing a clock. When a patient draws a house, study its general outline as well as specific details such as doors, windows, and chimneys. Patients who can draw the overall outline of the house but miss the details are more likely to have right hemisphere lesions, while those who draw a poorly outlined house with preserved details are more likely to have left hemisphere lesions. When analyzing a clock drawing, look first for evidence of poor planning such as crowding all the numbers on the right hand side of the circle. Evidence for perseveration (a sign of frontal lobe dysfunction) includes repeating the same number several times or continuing to number the clock beyond "12." Patients with visuospatial deficits may place the numbers outside the circle or draw the numbers in a spiral that closes in on itself. Visuospatial abilities and construction impairments tend to be more severe in patients with DLB than in those with other forms of dementia.

Mental flexibility

Mental flexibility, including the ability to switch quickly between different cognitive tasks, is governed largely by the frontal lobes. The Luria and Stroop tests are two useful bedside tests for patients with suspected frontal lobe disorders.

Luria test

The Luria test is a popular tool to evaluate metal flexibility. The patient is first asked to sequentially tap a table or other flat suface with the first, then with the palm, and then with the side of the hand. Instruct the patient to repeat this sequence several times in succession. Some patients with comprehension problems, apraxia, or severe frontal disorders have difficulty with even this first sequence. If the patient correctly learns and performs this sequence several times in succession, however, switch the sequence from fist–palm–side to fist–side–palm. Observe whether the patient is capable of switching to the second sequence, or whether they remain stuck in set and follow the original sequence.

Stroop test

This test exists in a variety of forms, one of which consists of a grid of 30–40 words written in different colors. The first several targets are color names written in the same color as the text. For example, the word "green" is written in the color green. After eight to ten such targets, the words are written in colors different from the text. For example, the word "green" is written in the color purple. To perform the Stroop test, first ask the patient to simply read the words. After they have read through the entire list, instruct them to read the list from start to finish again, this time saying not the written word, but rather its color. Patients with frontal dysfunction will remain stuck in set and continue to read the word rather than the color. Even after being corrected, they may continue to make the same kind of mistake.

Processing speed

Processing speed difficulties are signs of frontal lobe dysfunction and are often evident in the way the patient answers questions. A gestalt of processing speed may be estimated at the bedside by simple observation of the other parts of the mental status examination, particularly the "A" cancellation test described in Chapter 1 or by a Trails B-type test in which the patient is asked to "connect the dots" between alternating letters and numbers (Figure 4.2). A variety of formal tests performed during neuropsychological evaluation are superior at detecting and quantifying processing speed abnormalities.

Frontal release signs

The so-called frontal release signs or primitive reflexes are found in patients with moderate to severe dementia. The grasp sign is elicited by dragging a finger over the patient's opened palm, and is positive when the patient clutches at the finger. The palmomental sign is observed when the chin puckers slightly upon gently stroking the palm. The snout or rooting reflex is present when stroking the cheek at the corner of the mouth results in a twitching of the mouth or lips.

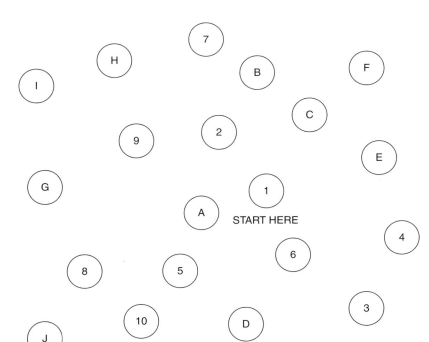

Figure 4.2 Example of a Trails B-type test. Instruct the patient to begin at the number "1" and then to connect the dots between alternating letters and numbers. The correct sequence is, therefore, 1–A–2–B–3–C–4–D, etc. Observe the speed at which the patient performs the test and whether they can follow the instructions or instead connects the dots between consecutive numbers or letters. This test is sensitive to frontal lobe dysfunction.

The glabellar sign is the failure to suppress continued blinking when the forehead is quickly tapped with an index finger.

The general neurological examination

The remainder of the neurological examination should focus on finding deficits that help to establish the diagnosis of a specific dementia. As a general rule, patients with AD and FTD have otherwise normal neurological examinations. The following is a brief summary of some of the more common and important examination abnormalities in demented patients.

Cranial nerve examination

A patient with FTD has difficulty following visual field examination instructions. When told to fix their attention on the examiner's nose, any stimulus such as wiggling fingers in the periphery will instantly draw their attention and prevent accurate visual field examination. Progressive supranuclear palsy leads to impaired downward saccade generation that corrects with oculocephalic maneuvers.

Motor examination

Parkinsonism is a core feature of DLB, but rigidity and bradykinesia may be minimal or absent at the time of initial presentation. Myoclonus, although classically associated with Creutzfeldt–Jakob disease, may be a feature of any advanced dementia. Paratonia is an increased involuntary resistance to passive movement that worsens despite instructions to relax, and is seen in frontal lobe disorders. Weakness, fasciculations, hyperreflexia, and other evidence of motor neuron disease are found in approximately 15% of patients with FTD.

Sensory examination

Because polyneuropathies are common in the elderly, any sensory abnormalities should be interpreted cautiously, as they are usually unrelated to the dementing process. Vitamin B_{12} deficiency may lead to impaired vibratory sensation and joint position in the lower extremities. Corticobasal ganglionic degeneration is accompanied by asymmetric loss of higher cortical sensory functions such as graphesthesia and stereognosis.

Gait

Normal pressure hydrocephalus results in a gait abnormality characterized by poor initiation and short, slow steps with the feet narrowly spaced. This pattern is also observed in some patients with vascular dementia. Elderly patients commonly have a multifactorial gait disorder that does not actually reflect any specific dementia and may confuse the diagnostic process.

Diagnostic testing

The diagnosis of dementia is made mostly from the history and mental status examination. Diagnostic testing is performed mainly to exclude reversible medical problems that masquerade as degenerative ones and, in some cases, to establish the diagnosis of a specific primary dementia.

Bloodwork

Every patient with dementia should undergo bloodwork including tests of thyroid stimulating hormone, vitamin B_{12}, folate, and rapid plasma reagin. While the yield of any of these studies is quite low, the associated abnormalities are all reversible causes of cognitive decline. Be cautious, however, when attributing cognitive dysfunction to any of these laboratory findings, as mild abnormalities are common and their presence does not necessarily exclude a degenerative dementia.

Structural neuroimaging

It is essential to perform a neuroimaging study in all patients with dementia to exclude structural lesions such as tumors, abscesses, subdural hematomas, and hydrocephalus. A noncontrast head CT is generally sufficient to demonstrate these problems. MRI, however, offers better neuroanatomic resolution and allows quantification of medial temporal lobe atrophy in AD (Figure 4.3) or frontal and anterior temporal lobe atrophy in FTD.[7,8] Changes consistent with vascular dementia including leukoaraiosis (Figure 4.4), cortical infarcts, and lacunar infarcts are also easier to visualize using MRI.

Functional neuroimaging

Functional neuroimaging studies include positron emission tomography (PET), single photon emission computed tomography (SPECT), functional MRI (fMRI), and magnetic resonance spectroscopy (MRS). These studies will likely play a more prominent role in the differential diagnosis and prognostication of dementia as they are refined and tested in larger groups of patients. For now, they are used mostly on a research

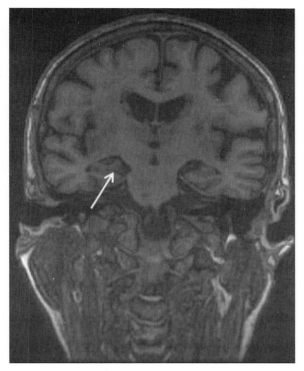

Figure 4.3 Coronal MRI of the brain demonstrating medial temporal lobe atrophy (arrow) in a patient with Alzheimer's disease.

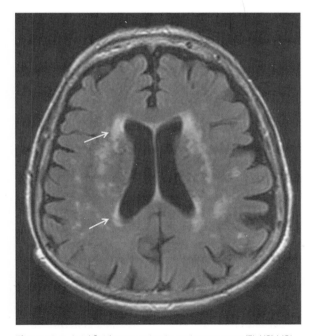

Figure 4.4 Axial fluid attenuation inversion recovery (FLAIR) MRI of the brain showing periventricular white matter hyperintensities (arrows) in a patient with vascular dementia.

basis or to help distinguish among AD, DLB, and FTD in difficult cases.[9–11]

Lumbar puncture

Lumbar puncture plays a limited role in evaluating dementia. It is particularly useful, however, for patients with rapid progression, as it may disclose infectious, inflammatory, or neoplastic causes of cognitive decline. Lumbar puncture and timed gait analysis is the essential test to evaluate for NPH. Spinal fluid showing decreased amyloid β_{42} and increased CSF-tau may be helpful to make a diagnosis in unclear cases of AD, although these tests are usually not required.[12]

Genetic testing

Genetic testing is available for several different dementias but is rarely employed in patients without clear familial histories of early-onset dementia.

Causes of dementia

Alzheimer's disease

Alzheimer's disease is the most common form of dementia. The typical patient with AD is 65 years or older and has a dementia characterized mainly by slowly progressive memory problems. Early-onset and rapidly progressive forms of AD, however, are uncommon but important variants. As the disorder progresses, memory deficits worsen, and essentially any cognitive domain may be affected. The diagnosis is established by history and mental status examination. Finding medial temporal atrophy on MRI may support the clinical diagnosis.[7]

The acetylcholinesterase inhibitors donepezil, rivastigmine, and galantamine (Table 4.2) are modestly effective in improving cognitive deficits but do not alter disease progression. The most common adverse effects of these medications are nausea, vomiting, and diarrhea: patients who do not tolerate one agent may find more success with a different one. The N-methyl-D-aspartate (NMDA) receptor antagonist memantine may be effective for patients with moderately severe disease, especially when used in combination with an acetylcholinesterase inhibitor. Side effects of memantine including dizziness and confusion are uncommon. As AD progresses, medications are of limited value, and treatment focuses on assistance with activities of daily living including bathing and eating, and control of behavioral symptoms. Ultimately, AD progresses

Table 4.2 Medications used to treat Alzheimer's disease

Medication	Starting dose	Titration instructions
Donepezil	5 mg	Increase to 10 mg qd in 4–6 weeks
Rivastigmine	1.5 mg bid	Increase by 1.5 mg bid every 2 weeks to maximum dose of 6 mg bid
Galantamine	4 mg bid	Increase by 4 mg bid every 4 weeks to maximum dose of 12 mg bid
Memantine	5 mg qd	Increase to 5 mg bid in 1 week, 5 mg qam and 10 mg qpm in 2 weeks, and 10 mg bid thereafter

and patients with advanced disease require nursing home placement.

Dementia with Lewy bodies

This is the second most common of the degenerative dementias and, like AD, tends to occur in older people. The three core clinical features of DLB are cognitive fluctuations (discussed above), visual hallucinations, and parkinsonism. Visual hallucinations are initially nonthreatening and may take the form of people, animals, or brightly colored objects. As the disease progresses, the hallucinations may become more threatening. Parkinsonism is often subtle or absent in the early stages of DLB: if it is present early in the course of the disease or is the main symptom, consider a form of parkinsonism other than DLB.[13] Development of REM sleep behavioral disorder, in which a patient acts out their dreams, may precede the development of other DLB symptomatology, often by many years.

On mental status examination, episodic memory is relatively preserved in the early stages of the disease. Both semantic and phonemic fluency may be affected. Visuospatial impairments are more prominent than in patients with AD. Extrapyramidal findings tend to involve axial more than appendicular musculature, and tremor is usually absent. Laboratory and radiological testing is of limited utility: ^{18}F-fluorodeoxyglucose PET scanning may demonstrate occipital lobe hypometabolism, but the diagnosis is still established by history and neurological examination.[14]

Treating DLB with acetylcholinesterase inhibitors may be effective. Levodopa is generally less useful for parkinsonism in DLB than it is in Parkinson's disease. Levodopa and dopamine agonists should be used cautiously as they may worsen hallucinations and other behavioral problems. In the early stages, hallucinations are not typically disturbing to the patient, and therefore do not require treatment. For patients with bothersome hallucinations, low-dose quetiapine (25 mg prn) is preferred, as it usually does not worsen extrapyramidal symptoms. Clozapine may also be used to treat hallucinations, although any patient who takes this medication requires periodic complete blood counts to monitor for agranulocytosis.

Frontotemporal dementia

Frontotemporal dementia is often first evaluated by a psychiatrist rather than a neurologist, as behavioral changes rather than memory impairment are usually the earliest symptoms of the disorder. Patients with FTD tend to be younger than those with AD and DLB, often developing symptoms in their 40s or 50s rather than in their 60s or later. Abnormal behaviors in FTD may be broadly clustered into socially inappropriate and withdrawn behaviors:

- Examples of socially inappropriate behavior include a reduced sense of social decorum including rude or often lewd comments and uncharacteristic risk-taking behaviors such as excessive gambling or alcohol consumption. Other features of FTD include bizarre preferences for certain types of foods (especially sweets), hoarding behaviors, and an obsession with generating artwork. The inappropriate patient is often evaluated and treated for bipolar or psychotic disorders before coming to neurological attention.
- The patient with the withdrawn phenotype of FTD is apathetic, showing little interest in work, family, or hobbies. They spend most of their time in bed, watching television, or simply staring into space. Personal hygiene is compromised. They may be evaluated and treated for depression before coming to neurological attention.

Examination shows impaired mental flexibility, slowed processing speed, and early frontal release signs. Episodic memory is generally preserved in the initial stage of the disease. Although a general neurological examination is usually normal, approximately 15% of patients with FTD also have motor neuron disease (Chapter 10). MRI may disclose disproportionate frontal and anterior temporal atrophy, which helps to distinguish FTD from AD.[8]

Treatment of FTD is often disappointing: acetylcholinesterase inhibitors are usually not effective and may actually worsen behavior.[15] Selective serotonin reuptake inhibitors may help to control some of the behavioral symptoms. Most patients with FTD, unfortunately, require close supervision and often need early nursing home placement.

Vascular dementia

The term "vascular dementia" encompasses three different disorders: multi-infarct dementia, subcortical white matter disease, and strategic-infarct dementia.

Multi-infarct dementia

Multi-infarct dementia is the condition that most neurologists would describe as vascular dementia. This form of dementia is characterized by the stepwise accumulation of neurological deficits from multiple, clinically apparent cerebral infarctions. While the strokes do not necessarily involve areas of the brain that are critical for memory, their cumulative effect is dementia. Although mental status testing in patients with multi-infarct dementia may resemble that of the other dementias (most commonly AD), abnormalities on the general neurological examination suggestive of prior infarctions such as hemiparesis and visual field cuts help to make the diagnosis. There is considerable overlap between multi-infarct dementia and AD, and distinguishing between the two on clinical or even radiological grounds is often difficult. From a treatment perspective, the distinction may not necessarily be crucial, as patients with multi-infarct dementia, like those with AD, benefit from acetylcholinesterase inhibitors.[16] Obviously, it is important to look for and treat risk factors for vascular disease such as hypertension, diabetes, and hyperlipidemia. While correcting these risk factors does not necessarily improve cognitive symptoms, it is important from a general health perspective.

Subcortical white matter disease

Subcortical white matter disease is known by a variety of names including Binswanger's disease, periventricular white matter disease, and leukoaraiosis. It is characterized by the progressive accumulation of multiple, often clinically silent infarctions in the subcortical white matter. Patients most commonly present with

bradyphrenia, impaired executive function, memory loss, and frontal gait abnormalities. Patients tend to resemble those with the withdrawn/abulic form of FTD or NPH. Typical risk factors for vascular disease such as hypertension, hyperlipidemia, and diabetes are present. In rare young patients, subcortical white matter disease may be a consequence of cerebral autosomal-dominant arteriopathy with subcortical infarcts and leukoencephalopathy (CADASIL) secondary to a *NOTCH3* gene mutation.[17] Unfortunately, subcortical white matter disease responds poorly to any treatments, and care is largely supportive.

Strategic infarct dementia

Strategic infarct dementia is produced by infarction of an area of the brain that is critical for memory. It is not strictly a dementia, as it is acute in onset and tends to be static rather than progressive. Nonetheless, the persistent memory deficits that occur as a consequence of strategic-infarct dementia force it to be considered here. Vascular territories associated with sudden-onset memory loss include the polar artery, paramedian thalamic artery, and the medial temporal branch of the posterior cerebral artery.[18] Patients with strategic infarct dementia may improve over time, unlike those with other dementias. The mainstay of treatment is preventing stroke recurrence.

Normal pressure hydrocephalus

The well-known clinical triad of NPH is dementia, urinary incontinence, and gait impairment. This simple summary, however, is misleading, and because the triad is rather nonspecific, it leads to many unnecessary referrals for "NPH evaluations." In brief, many demented patients will develop both urinary incontinence and gait impairment as their dementia progresses, and few of them will actually have NPH.

Although there is considerable heterogeneity in the clinical presentation of NPH, the features that are most consistent with the diagnosis are abulia (resembling FTD in some cases) and frontal gait abnormality. This frontal gait is characterized by slow initiation and shortened stride length to the point that the patient appears to be stuck to the floor by a magnetic force (Chapter 18). It is often incorrectly called ataxic or apraxic. This pattern is perhaps somewhat nonspecific, as it may also occur as a consequence of arthritic degeneration of the spine, hips, and knees, or parkinsonism. The urinary incontinence of NPH, while it tends to not be urge incontinence, has few features that distinguish it from incontinence of other causes.

Despite its relative rarity, consider NPH evaluation for patients with frontal dementia and frontal gait disorder, as the disorder may be treatable by CSF shunting. All patients with NPH should undergo a CT scan or MRI of the brain to document hydrocephalus (Figure 4.5) and to exclude ventricular system outflow obstruction. A modified version of the CSF tap test is the most common way to make the diagnosis:[19]

1. Admit the patient to the hospital.
2. Measure the amount of time and number of steps it takes to walk 60 feet. Repeat this walking test twice, encouraging the patient to do their best each time.
3. Remove 30–50 cc CSF by lumbar puncture.
4. Repeat the timed walking test immediately after and at 30-minute intervals up to 2 hours after lumbar puncture.

An improvement in the time and number of steps required to walk 60 feet predicts a positive response to CSF shunting. Although it is difficult to quantify what actually constitutes an improvement, a reduction in the time needed to cover 60 feet by 50% is strongly suggestive of the diagnosis. Monitoring mental status testing before and after lumbar puncture is less reliable than timed gait analysis.

Consider ventriculoperitoneal shunting in a patient with a disease duration of <2 years, a positive CSF tap test, and a low burden of both cortical atrophy and periventricular white matter disease. Prior to surgery, it is important to inform the patient and their family about possible complications from an indwelling shunt including meningitis, subdural hygroma or hematoma formation, and chronic headache.

Primary progressive aphasia

Aphasia is a feature of many dementias, including AD, FTD, and corticobasal degeneration. Primary progressive aphasia (PPA) is a progressive dementia characterized by language deficits that are out of proportion to other deficits, and dominate the first 2 years of disease.[20] While our understanding of this disorder is still in its relative youth compared with other types of dementia, there are three generally recognized forms of PPA:[21]

- Nonfluent progressive aphasia, characterized by a lack of fluency, poor syntax, and comprehending difficulties with complex structures. Atrophy is

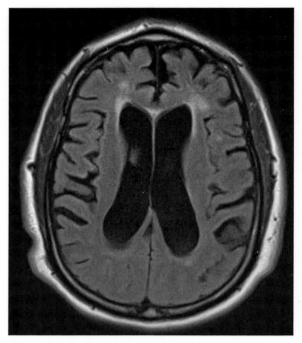

Figure 4.5 Axial fluid attenuation inversion recovery (FLAIR) MRI showing ventricular dilation in a patient with normal pressure hydrocephalus.

usually seen in the left inferior frontal and insular cortices.
- Semantic dementia, characterized by a fundamental loss of word meanings. Fluency is preserved and comprehension is poor. Atrophy tends to affect the left anterior temporal lobe.
- Logopenic progressive aphasia, characterized by decreased fluency with relatively good but simple syntax. Comprehension is good. Atrophy characteristically involves the left inferior parietal lobule and posterior temporal cortex.

Alcohol and dementia

Chronic alcohol abuse may result in rather nonspecific long-term cognitive changes. The classical alcohol-related dementia, however, is Korsakoff's dementia, in which anterograde and retrograde amnesia are profound and out of proportion to other cognitive deficits. Korsakoff's dementia often develops in a patient recovering from Wernicke's encephalopathy. Because patients with Korsakoff's dementia have severe memory deficits but preserved attention, they are prone to confabulation. They will fabricate explanations as to why they are in hospital, relationships to the examiner, and current events. They actively seek environmental clues that sustain the impression that their memory is preserved. Mammillary body atrophy visualized on MRI helps to establish the diagnosis of Korsakoff's syndrome. Unfortunately, the memory deficits do not tend to improve, even with alcohol discontinuation and thiamine supplementation.

Human immunodeficiency virus dementia

Human immunodeficiency virus (HIV) patients develop dementia with an incidence of approximately 1% per year, a figure that is decreasing with more widespread use of highly active antiretroviral therapy (HAART).[22] Presenting symptoms include psychomotor slowing and memory deficits, but as the disease progresses any cognitive domain may be affected. The diagnosis is confirmed radiologically by finding cortical and subcortical atrophy and confluent, subcortical white matter hyperintensities. Other sources of dementia specific to patients with AIDS, such as progressive multifocal leukoencephalopathy, toxoplasmosis, and CNS lymphoma, must be excluded. Treatment with HAART may improve cognitive symptoms or slow their progression.

Neurosyphilis

General paresis of the insane (GPI), a form of tertiary neurosyphilis, was a common cause of dementia in the preantibiotic era. It is now vanishingly rare, but should be considered as a possible source of dementia in patients with a history of syphilis (which usually precedes the dementia by 5–20 years) and in HIV-positive patients. Finding an abnormal CSF venereal disease research laboratory (VDRL) confirms the diagnosis. If the index of suspicion is high and the VDRL is negative, check the fluorescent treponemal antibody absorption (FTA-ABS) test.[23] The standard treatment of GPI is penicillin (3–4 g IV q6h for 14 days). This treatment, however, may not result in a cognitive recovery.

Dementia and movement disorders

Dementia frequently accompanies movement disorders, especially corticobasal ganglionic degeneration, progressive supranuclear palsy, and Parkinson's disease (Chapter 13). In general, these dementias are of the subcortical type, characterized by slow processing speed and difficulty with switching sets. Corticobasal ganglionic degeneration, however, may produce a dementia with prominent cortical features, especially asymmetric limb apraxia.

Mild cognitive impairment

Mild cognitive impairment (MCI) occupies the transitional state between normal cognitive function and overt dementia. In MCI, cognitive abnormalities are present but do not yet meaningfully impact on activities of daily living. Approximately 10% of patients with MCI will progress to AD (amnestic MCI) or to one of the other dementias (nonamnestic MCI) per year, far exceeding the 1% annual conversion rate of otherwise normal adults older than 65.[24] Acetylcholinesterase inhibitors do not clearly delay the progression of MCI to dementia, although they are commonly prescribed.[25]

Pseudodementia

Several conditions may lead to progressive cognitive deficits that may resemble dementia. When a patient presents with progressive cognitive decline, it is important to consider these mimics of dementia, as they generally respond better to treatment than do the degenerative processes discussed above.

Depression

Cognitive complaints, especially memory loss, are common in patients with depression. It is a classical teaching but not a universal truth that patients with depression are aware of their memory problems, unlike patients with dementia who lack awareness. Separating patients with dementia from those with depression by mental status examination is often challenging. Inquiring directly about depression may bring the problem to light in some cases. In others, a screening questionnaire such as the Beck Depression Inventory or similar tool may be helpful.[26] Psychiatric consultation and antidepressants may improve symptoms of depression and the associated cognitive complaints.

Obstructive sleep apnea and other sleep disorders

Patients with obstructive sleep apnea (OSA) complain of difficulty concentrating during the daytime, an urge or need to take naps, snoring, and morning headaches. In some cases, memory difficulties or other cognitive complaints may be the chief complaint. Although cognition is often impaired in patients with OSA, it is not clear whether OSA is actually the cause of the problem.[27] Physical examination findings suggestive of OSA include obesity, increased neck circumference, and a crowded oropharynx. Patients with unexplained cognitive complaints should undergo screening for OSA or other sleep disorders with a polysomnogram and formal sleep medicine consultation. Mask ventilation, if used properly, may reverse many of the cognitive complaints associated with OSA.

Pain

Patients may find it difficult to sleep or concentrate due to chronic, unresolved pain, or may have cognitive difficulties as a result of excessive pain medications. Because successful pain treatment or modification of existing pain treatment regimens may lead to an improvement in mental status, it is a good idea to review any ongoing pain symptoms and medications with all patients referred for cognitive complaints.

Adult attention deficit hyperactivity disorder

Although adult attention deficit hyperactivity disorder (ADHD) is a disorder that begins in childhood, it may go undiagnosed until adulthood, especially in people who grew up before the diagnosis was recognized with any frequency. Attention deficit hyperactivity disorder is perhaps the most common diagnosis in patients who are evaluated for cognitive dysfunction in their 20s and 30s. Patients with ADHD are impulsive, disorganized, and have difficulty concentrating. They may complain of memory problems, but their real problem is with sustaining attention. Stimulants including methylphenidate (started at 10 mg bid), dextroamphetamine (started at 5 mg bid), and atomoxetine (started at 40 mg qd) are the mainstays of pharmacological treatment for ADHD. Cognitive–behavioral therapy also plays an important role.

Conversion disorders and malingering

These two psychiatric disorders may mimic any neurological symptom and, unless you maintain a high degree of suspicion, they may be difficult to detect. In many cases, neuropsychological evaluation is necessary to tease apart these psychiatric disorders from organic dementia.

Postconcussion syndrome

Mild traumatic brain injury (TBI), defined as a head injury that produces a loss of consciousness of <30 minutes in duration or a Glasgow Coma Scale ≤13 (Chapter 21, Table 21.4), is associated with a variety of neuropsychological complaints.[28] Three months after TBI, approximately 60–80% of patients will complain of one or more neurological problems including headache, dizziness, memory loss, irritability, and inattention. The term postconcussion syndrome is often used to describe this cluster of complaints, although most patients lack one or more elements of the complete "syndrome." Complaints lasting for more than a year are less frequent, occurring in perhaps 10% of patients. The mechanism of postconcussive symptoms is unclear, but axonal injury, secondary gain including unresolved legal disputes, and preexisting or superimposed psychiatric disorders such as anxiety and depression all contribute.[28] Fortunately, many of the problems resolve spontaneously in a few weeks to months after TBI. Although cognitive rehabilitation may help, there is no single treatment for postconcussion syndrome, and the individual complaints must be isolated from each other and treated independently.

Subacute and rapidly progressive dementias

Although dementia is operationally defined as a disorder lasting for at least 6 months, a subpopulation of patients declines more rapidly over a period of weeks to just a few months. The diagnosis may ultimately prove to be one of the more common degenerative dementias such as AD or vascular dementia, but the following conditions must be considered first when evaluating a patient with rapidly progressive dementia:

Creutzfeldt–Jacob disease

The prion disease Creutzfeldt–Jacob disease (CJD) is the prototypical rapidly progressive dementia. In addition to producing any pattern of cognitive deficits, patients with CJD may have a variety of other signs and symptoms including seizures and abnormalities of the cerebellar, pyramidal, and extrapyramidal systems. Creutzfeldt–Jacob disease develops years to decades after exposure to infected brain tissue such as dural grafts, human pituitary hormones, or improperly sterilized neurosurgical equipment. In most patients, however, the source cannot be identified. Beyond the cognitive deficits, the best-known sign of CJD is myoclonus (see Chapter 14). If it is not visible at rest, myoclonus or an enhanced startle response may be elicited by suddenly clapping your hands or dropping your keys on the ground. Bear in mind, though, that myoclonus may be a feature of any dementia in its advanced stages and is not pathognomonic for CJD. The single best noninvasive diagnostic test for evaluating CJD is diffusion-weighted MRI of the brain that shows cortical and basal ganglionic hyperintensities (slowed diffusion).[29] Other laboratory findings of CJD include EEG showing periodic sharp waves with a biphasic or triphasic morphology, elevated 14-3-3 protein in the CSF, and elevated neuron-specific enolase in the CSF. Brain biopsy showing spongiform changes and abnormal prion protein histochemistry make the diagnosis when noninvasive tests fail to do so. Unfortunately, there is no effective treatment for CJD, and patients have a uniformly fatal outcome, generally within several weeks to months of diagnosis.

Hashimoto's encephalopathy

Hashimoto's encephalopathy is a rapidly progressive, somewhat controversial dementia that clinically resembles CJD in many ways. Originally described in patients with hypothyroidism, the symptoms are not actually the result of thyroid hormone abnormalities, but are more likely secondary to an autoimmune process.[30] Systemic symptoms suggestive of thyroid dysfunction are usually not present, and the degree of cognitive dysfunction is not correlated with serum thyroxine or thyrotropin levels. The diagnosis of Hashimoto's encephalopathy is established by finding antithyroid peroxidase or antithyroglobulin antibodies. MRI may show nonspecific atrophy. CSF analysis characteristically shows elevated protein, with a small proportion of patients demonstrating a lymphocytic pleocytosis. Hashimoto's encephalitis responds to treatment with corticosteroids, often dramatically.

Leptomeningeal metastasis and limbic encephalitis

Cancer may produce subacutely progressive cognitive dysfunction by direct infiltration of the nervous system or via a paraneoplastic mechanism, as discussed in Chapter 1.

References

1. American Psychiatric Association. *Diagnostic and Statistical Manual of Mental Disorders*. Washington: American Psychiatric Association; 1994.

2. Ferman TJ, Smith GE, Boeve BF, et al. DL fluctuations: specific features that reliabl DLB from AD and normal aging. *Neurol* 2004;**62**:181–187.

3. Tombaugh TN, McIntyre NJ. The mini-mental state examination: a comprehensive review. *J Am Geriatr Soc* 1992;**40**:922–935.

4. Tombaugh TN, Kozak J, Rees L. Normative data stratified by age and education for two measures of verbal fluency: FAS and animal naming. *Arch Clin Neuropsychol* 1999;**14**:167–177.

5. Levy JA, Chelune GJ. Cognitive-behavioral profiles of neurodegenerative dementias: beyond Alzheimer's disease. *J Geriatr Psychiatry Neurol* 2007;**20**:227–238.

6. Ochipa C, Gonzalez Rothi LJ. Limb apraxia. *Semin Neurol* 2000;**20**:471–478.

7. Wahlund LO, Julin P, Johansson S-E, Scheltens P. Visual rating and volumetry of the medial temporal lobe on magnetic resonance imaging in dementia: a comparative study. *J Neurol Neurosurg Psychiatry* 2000;**69**:630–635.

8. Likeman M, Anderson VM, Stevens JM, et al. Visual assessment of atrophy on magnetic resonance imaging in the diagnosis of pathologically confirmed young-onset dementias. *Arch Neurol* 2005;**62**:1410–1415.

9. Johnson KA, Jones K, Holman BL, et al. Preclinical prediction of Alzheimer's disease using SPECT. *Neurology* 1998;**50**:1563–1571.

10. Ibach B, Poljansky S, Marienhagen J, et al. Contrasting metabolic impairment in frontotemporal degeneration and early onset Alzheimer's disease. *NeuroImage* 2004;**23**:739–743.

11. Gilman S, Koeppe RA, Little R, et al. Differentiation of Alzheimer's disease from dementia with Lewy bodies utilizing positron emission tomography with 18-flurodeoxyglucose and neuropsychological testing. *Exp Neurol* 2005;**191**:S95–S103.

12. Sonnen JA, Montine KS, Quinn JF, et al. Biomarkers for cognitive impairment and dementia in elderly people. *Lancet Neurol* 2008;**7**:704–714.

13. McKeith IG, Dickson DW, Lowe J, et al. Diagnosis and management of dementia with Lewy bodies: third report of the DLB consortium. *Neurology* 2005;**65**:1863–1872.

14. Minoshima S, Foster NL, Sima AAF, et al. Alzheimer's disease versus dementia with Lewy bodies: cerebral metabolic distinction with autopsy confirmation. *Ann Neurol* 2001;**50**: 358–365.

15. Vossel KA, Miller BL. New approaches to the treatment of frontotemporal lobar degeneration. *Curr Opin Neurol* 2008;**21**:708–716.

39

16. Malouf R, Birks J. Donepezil for vascular cognitive impairment. *Cochrane Database Syst Rev* 2004:(1):CD004395.

17. Tournier-Lasserve E, Joutel A, Melki J, et al. Cerebral autosomal dominant arteriopathy with subcortical infarcts and leukoencephalopathy maps to chromosome 19q12. *Nature Gen* 1993;**3**:256–259.

18. Leys D, Pasquier F. Poststroke dementia. In: Bogousslavsky J, Caplan L, eds. *Stroke Syndromes*. Cambridge: Cambridge University Press; 2001; 273–284.

19. Wikkelso C, Andersson H, Blomstrand C, Lindqvist, G. The clinical effect of lumbar puncture in normal pressure hydrocephalus. *J Neurol Neurosurg Psych* 1982;**45**:64–69.

20. Mesulam MM. Primary progressive aphasia: a 25-year retrospective. *Alzheimer Dis Assoc Disord* 2007;**21**:S8–S11.

21. Gorno-Tempini ML, Dronkers NF, Rankin KP, et al. Cognition and anatomy in three variants of primary progressive aphasia. *Ann Neurol* 2004;**55**:335–346.

22. McArthur JC. HIV dementia: an evolving disease. *J Neuroimmunol* 2004;**157**:3–10.

23. Timmermans M, Carr J. Neurosyphilis in the modern era. *J Neurol Neurosurg Psych* 2004;**75**:1727–1730.

24. Petersen RC, Smith GE, Waring SC, et al. Mild cognitive impairment: clinical characterization and outcome. *Arch Neurol* 1999;**56**:303–308.

25. Petersen RC. Mild cognitive impairment: current research and clinical implications. *Semin Neurol* 2007;**27**:22–31.

26. Beck AT, Ward CH, Mendelson M, Erbaugh J. An inventory for measuring depression. *Arch Gen Psychiatry* 1961;**4**:561–571.

27. Bédard M-A, Montplaisir J, Richer F, Rouleau I, Malo J. Obstructive sleep apnea syndrome: pathogenesis of neuropsychological deficits. *J Clin Exp Neuropsychol* 1991;**13**:950–964.

28. McAllister TW, Arciniegas D. Evaluation and treatment of postconcussive symptoms. *NeuroRehab* 2002;**17**:265–283.

29. Shiga Y, Miyazawa K, Sato S, et al. Diffusion-weighted MRI abnormalities as an early diagnostic marker for Creutzfeldt–Jakob disease. *Neurology* 2004;**63**:443–449.

30. Chong JY, Rowland LP, Utiger RD. Hashimoto encephalopathy. Syndrome or myth? *Arch Neurol* 2003;**60**:164–171.

Chapter 5

Visual loss

Neuroanatomy

A brief discussion of the neuroanatomy of the visual system (Figure 5.1) is necessary to understand how to approach a patient with visual loss. Light enters the eye through the cornea, passes through the anterior chamber, the lens, and the vitreous to reach the retina. Images are projected upside down and backwards onto the retina: the inferior temporal retina, therefore, contains the image of the superior nasal part of space. The optic nerve enters the retina at the optic disc. Lateral to the optic disc is the macula, the center of which is the fovea, the area of greatest visual acuity. The optic nerve projects posteriorly: nasal optic nerve fibers (those that see the temporal field of vision) decussate in the optic chiasm while the temporal optic nerve fibers remain uncrossed. The optic chiasm gives rise to the optic tracts. The optic tract contains the representation of the contralateral half of visual space: the left optic tract therefore "sees" the temporal field of the right eye and the nasal field of the left eye. The optic tracts send fibers to the lateral geniculate body of the thalamus and to the pretectal nucleus of the midbrain. These pretectal fibers synapse with the Edinger–Westphal nucleus of the oculomotor nerve (which mediates pupilloconstriction; see Chapter 7) and decussate in the posterior commissure to reach the contralateral pretectal nucleus. The lateral geniculate body sends fibers to the occipital cortex via the optic radiations. The temporal optic radiations contain fibers from the superior visual fields and are known as Meyer's loop, while the parietal optic radiations contain fibers from the inferior visual fields. The posterior occipital cortex contains the representation of macular vision. Progressively more anterior parts of the occipital cortex contain progressively more peripheral representations of visual space. The anterior part of the visual cortex contains a representation of the extreme temporal periphery in the contralateral eye (the temporal crescent) but lacks a homonymous nasal representation

from the ipsilateral eye. The occipital cortex sends projections to the ipsilateral visual association cortices. These may be roughly divided into the "where" cortex of the parietal lobe, which processes spatial information, and the "what" cortex of the temporal lobe, which processes content.

History

Most patients with visual loss have ophthalmological problems such as cataracts, glaucoma, and macular degeneration. With some exceptions such as angle-closure glaucoma and retinal detachment, most of these conditions tend to develop slowly over months to years. The neurological conditions that affect vision, on the other hand, generally develop over a course of minutes, hours, or days, and often lead to evaluation in the emergency room. Similar to all other neurological processes, the key task in evaluating a patient with visual loss is to localize the problem. The most important elements of the history, beyond the tempo of symptom development, are whether pain accompanies visual loss and the exact pattern of visual field loss. This may be established to some degree by the history, but in most cases, the examination is more helpful. In some instances, it may be useful to "cheat" slightly by beginning with a brief examination in order to tailor the history appropriately.

Examination of the visual system

Visual acuity

The first step in examining the visual system is to measure visual acuity in each eye. In order to eliminate refractive errors, the patient should wear their eyeglasses or contact lenses when their acuity is tested. If they do not have their glasses, eliminate refractive errors by using a pinhole occluder or by poking tiny holes through an index card.

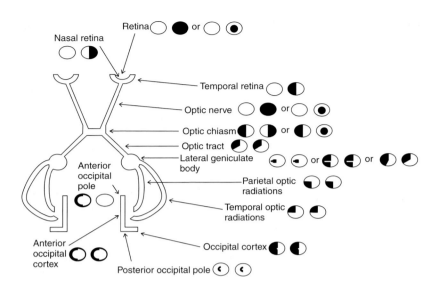

Figure 5.1 Schematic of visual system neuroanatomy and common visual field defects. See text for more details.

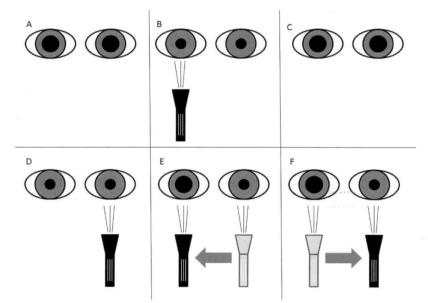

Figure 5.2 Testing for a right relative afferent pupillary defect. Note that in (E) and (F), the consensual light reaction is not shown. See text for more details.

Pupillary reactions

The anatomy of pupillary reactions is discussed in Chapter 7. In a patient with visual loss, examine the pupils in both light and dark. Make note of their size and regularity. Use a sufficiently bright flashlight when examining pupillary reactions: if the patient's pupils constrict and then dilate quickly (hippus), the intensity of the light is probably too low. Observe for both the direct (pupillary reaction in the eye in which the light is shined) and consensual (pupillary reaction in the eye in which the light is not shined) reactions.

Relative afferent pupillary defect

Relative afferent pupillary defect (RAPD) almost always indicates an ipsilateral optic nerve lesion (Figure 5.2). To test for RAPD, examine the patient in a dimly lit room with a bright flashlight. Instruct the patient to focus on a distant target and shine the light into the eye that is being tested from below eye level. For a patient with a right RAPD:

1. At rest, both pupils should be equal (Figure 5.2A).
2. Shine the light in the right eye for approximately 3 seconds and observe the direct and consensual pupillary reactions (Figure 5.2B).
3. Remove the light and allow the pupils to dilate (Figure 5.2C).
4. Shine the light in the left eye for approximately 3 seconds and observe the direct and consensual pupillary reactions (Figure 5.2D).
5. Swing the light to the right eye and watch its reaction. If the pupil dilates even slightly on the right, the patient has a right RAPD (Figure 5.2E). The left pupil should also dilate (not shown).
6. Swing the light back to the left eye and look for constriction of the left pupil (Figure 5.2F). The right pupil should also constrict (not shown).

It is important to swing the flashlight back and forth several times in order to verify that RAPD is indeed present.

Color discrimination

The next step in assessing visual loss is to test color discrimination, as color vision is often lost early in patients with optic nerve disease. The most sensitive way to do this at the bedside is with Ishihara color plates. Because these are often not readily available, a simple way to examine for gross color vision defects is to test for red desaturation. Hold a bright red object in front of each eye in sequence and ask the patient to describe the color of the object and to note any color differences between the eyes. A patient with an optic neuropathy will perceive a bright red object as pink, black, brown, or washed out in appearance.

Visual field examination

Most gross visual field defects that bring a patient to acute neurological attention are detectable with bedside confrontation testing. Perimetry may be required, however, to detect more subtle deficits.

Central visual fields

Examine the visual fields in each eye independently. First, instruct the patient to look directly at your nose and test their central visual fields by asking them whether any parts of your face appear to be missing or blurred. Another good test of central vision is to ask the patient to trace their visual field deficit onto an Amsler grid or piece of graph paper.

Peripheral visual fields

Start by placing yourself approximately 2–3 feet away from the patient. Instruct them to close one eye and to look directly at your nose. For the first part of the examination, tell them that you will show them one or two fingers, and that it is their job to tell you how many they see. Quickly flash one or two fingers in each of the four quadrants of the visual field in succession. This is a gross test of each of the peripheral visual fields. Next, map out the visual fields using a red pinhead. Remind the patient yet again that they should be focusing on your nose and tell them to report the exact instant at which they perceive the redness of the pin. Sweep the pin from the periphery to the center of the visual field. If the pin is halfway between their viewing perspective and your own, you should both appreciate its redness at approximately the same time.

Common patterns of visual field deficits

Visual field examination is often time-consuming and subtle deficits may be missed if the fields are examined too hastily. Conversely, most visual field defects indicative of serious neurological disease are quite obvious. It may be helpful to screen for the following common patterns (Figure 5.1) of visual field loss:

*   Monocular visual loss. This is the expected pattern of visual field loss in a patient with dysfunction of the eye or optic nerve.
*   Central scotoma. In this pattern, the central portion of vision is lost while the periphery is preserved. This too implies dysfunction of the retina or optic nerve.
*   Monocular altitudinal defect (not shown). Either the top or bottom half of vision is lost. This pattern suggests disease of the retinal vessels.
*   Bitemporal hemianopsia. The temporal half of vision is lost in both eyes. This is the classical pattern produced by disorders of the chiasmal region such as pituitary adenomas and craniopharyngiomas.
*   Junctional scotoma. A junctional scotoma occurs when a mass at the optic chiasm compresses the ipsilateral optic nerve and the decussating fibers from the contralateral nasal portion of the optic nerve. The result is ipsilateral monocular visual loss (or a central scotoma) and a contralateral temporal field cut.

- Homonymous hemianopsia. This is the typical pattern of postchiasmatic lesions: the same "half" of vision (e.g. right nasal field and left temporal field) is affected in both eyes. Postchiasmatic lesions that are relatively more anterior (e.g. in the optic tracts and anterior radiations) tend to be less symmetric than those that are more posterior (e.g. the posterior radiations and occipital lobes).
- Lateral geniculate lesions. These lesions may produce contralateral homonymous hemianopia. However, lesions of the anterior choroidal artery may produce a homonymous hemianopia with a spared horizontal central wedge, while lesions of the posterior choroidal artery may cause loss of the central wedge with sparing of the periphery. These deficits are present inconsistently and are often difficult to map out at the bedside.
- Upper quadrantanopsia. This is the loss of the superotemporal field in the contralateral eye and the superonasal field in the ipsilateral eye. It is the characteristic field cut produced by lesions of the temporal optic radiations.
- Lower quadrantanopsia. Loss of the inferotemporal field in the contralateral eye and the inferonasal field in the ipsilateral eye is the characteristic field cut of the optic radiations within the parietal lobe.
- Macular-sparing homonymous hemianopsia. Occipital lesions classically lead to homonymous hemianopsia with sparing of macular vision. The exact explanation as to why the macula is spared is uncertain. Possible but not completely satisfactory explanations include a dual blood supply (posterior cerebral and middle cerebral arteries) of the occipital cortex subserving foveal vision and bilateral representation of foveal vision in the occipital cortex.
- Temporal crescent defects. Anterior occipital lesions produce loss of vision in the extreme temporal periphery of the contralateral eye while sparing vision in the ipsilateral eye.

Funduscopic examination

The final step in evaluating the patient who complains of visual loss is funduscopic examination. Accurate funduscopic examination is essential to the diagnosis of monocular visual loss and may also be helpful in patients with binocular visual loss. It is important to visualize the fundi in the dark or to dilate the pupils pharmacologically. Important funduscopic abnormalities include:

- Central retinal artery occlusion. In the hyperacute setting, the optic disc appears normal or may show boxcar segmentation of blood within the retinal vessels. After approximately 1 hour, the retina takes on a white appearance. The vascular choroid (supplied by the posterior ciliary artery) shines through at the fovea, producing the classical cherry-red spot at the macula. Dull white (platelet–fibrin embolus) or bright yellow (cholesterol or Hollenhorst plaque) retinal emboli may be detected in the branches of the central retinal artery.
- Central retinal venous occlusion. The funduscopic appearance of central retinal venous occlusion is difficult to miss: the disc is blurred and the periphery of the fundus is smeared with hemorrhages.
- Optic disc pallor. This pattern reflects chronic disease of the optic nerve.
- Papilledema. Papilledema reflects increased intracranial pressure. In the earliest stages, papilledema is manifest by disc hyperemia and loss of venous pulsations. As the papilledema worsens, the disc becomes elevated and peripapillary vessel engorgement and hemorrhages develop. Chronic increased intracranial pressure leads to disc atrophy.

Monocular visual loss

The most common neurological etiologies of monocular visual loss are inflammatory and ischemic processes. It is important to consider these problems not only in patients with unilateral visual loss but also in patients with sequential bilateral visual loss.

Optic neuritis

Idiopathic optic neuritis

Optic neuritis is a common cause of acute to subacute visual loss in young people, especially young women. It is characterized by monocular vision loss associated with mild periocular pain upon eye movement. Visual loss occurs over a period of several days, and ranges from mildly reduced acuity to complete blindness with no light perception. Funduscopic examination is usually unremarkable in the acute setting. The vast majority of patients with optic neuritis have a complete or near-complete recovery of vision within a month. Further evaluation and treatment of optic neuritis is discussed in Chapter 22.

Atypical optic neuritis

Less common inflammatory and autoimmune causes of optic neuritis include sarcoidosis, Sjögren's syndrome, systemic lupus erythematosus, and Behçet's disease. These conditions may be distinguished from typical optic neuritis by the accompanying systemic symptoms. Devic's disease (neuromyelitis optica) is characterized by bilateral optic neuritis and transverse myelitis, and is discussed further in Chapter 22.

Ischemic optic neuropathies

Temporal arteritis

Temporal arteritis is a systemic vasculitis that may result in blindness due to ischemia of the retina, choroid, or optic nerve. Patients with temporal arteritis are always older than 50, with a mean age of onset of about 70. Symptoms in addition to visual loss that suggest the diagnosis include headache, jaw claudication (pain with chewing), and scalp tenderness. Polymyalgia rheumatica, characterized by fever and aches in the shoulders and hips, accompanies temporal arteritis about half the time. Visual loss occurs in both eyes in up to 50% of patients: in approximately one-third of these, visual loss affects the fellow eye within 1 day, in another one-third within 1 week, and in the remaining one-third within 1 month. In patients with suspected temporal arteritis, check the erythrocyte sedimentation rate (ESR) and C-reactive protein (CRP) immediately.[1] A normal ESR for a man is his age divided by two, and for a woman, her age plus ten divided by two.[2] Unfortunately, recovery from visual loss related to temporal arteritis is rare, and the main purpose of treatment is to prevent visual loss in the fellow eye and other systemic symptoms. In order to give the patient the best chance of preserving their vision, start prednisone at 60–80 mg as soon as you consider the diagnosis. Because the morbidity of chronic steroid administration is high, it is advisable to arrange for temporal artery biopsy to confirm the diagnosis in almost all cases. Pathological changes of temporal arteritis remain visible on biopsy for as long as 2 weeks after initiating steroids.[3] In patients with confirmed temporal arteritis, begin a slow steroid taper approximately 1 month after initiating therapy. Most patients require at least a low dose of steroids for approximately 1 year after starting treatment. Frequent examinations and ESR measurements are required for long-term monitoring purposes.

Nonarteritic ischemic optic neuropathy

Nonarteritic ischemic optic neuropathy (NAION) is a disorder of unclear etiology, which typically presents in older patients with painless monocular visual loss that develops over hours to days.[4] Obviously, this presentation is similar to temporal arteritis, and several clinical clues must be used to distinguish between the two conditions. The degree of visual loss is typically milder in NAION than it is in patients with temporal arteritis. Patients lack headache or other symptoms of systemic disease. Binocular visual loss occurs in approximately 20% of patients, a much lower frequency than in temporal arteritis. ESR and CRP are normal. Unfortunately, there is no clearly proven therapy for NAION. Visual loss is usually permanent, but a minority of patients may improve spontaneously. Because the presumed mechanism of NAION involves ischemia of the posterior ciliary arteries, it is important to address risk factors for vascular disease to prevent systemic disease.

Less common optic neuropathies

Structural optic neuropathies

Compressive or infiltrative causes of optic neuropathies include trauma, tumor, abscess, or inflammatory lesions. It is important to recognize these causes of monocular visual loss quickly, as they require immediate consultation with an orbital surgeon.

Toxic and nutritional optic neuropathies

Methanol and ethylene glycol intoxication produce fulminant encephalopathies associated with bilateral severe optic neuropathies and a variety of systemic symptoms. Management of patients intoxicated with these substances usually requires consultation with multiple specialists including toxicologists and nephrologists. Ethambutol, disulfiram, and amiodarone are the most common medications that produce optic neuropathies. Vitamin B_1 and B_{12} deficiencies may also cause optic neuropathies.

Inherited optic neuropathies

Autosomal dominant and recessive optic neuropathies generally come to clinical attention in children. Leber's hereditary optic neuropathy (LHON) is a mitochondrial disorder that affects mostly men, and may develop in adulthood.[5] It is passed down from mothers to their children in the mitochondrial DNA, and is characterized by painless, subacutely progressive visual loss. Visual loss becomes bilateral in almost all patients within several weeks to months. Some patients with LHON develop other CNS abnormalities, which may lead to a clinical picture resembling multiple sclerosis. Commercial testing is available for the most common mutations that cause LHON. The mainstays of therapy include cocktails of antioxidants (vitamin C, vitamin E, and coenzyme Q) and avoidance of tobacco and foods that contain high levels of cyanide such as cassavas. In some patients, vision may improve spontaneously.

Retinal ischemia and infarction

The ophthalmic artery is the first intracranial branch of the internal carotid artery. It gives rise to several branches including the central retinal and posterior ciliary arteries. The central retinal artery supplies blood to the retina via smaller branch arteries. The posterior ciliary arteries supply blood to the choroid, ciliary body, and iris. Reduced blood flow to the ophthalmic, central retinal, or branch retinal arteries may result in acute visual loss.

Central retinal artery occlusion is characterized by acute, painless, monocular visual loss. Transient ischemic attack involving the central retinal artery produces amaurosis fugax, in which the patient experiences visual blurring as if a shade is being pulled over the eye. This usually lasts between 5 and 20 minutes and resolves spontaneously. Branch retinal artery infarction causes visual loss in a sector of the visual field.

Ophthalmic artery infarction is clinically quite similar to central retinal artery occlusion, but may be associated with orbital pain and mydriasis due to infarction of the ciliary ganglion or iris sphincter. Because the choroid is also infarcted, the cherry-red spot (see above) is usually absent in ophthalmic artery infarction.

Unfortunately, there is no clearly effective treatment to reverse or reduce visual loss from central retinal or ophthalmic artery occlusion.[6] Evaluation and treatment focuses on preventing cerebral ischemia secondary to ipsilateral carotid artery or cardiac disease (Chapter 21).

Migraine aura without headache

Approximately half of patients with migraine aura (Chapter 19) will have some element of visual loss.[7] In a small minority of these patients, aura occurs without a subsequent headache. The aura typically develops over a few minutes and lasts for up to half an hour. Migraine aura without headache should be considered a diagnosis of exclusion unless the patient has a strong prior history of migraine with visual aura: all patients require a detailed evaluation for other, more serious causes of visual loss.

Angle-closure glaucoma

Although the diagnosis of angle-closure glaucoma should be fairly obvious to emergency room physicians and internists, it occasionally comes to the attention of a neurologist. A patient with angle-closure glaucoma usually has a red eye and appears to be in acute distress, clutching and covering the affected eye. Visual acuity is markedly decreased and the pupil is unreactive and in midposition. Measure the intraocular pressure and obtain an ophthalmological consultation as soon as angle-closure glaucoma is suspected.

Bitemporal hemianopsia and junctional scotoma

Bitemporal hemianopsia and junctional scotoma are caused by extension of pathology in the sella turcica into the adjacent optic chiasm. In many cases, visual loss is gradual and the patient may not report any problems beyond slight visual blurring. Headaches from mass lesions in this region are also common, and result from stretching of the diaphragma sellae. Because most of the pathology that involves the optic chiasm also involves the pituitary gland, accompanying endocrine disturbances are frequent. Common causes of sellar lesions in adults include pituitary adenoma, craniopharyngioma, and meningioma (Chapter 23). Uncommon sellar lesions include aneurysms of the circle of Willis, adenohypophysitis (classically secondary to sarcoidosis or tuberculosis), and pituitary abscess. Sellar region tumors sufficient to produce bitemporal hemianopsia almost always require the assistance of a neurosurgeon and an endocrinologist. Pituitary apoplexy is a rapidly developing, life-threatening syndrome discussed further in Chapter 19.

Homonymous upper quadrantanopsia

Lesions of the optic radiations within the temporal lobe (Meyer's loop) produce visual field loss in the contralateral superotemporal quadrant and the ipsilateral superonasal quadrant. The classic setting in which this occurs is following anterior temporal lobectomy for refractory epilepsy. Although there are differing opinions concerning the degree of field cut produced by temporal lobectomy, a general rule of thumb is that resection produces no field defects if it is performed within 4 cm of the anterior temporal tip, a homonymous upper quadrantanopsia is the most likely defect with resections between 4 and 8 cm of the temporal tip, and a homonymous hemianopsia is most likely when the resection extends more than 8 cm posterior to the temporal tip.[8] Other lesions in the temporal lobe that may produce homonymous upper quadrantanopsia include hemorrhages, arteriovenous malformations, and tumors. Any patient with this pattern of visual field deficits without a history of temporal lobectomy should undergo MRI of the brain with and without contrast to define the lesion.

Homonymous hemianopsia
Posterior cerebral artery infarction

Posterior cerebral artery (PCA) infarction is the most common cause of macular-sparing homonymous hemianopsia. Many patients with PCA infarctions do not recognize their deficits because central vision is spared or they may be able to compensate for their visual loss by simply moving their eyes. Some patients, however, note problems with reading or driving. In some cases, the deficits produced by PCA infarction that bring patients to clinical attention are confusional states or memory problems rather than visual field loss (Chapter 21).

Alexia without agraphia

Alexia without agraphia results from a lesion (usually a PCA infarction) of the left occipital lobe and the splenium of the corpus callosum. The patient can write but cannot read – even something that they themselves have just written! The explanation for this peculiar syndrome is as follows:

- The left occipital lobe lesion produces a right homonymous hemianopsia. Thus, there is no perception of written material in the right half of space.
- The callosal lesion disconnects the intact right visual cortex, which perceives written material in the left half of space from the language centers in the left hemisphere.

- The ability to write is retained because the language centers in the left hemisphere are still connected to the motor centers that govern the physical act of writing.

Cortical blindness
Bilateral occipital lobe infarction

Bilateral PCA infarction leads to complete blindness. Because funduscopic examination and pupillary reactions are normal, a patient with cortical blindness may be diagnosed as a malingerer. This is especially true when cortical blindness is accompanied by Anton's syndrome, in which the patient fabricates a detailed, often preposterous visual environment.

Posterior reversible encephalopathy syndrome

Posterior reversible encephalopathy syndrome (PRES) is a severe encephalopathy produced by vasogenic edema, and is discussed further in Chapter 1.[9] Patients with PRES rapidly develop an encephalopathy, blindness related to edema of the parietal and occipital lobes, and seizures.

Functional visual loss

Visual loss secondary to malingering or conversion disorders may be difficult to diagnose with routine bedside examination. Patients with psychogenic visual loss frequently wear sunglasses indoors, modeling their "blind person behavior" on those of well-known blind celebrities such as Ray Charles and Stevie Wonder. Pupillary reactions and funduscopic examination are normal in patients with functional visual loss. Psychiatric disease may mimic any organic pattern of visual loss, but common patterns include tunnel vision, complete blindness, and subtle bilateral visual loss. In tunnel vision, visual field constriction is identical regardless of the distance from which the patient is examined: a patient with tunnel vision describes the same field defect at 1 foot as at 20 feet. The patient with functional complete blindness will not fall or injure himself when attempting to traverse a path strewn with obstacles. Optokinetic drums or tapes may also be used to demonstrate preserved acuity in the patient who feigns blindness. The most difficult functional visual loss scenario to prove is the patient who complains of subtle bilateral visual loss.

Diagnosing functional visual loss is often challenging, and formal ophthalmological evaluation is required in many cases.

References

1. Hayreh SS, Podhajsky PA, Raman R, Zimmerman B. Giant cell arteritis: validity and reliability of various diagnostic criteria. *Am J Ophthalmol* 1997;**123**: 285–296.

2. Miller A, Green M, Robinson D. Simple rule for calculating normal erythrocyte sedimentation rate in the elderly. *Br Med J* 1983;**286**:266.

3. Achkar AA, Lie JT, Hunder GG, O'Fallon WM, Gabriel ME. How does previous corticosteroid treatment affect the biopsy findings in giant cell (temporal) arteritis. *Ann Int Med* 1994;**120**: 987–992.

4. Arnold AC. Ischemic optic neuropathy. In: Miller NR, Newman NJ, eds. *Walsh & Hoyt's Clinical Neuro-Ophthalmology*. Philadelphia: Lippincott Williams & Wilkins; 2005:349–384.

5. Newman NJ. Hereditary optic neuropathies: from the mitochondria to the optic nerve. *Am J Ophthalmol* 2005;**140**:517–523.

6. Fraser SG, Adams W. Interventions for acute non-arteritic central retinal artery occlusion. *Cochrane Database Syst Rev* 2009;(1):CD001989.

7. Russell MB, Olesen J. A nosographic analysis of the migraine aura in a general population. *Brain* 1996;**119**:355–361.

8. Levin L. Topical diagnosis of chiasmal and retrochiasmal disorders. In: Miller NR, Newman NJ, eds. *Walsh and Hoyt's Clinical Neuro-Ophthalmology*. Philadelphia: Lippincott Williams & Wilkins; 2005:503–573.

9. Lee VH, Wijdicks EFM, Manno EM, Rabinstein AA. Clinical spectrum of reversible posterior leukoencephalopathy syndrome. *Arch Neurol* 2008;**65**:205–210.

Chapter 6

Diplopia

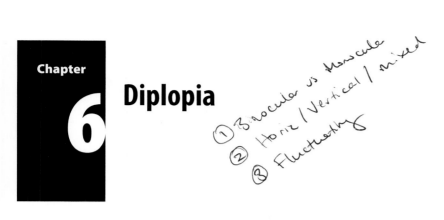

Establishing binocularity and direction of diplopia

Patients with a variety of neurological, ophthalmological, and psychiatric disorders complain of diplopia. The first step in diagnosing diplopia is to determine whether the problem occurs only when both eyes are viewing the target (binocular) or if it persists when one eye is closed (monocular). Binocular diplopia is usually secondary to nervous system dysfunction and therefore will be the focus of this chapter. Monocular diplopia is usually secondary to intraocular pathology and should prompt appropriate referral to an ophthalmologist. In some cases, monocular diplopia is due to psychogenic disease – only rarely is it due to CNS disease such as head trauma.[1] All patients with monocular diplopia also have binocular diplopia – monocular diplopia that disappears when both eyes are opened is almost always secondary to psychogenic disease. If it is not clear from the history whether diplopia is monocular or binocular, ask the patient to close or cover each eye in sequence. If the diplopia disappears when one eye is covered, it is binocular.

After establishing that diplopia is binocular, the next step is to determine whether it is horizontal, vertical, mixed (diagonal or oblique), or fluctuating. Ask the patient whether the images are stacked on top of each other, are side by side, or are diagonal to each other. For horizontal diplopia, it may be helpful to ask whether the images are worse when viewing objects near (e.g. reading a book) or far away (e.g. watching television): horizontal diplopia worse with near viewing suggests an adduction deficit, while horizontal diplopia worse with distant viewing suggests an abduction deficit. For patients with vertical diplopia, ask about difficulty with reading or descending stairs, both of which suggest difficulty with depressing or intorting the eyes. It is also important to ask about fluctuating symptoms. Double vision that changes from the horizontal to the vertical plane, gets worse as the day progresses, or disappears and reappears later is

consistent with neuromuscular junction dysfunction, specifically myasthenia gravis.

Inspecting ocular misalignment

Inspecting the eyes before starting the formal examination often provides valuable information about ocular misalignment. In some cases, eye deviation is obvious at rest. For example, an oculomotor nerve lesion puts the eye in a "down-and-out" position due to the unopposed actions of the superior oblique and lateral rectus muscles, while a severe abducens nerve lesion leads to medial deviation of the eye in the orbit. Shining a flashlight onto both eyes from a distance may uncover subtle diplopia: if the eyes are misaligned, light will reflect from different spots on the two corneas. Examine patients who complain of diplopia for a head tilt indicating a torsional deficit, which is especially common in patients with fourth-nerve palsies and brainstem abnormalities. Finally, look for abnormalities in the pupils and eyelids: a large or blown pupil or ptosis both point to dysfunction of the ipsilateral third nerve.

Localizing the dysfunctional eye movement

In order to localize the cause of binocular diplopia to a particular site in the nervous system, the dysfunctional eye movement must be identified. Figure 6.1 shows the two-step testing schematic for localizing horizontal diplopia, while Figure 6.2 shows the three-step testing schematic for vertical eye movements. In most cases of dysfunction of a single eye movement, these rules are effective. This testing scheme may be less useful when multiple eye movements are abnormal or when the patient has a prenuclear defect such as a skew deviation.

- Step 1: Find the direction of maximal image separation. Ask the patient to follow your finger to the left, right, up, and down, observing for weakness of eye movements in each direction and

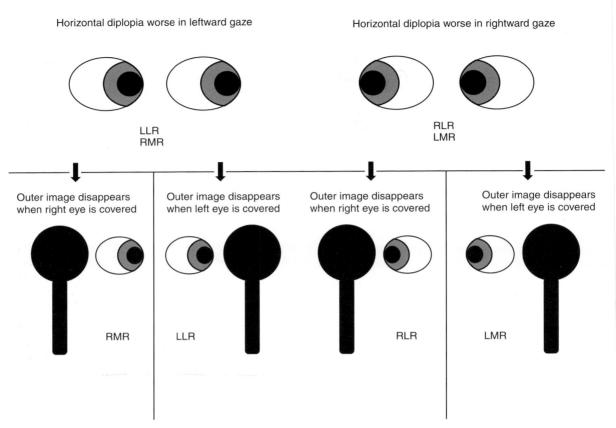

Figure 6.1 Testing schematic for horizontal diplopia. LLR = left lateral rectus, LMR = left medial rectus, RLR = right lateral rectus, RMR = right medial rectus. See text for further details.

inquiring specifically about worsening of double vision in each direction of gaze.

- Step 2: Determine which eye is seeing the false image. After the patient identifies the direction of maximal diplopia, point out to them that there is one image on the outside (e.g. to the right when looking to the right) and one image on the inside (e.g. to the left when looking to the right). Once they verify that there is an inner and an outer image, instruct them to cover one eye and ask which image disappears. The outer image will disappear when the abnormal eye is covered. *To state this differently, the eye that sees the false image will always see it as the outer one.* Steps 1 and 2 will localize the dysfunctional eye movement for patients with horizontal diplopia.
- Step 3 (for vertical diplopia): Steps 1 and 2 will localize the source of vertical diplopia to an oblique muscle or to a rectus muscle in one eye. The oblique muscles are the primary elevators and

depressors of the eye in the adducted position, while the rectus muscles are the primary elevators and depressors of the eye in the abducted position. If vertical image separation is greater in adduction, the oblique muscle is dysfunctional. If it is greater in abduction, the rectus muscle is dysfunctional.

Localizations of horizontal diplopia

Abducens nerve palsy

Nuclear lesions

The abducens nucleus, found in the pons, gives rise to both the abducens nerve, which innervates the ipsi-lateral lateral rectus, and to fibers that ascend in the medial longitudinal fasciculus (MLF) and synapse with the contralateral oculomotor nucleus, thereby yoking horizontal eye movements. Because lesions of the abducens nucleus affect fibers of both the

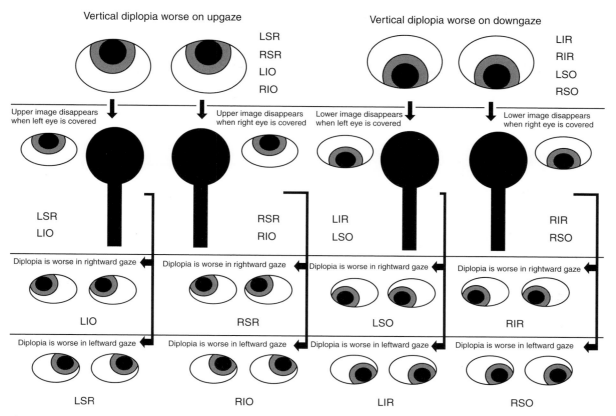

Figure 6.2 Testing schematic for vertical diplopia. LIO = left inferior oblique, LIR = left lateral rectus, LSO = left superior oblique, LSR = left superior rectus, RIO = right inferior oblique, RIR = right inferior rectus, RSO = right superior oblique, RSR = right superior rectus. See text for further details.

abducens nerve and the MLF, lesions at this site lead to gaze palsy towards the side of the lesion rather than simply restricting lateral movement of the ipsilateral eye. Nuclear lesions usually also affect the facial nerve fascicles as they sweep around the abducens nucleus, leading to ipsilateral gaze palsy and ipsilateral facial paresis.

Fascicular lesions

The abducens nerve fascicles project ventrally through the pons and cross the corticospinal tract, leading to ipsilateral abducens nerve palsy and contralateral hemiparesis. The most common causes of abducens fascicle lesions are demyelination and ischemia.

Prepontine segment lesions

The abducens nerve emerges from the brainstem in the prepontine cistern, and enters the cavernous sinus via Dorello's canal. The most important cause of abducens nerve palsy in the prepontine cistern is increased intracranial pressure, which often affects

both abducens nerves simultaneously. In some cases, decreased intracranial pressure, as may occur after a lumbar puncture or as a consequence of spontaneous intracranial hypotension, may stretch the abducens nerve as it enters Dorello's canal. Gradenigo syndrome is characterized by ipsilateral facial pain and eye abduction weakness caused by simultaneous involvement of the fifth and sixth nerves at the tip of the petrous bone, usually by spread of infection from the inner ear.

Cavernous sinus and orbit lesions

Within the cavernous sinus, the abducens nerve may be involved in isolation, although the other cranial nerves that travel through the cavernous sinus are usually also involved (see below). The abducens nerve emerges from the cavernous sinus, enters the orbit via the superior orbital fissure, and innervates the lateral rectus muscle. Important causes of abducens nerve lesions within the orbit include trauma, infection, and neoplasm.

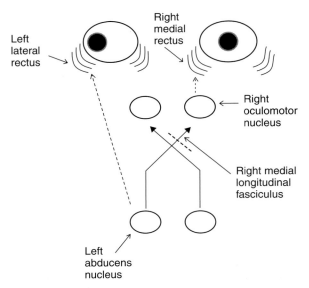

Figure 6.3 Illustration of right internuclear ophthalmoplegia. A lesion of the right medial longitudinal fasciculus prevents adduction of the right eye. Abduction of the left eye is preserved.

Partial oculomotor (cranial nerve III) palsy

A more detailed discussion of the anatomy and pathology of the third nerve is provided below. Because it innervates four extraocular muscles, isolated eye adduction weakness is not a common presentation of an oculomotor nerve lesion. Isolated adduction weakness is more commonly secondary to lesions of the MLF or neuromuscular junction.

Internuclear ophthalmoplegia

Internuclear ophthalmoplegia (INO) is caused by a lesion of the MLF, the pathway that connects the abducens nucleus to the contralateral oculomotor nucleus (Figure 6.3). On examination, patients with INO cannot adduct the ipsilateral eye and have nystagmoid movements in the contralateral eye. Internuclear ophthalmoplegia often occurs in combination with other ocular motor abnormalities including vertical nystagmus and skew deviation. Common causes of INO include multiple sclerosis, in which case it tends to be bilateral, and stroke, in which case the INO is more often unilateral. When bilateral, the term wall-eyed bilateral INO (WEBINO) is often used, as neither eye is capable of adducting. The one-and-a-half syndrome is caused by a pontomesencephalic lesion of one abducens nucleus and both MLF pathways. The patient with one-and-a-half syndrome is unable to abduct the eye ipsilateral to the lesion or to adduct either eye.

Localizations of vertical diplopia

Trochlear nerve palsy

Trochlear nerve lesions produce vertical or oblique (diagonal) diplopia. One clue to the presence of trochlear nerve palsy is that the patient will tilt their head to the side opposite to the lesion in order to reduce the diplopia.

Nuclear, fascicular, and cisternal segment lesions

The trochlear nucleus is found in the midbrain, contralateral to the superior oblique muscle that it innervates. Ischemic or demyelinating lesions may affect the nerve or its fascicles within the brainstem. The fibers of the trochlear nerve decussate in the anterior medullary velum and emerge posteriorly from the midbrain. Along this segment, the trochlear nerve is most often affected by trauma. The trochlear nerve then runs anteriorly along the lateral aspect of the brainstem and enters the cavernous sinus.

Cavernous sinus and orbit lesions

Lesions within the cavernous sinus are likely to affect the trochlear nerve in conjunction with the other cranial nerves that pass through it. The trochlear nerve emerges through the superior orbital fissure to innervate the superior oblique muscle, a muscle that depresses and intorts the eye.

Skew deviation

Skew deviation is vertical ocular misalignment produced by disruption of prenuclear vestibular inputs to the ocular motor nuclei. Discussing the neuroanatomy and physiology of skew deviation is beyond the scope of the text, and I will direct the interested reader to the review by Brodsky et al.[2] Briefly, skew deviation should be considered as the cause of vertical diplopia under the following circumstances:

- when vertical diplopia is comitant (of the same magnitude) with both left and right gaze
- when examination suggests dysfunction isolated to the inferior rectus, superior rectus, or inferior oblique
- when internuclear ophthalmoplegia is present
- in patients with known brainstem disease

Lesions in a variety of locations within the brainstem, cerebellum, and sometimes the peripheral vestibular system may lead to skew deviation.

Approximately one-third of patients with brainstem infarction will have skew deviation, which is often explained incorrectly as a "partial third-nerve palsy."[3] Other causes include hemorrhage, trauma, neoplasm, and demyelination.

Partial third-nerve palsy

Damage to the third-nerve fibers that supply either the superior rectus or inferior oblique muscles without involvement of other muscles innervated by the third nerve may produce vertical diplopia. The selective involvement of these specific muscles, however, is uncommon.

Localizations that produce diplopia in more than one direction

Oculomotor nerve palsy

Nuclear lesions

The oculomotor nucleus actually consists of a cluster of subnuclei in the dorsal midbrain. The medial rectus, inferior rectus, and inferior oblique subnuclei are all ipsilateral to the muscles that they innervate. The superior rectus subnuclei are contralateral to the muscles that they innervate, while the levator palpebrae are innervated by a shared midline subnucleus. Thus, a lesion of one side of the oculomotor nuclear complex will affect the:

- ipsilateral medial rectus
- ipsilateral inferior rectus
- ipsilateral inferior oblique
- contralateral superior rectus
- bilateral levator palpebrae

Pupilloconstrictor fibers are found in the Edinger–Westphal nucleus, as discussed in Chapter 7.

Fascicular lesions

The oculomotor nerve arises from its nucleus in the midbrain and runs anteriorly in the brainstem as the oculomotor nerve fascicles. It contains fibers to the ipsilateral:

- medial rectus
- inferior rectus
- inferior oblique
- superior rectus
- levator palpebrae
- pupilloconstrictor muscles

Fascicles of the third nerve run anteriorly in the midbrain, adjacent to several important structures (Figure 6.4). A third-nerve lesion that involves the adjacent red nucleus produces Claude's syndrome, characterized by oculomotor dysfunction and contralateral limb ataxia. More anteriorly within the midbrain, a lesion of the third nerve and cerebral peduncle produces Weber's syndrome, characterized by oculomotor dysfunction and contralateral hemiparesis.

Cisternal segment lesions

The third nerve emerges from the ventral midbrain in the interpeduncular cistern. It passes between the posterior cerebral and superior cerebellar arteries before penetrating the cavernous sinus. A mass lesion in the interpeduncular cistern affects the dorsally located pupilloconstrictor fibers first, leading to a dilated, unreactive pupil, while sparing extraocular motor and lid levator fibers.[4] Complete palsy of the third nerve will develop if this mass lesion, most commonly an aneurysm of the posterior communicating artery or

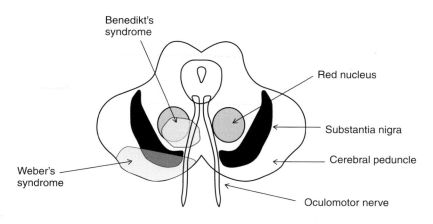

Figure 6.4 Important lesions affecting the oculomotor nerve in the midbrain. Claude's syndrome is characterized by an ipsilateral third-nerve palsy and contralateral limb ataxia. Weber's syndrome is characterized by an ipsilateral third-nerve palsy and contralateral hemiparesis.

Benedikt's syndrome

Red nucleus

Substantia nigra

Cerebral peduncle

Weber's syndrome

Oculomotor nerve

herniating uncus, is left untreated. Pupil-involving third-nerve palsies are discussed in further detail in Chapter 7.

Cavernous sinus lesions

The third nerve enters the cavernous sinus, where it is usually affected in combination with the other ocular motor nerves and the first two divisions of the trigeminal nerve. In the anterior cavernous sinus, the nerve divides into superior (which innervates the superior rectus and levator palpebrae) and inferior (which innervates the medial rectus, inferior rectus, inferior oblique, and pupilloconstrictors) divisions. Either division may be affected in isolation.

Pupil-sparing third-nerve lesions

The typical clinical history of the pupil-sparing third-nerve lesion is that of an older patient with diabetes or other risk factors for vascular disease who develops the acute onset of retro-orbital pain and weakness of the extraocular muscles and the levator palpebrae. It is often called a "diabetic third" or an "ischemic third." The precise localization of the pupil-sparing third-nerve lesion is unclear, and may lie within the midbrain fascicles or in the nerve proper after its emergence from the brainstem.

Wernicke's encephalopathy

Wernicke's encephalopathy is the clinical triad of ataxia, ophthalmoplegia, and confusion in patients with thiamine deficiency, usually secondary to chronic alcohol use. Only a small minority presents with the complete triad, with confusion being the most consistent element.[5] Eye movement in any direction may be affected, although the sixth nerve is involved most frequently.[6] Treat patients with Wernicke's encephalopathy with a 5-day course of thiamine (100 mg IV). Timely vitamin supplementation usually reverses the ocular motor deficits within hours to days.

Cavernous sinus lesions

Deficits of multiple extraocular movements should always prompt consideration of cavernous sinus lesions, as the oculomotor, trochlear, and abducens nerves lie in close proximity within the cavernous sinus. Other clues to a cavernous sinus lesion include ipsilateral facial and retro-orbital pain due to involvement of the first two divisions of the trigeminal nerve and visual field defects due to involvement of the adjacent optic chiasm (Chapter 5). The most important cause of cavernous sinus syndrome is septic cavernous sinus thrombosis, a life-threatening emergency that must be treated quickly. Patients usually have a preceding history of a sinus infection and may be immunocompromised. The clinical syndrome develops over hours to days and includes fever, proptosis, ptosis, chemosis, and external ophthalmoplegia. Untreated cavernous sinus thrombosis leads to blindness and clot propagation, which may be fatal. Diagnosis of septic cavernous sinus thrombosis is confirmed with a CT scan or magnetic resonance venography (MRV). Treat patients with a combination of vancomycin, metronidazole, and ceftriaxone. Controversy surrounds anticoagulation with heparin as an adjunct to antibiotics. It may prevent thrombus extension and promote recanalization at the risk of increasing the chance for hemorrhage and allowing the infection (which is theoretically walled off by the clot) to spread. Limited data suggest that anticoagulation may reduce the risk for long-term complications.[7] Noninfectious cavernous sinus thrombosis, intracavernous carotid artery aneurysmal rupture, and neoplasms are the other important causes of cavernous sinus syndrome.

Tolosa–Hunt syndrome

Tolosa–Hunt syndrome is characterized by the acute to subacute development of painful ophthalmoplegia.[8] The first symptom is usually retro-orbital pain, which is followed several days later by ophthalmoplegia secondary to dysfunction of any of the ocular motor nerves. Ipsilateral facial pain, tingling, and numbness are secondary to involvement of the first and second divisions of the trigeminal nerve. Visual loss may occur as a result of optic nerve compression. As the symptoms suggest, Tolosa–Hunt syndrome is caused by a mass lesion within the cavernous sinus or the orbit. Most commonly, this is an idiopathic granulomatous process, but the syndrome may also be caused by other pathologies including neoplasm, sarcoidosis, or tuberculosis. All patients require MRI of the orbit and cavernous sinus in an attempt to find a cause. Tolosa–Hunt syndrome is usually steroid responsive within 72 hours, but the response may be incomplete and the symptoms may recur after steroid withdrawal. One of the challenges of Tolosa–Hunt syndrome is that both the idiopathic granulomatous form and the more dangerous processes that produce it are steroid sensitive. Patients with ongoing or recurrent symptoms should be re-imaged every 3 months to assure that any responsible mass is not growing. Biopsy and resection of neoplastic or granulomatous masses must be considered with extreme caution.

Orbital lesions

Orbital lesions, usually secondary to trauma, neoplasm, or infection, may affect any of the extraocular muscles, either alone or in combination. These are usually evaluated and treated by ophthalmologists and therefore will not be discussed further.

Miller Fisher syndrome and brainstem encephalitis

The clinical triad of Miller Fisher syndrome (MFS) is ataxia, ophthalmoplegia, and areflexia. It is often considered a variant of Guillain–Barré syndrome (Chapter 12), as it is also a subacutely progressive autoimmune demyelinating disorder that affects the peripheral nervous system. Miller Fisher syndrome also overlaps with Bickerstaff's brainstem encephalitis, a disorder also characterized by ophthalmoplegia and ataxia, but also by signs of CNS dysfunction including encephalopathy and hyperreflexia. The diagnosis of MFS is confirmed by finding GQ1b antibodies in the serum. MRI is usually normal. There is no consensus as to the best treatment of MFS. It is usually self-limiting, but for patients with severe symptoms, a trial of intravenous immunoglobulin or plasmapheresis (using protocols similar to those used for Guillain–Barré syndrome) may be warranted.

Cranial polyneuropathy

A small number of conditions may affect multiple cranial nerves simultaneously. These are generally associated with meningeal inflammation, and include carcinomatous meningitis, bacterial meningitis, tuberculosis, sarcoidosis, and Lyme disease. MRI with contrast of the brainstem and lumbar puncture are indicated to evaluate patients with cranial polyneuropathy.

Restrictive disorders

Restrictive extraocular muscle disease prevents movement of the eye in the direction of the involved extraocular muscle. For example, restriction of the medial rectus keeps the eye in the adducted position, and therefore resembles an abduction deficit. The most common causes of restrictive ophthalmopathy are Graves' disease, which usually affects the inferior and medial recti, and connective tissue disorders. Restrictive disorders are diagnosed by the forced duction test, in which an ophthalmologist finds restricted movement of the anesthetized globe when attempting to move the eyeball with a pair of forceps.

Fluctuating diplopia – ocular myasthenia gravis

Myasthenia gravis is a disorder of postsynaptic neuromuscular function discussed further in Chapter 10. Ocular myasthenia gravis is characterized by diplopia and ptosis without other muscular weakness. Patients with ocular myasthenia classically report that their diplopia is fatigable, initially appearing after long sessions of reading or looking at a computer screen, or towards the end of the day. The fluctuating examination in myasthenia gravis is almost diagnostic: diplopia localizes to different muscles at different times. For example, in the morning, the patient may have diplopia that localizes to the left inferior oblique, while in the afternoon the diplopia localizes to the right medial rectus. Fixed, nonfatigable diplopia that persists for days is less characteristic of myasthenia gravis, but does not exclude the diagnosis.

To demonstrate fatigability, ask the patient to look upwards for 1–2 minutes and observe for worsening diplopia or visible ocular deviation. Two provocative tests may help to establish fatigability and therefore a diagnosis of ocular myasthenia gravis:

- The ice test requires a patient with active diplopia or ptosis. Instruct the patient to close the affected eye and place a plastic bag filled with ice over that eyelid for 1–2 minutes. An improvement in diplopia or ptosis immediately after the ice is removed is often clearly visible.
- The edrophonium (tensilon) test also requires a patient with active diplopia or ptosis. Edrophonium is a short-acting acetylcholinesterase inhibitor, which may be given intravenously. Because edrophonium may cause bradycardia, the patient should be placed on cardiac telemetry and atropine should be available at the bedside. First, inject a 2 mg test dose of edrophonium over 1 minute to assure that the patient tolerates it. Next, inject an 8 mg dose of edrophonium over 2 minutes and observe for an improvement in ptosis or diplopia. Should the patient become bradycardic,

inject atropine (0.5 mg × 1, up to a total dose of 3 mg) and continue cardiac telemetry for at least 30 minutes (by which point all the edrophonium will be metabolized). It is usually best to perform the edrophonium test with a blinded observer. Truly blinding an observer may be challenging, however, as the side effects of edrophonium including lacrimation and rhinorrhea are often obvious.

Diagnostic testing for myasthenia gravis is discussed further in Chapter 10. It is important to note that only half of patients with ocular myasthenia will have acetylcholine receptor antibodies.

I attempt to treat most ocular myasthenics with the acetylcholinesterase inhibitor pyridostigmine at a dose of 30–60 mg tid–qid. Side effects include gastrointestinal cramping, lacrimation, and rhinorrhea. There is little benefit in increasing the total daily dose of pyridostigmine beyond 240 mg, so if the diplopia persists after more than a week of pyridostigmine treatment, then initiate corticosteroids as outlined in Chapter 10.

Diagnostic testing

Unless there is obvious evidence for myasthenia gravis, almost all patients with diplopia of neurological origin require a brain imaging study, usually MRI with diffusion-weighted imaging and contrast. Thin cuts through the brainstem, cavernous sinus, and orbits should be performed as indicated by the history and physical examination. Vascular imaging is necessary in patients with suspected aneurysms. Lumbar puncture is useful when infectious, inflammatory, or neoplastic disorders are suspected.

Treatment

Obviously, treating the underlying disorder offers the best chance of reversing diplopia. Many patients start to wear an eye patch (sometimes over the wrong eye) before even seeing a doctor. Patches may be helpful for diplopia of short duration. Most patients with chronic, persistent diplopia require referral to an ophthalmologist for consideration of prisms or, in some cases, corrective surgery.

References

1. Bender MB. Polyopia and monocular diplopia of cerebral origin. *Arch Neurol Psych* 1945;**54**:323–338.

2. Brodsky MC, Donahue SP, Vaphiades M, Brandt T. Skew deviation revisited. *Surv Ophthalmol* 2006;**51**:105–128.

3. Brandt T, Dieterich M. Skew deviation with ocular torsion: a vestibular brainstem sign of topographic diagnostic value. *Ann Neurol* 1993;**33**:528–534.

4. Kerr FW, Hallowell OW. Localization of the pupillomotor and accommodation fibers in the oculomotor nerve: experimental observations on paralytic mydriasis. *J Neurol Neurosurg Psychiatry* 1964;**27**:473–481.

5. Harper CG, Giles M, Finlay-Jones R. Clinical signs in the Wernicke–Korsakoff complex: a retrospective analysis of 131 cases diagnosed at necropsy. *J Neurol Neurosurg Psychiatry* 1986;**49**:341–345.

6. Cogan DG, Victor M. Ocular signs of Wernicke's disease. *Arch Ophthalmol* 1954;**51**:204–211.

7. Levine SR, Twyman RE, Gilman S. The role of anticoagulation in cavernous sinus thrombosis. *Neurology* 1988;**38**:517–522.

8. La Mantia L, Curone M, Rapoport AM, Bussone G, International Headache Society. Tolosa–Hunt syndrome: critical literature review based on IHS 2004 criteria. *Cephalalgia* 2006;**26**:772–781.

Disorders of the eyelids and pupils

Ptosis and lid retraction

Drooping eyelids may come to clinical attention independently, but are more often part of a larger neurological syndrome. Understanding the potential sites of pathology is essential to localizing the responsible lesion correctly (Figure 7.1).

Supranuclear lesions

The supranuclear control of lid position is incompletely understood. Hemispheric strokes or other large hemispheric lesions, however, may lead to contralateral, or in some cases bilateral, ptosis.[1] Because these lesions are generally large and produce hemiparesis among other neurological symptoms, ptosis is often overlooked on examination.

Nuclear and nerve lesions

Oculomotor nuclear and nerve lesions

The Edinger–Westphal subnuclei of the oculomotor nuclear complex, which control eyelid elevation, are located within a shared midline complex in the midbrain. The oculomotor nerve innervates the levator palpebrae, the main elevator of the lid. Oculomotor nuclear lesions produce bilateral ptosis. Oculomotor nerve lesions cause eyelid dysfunction in combination with extraocular muscle dysfunction, described in Chapter 6. Lesions within the anterior cavernous sinus or orbit, however, may produce deficits restricted to the levator palpebrae and superior rectus.

Oculosympathetic nerves

The oculosympathetic fibers innervate Muller's muscle, a minor elevator of the lid (see Figure 7.2 and "Anisocoria" below). Ptosis that arises from oculosympathetic dysfunction is milder than ptosis due to oculomotor nerve dysfunction. Unlike oculomotor nerve dysfunction, however, ptosis is often the main or only finding in oculosympathetic dysfunction (i.e. a partial Horner's syndrome). Oculosympathetic dysfunction

may also lead to inverted ptosis in which the lower eyelid is slightly elevated.

Facial nerve

The facial nerve innervates the frontalis, the least important of the lid elevators: dysfunction of the facial nerve usually does not lead to clinically important ptosis.

Neuromuscular junction lesions

Myasthenia gravis is the most important cause of ptosis localized to the neuromuscular junction. Problems tend to fluctuate or worsen towards the end of the day. Ptosis is common in patients with both ocular and generalized myasthenia gravis (Chapters 6 and 10). Botulism is the other neuromuscular junction disorder that may lead to ptosis (Chapter 12). Ptosis in foodborne botulism is almost always overshadowed by bulbar dysfunction or generalized weakness. Iatrogenic botulism, however, may lead to isolated ptosis: patients who receive botulinum toxin injections in the forehead or around the eyes for cosmetic purposes, tension headaches, or blepharospasm may develop symptoms several hours to days after the injection as a result of diffusion of the toxin into the levator palpebrae or Muller's muscle. Because many patients do not spontaneously reveal that they are using botulinum toxin, it is important to ask about an exposure history in patients with undiagnosed ptosis.

Muscle lesions

Myopathies produce ptosis, which is usually bilateral, symmetric, and fixed. Oculopharyngeal muscular dystrophy (OPMD) is inherited in an autosomal-dominant fashion and is usually associated with swallowing dysfunction or other signs of extraocular muscle dysfunction (Chapter 8). Chronic progressive external ophthalmoplegia (CPEO) is a mitochondrial myopathy that also produces fixed bilateral ptosis. Patients with CPEO also

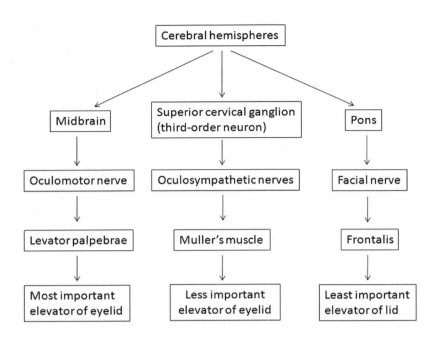

Figure 7.1 Schematic of the three pathways that control elevation of the eyelids.

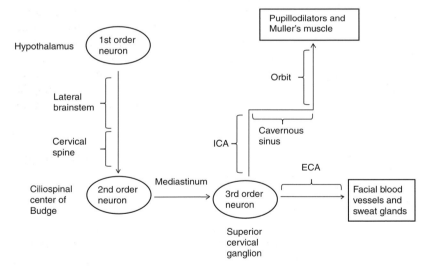

Figure 7.2 Schematic of the oculosympathetic pathway. Lesions of this pathway result in Horner's syndrome. ECA = external carotid artery, ICA = internal carotid artery.

usually have weakness of eye movement, but rarely complain of diplopia.

Soft tissue lesions

As a neurologist, it is easy to overlook non-neurological causes of ptosis. Soft tissue problems are often responsible for isolated ptosis. Degeneration of the aponeurosis of the levator palpebrae results in involutional ptosis. This is common in older patients, but may also occur as a result of trauma. Dermatochalasis is also a disorder of older patients, and results from drooping of redundant skin and other soft tissue over the eyes. Peeling back this excess skin reveals that eyelid elevation is actually normal.

Lid retraction

In some cases, the eye with the widened palpebral fissure is actually the abnormal one because the eyelid is retracted. Although lid retraction is often bilateral (as in Graves' disease and dorsal midbrain or Parinaud's syndrome), it may be unilateral, as in Bell's palsy.

Treatment of ptosis and lid retraction

Many patients with ptosis and lid retraction have mild symptoms that do not necessarily require treatment. Some causes, such as myasthenia gravis, Bell's palsy, and Graves' disease, are directly treatable. Others, such as iatrogenic botulism, resolve over time. Patients with disabling, irreversible ptosis may require referral to an orbital surgeon for consideration of eyelid crutches or lid surgery.

Other disorders of the eyelids

Blepharospasm

Blepharospasm is a focal dystonia characterized by intermittent sustained contraction of the orbicularis oculi muscles resulting in tight eye closure. Although it may affect only one eye at onset, almost all patients eventually develop bilateral symptoms.[2] Blepharospasm may be a mild problem or may be severe and frequent enough to cause functional blindness. Eye strain tends to worsen symptoms. Similar to other dystonias (Chapter 14), blepharospasm may improve with sensory tricks such as gently stroking the eyelids or forehead. When blepharospasm is associated with oromandibular dystonia, it is known as Meige's syndrome. In most cases, blepharospasm is an idiopathic condition, but it may also be associated with Parkinson's disease, other extrapyramidal disorders, or neuroleptic exposure. Blepharospasm responds best to local treatment with botulinum toxin injections. Anticholinergic agents such as trihexyphenidyl and dopaminergic agents including levodopa are only modestly effective.

Eyelid-opening apraxia

Eyelid-opening apraxia is a disorder defined by the combination of:[3]
- inability to open the eyes
- *excessive frontalis contraction* during attempted eyelid opening
- *no evidence of orbicularis oculi contraction* to suggest blepharospasm
- no evidence of oculomotor or oculosympathetic dysfunction
- no evidence of ocular myopathy

It may be present in isolation, but is often associated with an extrapyramidal disorder, particularly progressive supranuclear palsy or Parkinson's disease. Symptomatic improvement with levodopa or focal botulinum toxin injection is typically modest.[4]

Anisocoria

Because of its association with ominous disorders such as posterior communicating artery aneurysm and uncal herniation, anisocoria often leads to urgent neurological consultation. With the possible exception of mild photophobia produced by an abnormally dilated pupil, isolated anisocoria is unlikely to cause specific symptoms. If old photographs of the patient are available, examine them carefully to determine whether the anisocoria is longstanding (and likely benign) or more recent in onset. An important sign of chronic developmental anisocoria is hypochromia iridis, a bluish or grayish discoloration of the iris associated with a small pupil.

The first step in determining the source of anisocoria is to figure out which pupil is abnormal: the big one (mydriasis) or the small one (miosis). This is accomplished by examining the pupils in light and dark. Anisocoria that is worse in light points to an abnormality of the large pupil and the parasympathetic system. Anisocoria that is worse in the dark implies a problem with the smaller pupil and, therefore, the sympathetic system.

Anisocoria worse in light (parasympathetic dysfunction)

Nuclear lesions

The paired Edinger–Westphal nuclei lie in the oculomotor complex of the midbrain and give rise to pupilloconstricting fibers. Because lesions of the Edinger–Westphal nuclei are bilateral, they should cause symmetric pupillary dilation and should not lead to anisocoria.

Fascicular and subarachnoid lesions

The pupilloconstrictor fibers travel anteriorly through the midbrain with the fascicles of the oculomotor nerve. Fascicular lesions, therefore, produce pupillary dilation accompanied by extraocular muscle weakness (Chapter 6). As they emerge from the anterior aspect of the midbrain in the interpeduncular fossa, the superficial pupilloconstricting fibers of the third nerve are susceptible to compression by structural lesions. The two most important of these are expanding aneurysms of the posterior communicating artery (PCOM) and the herniating uncus of the temporal lobe, both of which are neurological emergencies. Although anisocoria secondary to a PCOM aneurysm may be isolated, anisocoria secondary to uncal herniation must be accompanied by altered mental status, coma, and other focal neurological findings (Chapter 1).

Cavernous sinus lesions

The pupilloconstricting fibers course through the cavernous sinus in the oculomotor nerve (Chapter 6). Adjacent structures include the trochlear, ophthalmic, maxillary, and abducens nerves. Isolated anisocoria is therefore unlikely in cavernous sinus lesions.

Ciliary ganglion lesions

The oculoparasympathetic fibers pass through the ciliary ganglion within the orbit. Lesions at this site result in a large, dilated, unreactive pupil. The classical ciliary ganglion lesion is Adie's tonic pupil, an idiopathic condition that is most common in young to middle-aged women. Adie's pupil is diagnosed by finding denervation supersensitivity of the pupilloconstricting fibers: a dilute (0.1%) solution of the cholinergic agent pilocarpine causes brisk pupilloconstriction.

Iris lesions

The pupilloconstricting fibers in the iris are susceptible to damage during ocular surgery or other trauma. The oculoparasympathetic fibers may also be blocked by anticholinergic medications such as atropine or scopolamine. These agents are used to treat bradycardia, reactive airway disease, and motion sickness, and may accidentally be splashed in the eye. In some cases, these medications are placed into the eye intentionally by malingerers. The key finding of a pharmacologically dilated pupil is that it will not constrict, even in response to concentrated (1%) pilocarpine.

Clinical approach

Obviously, the first step in evaluating oculoparasympathetic dysfunction is to perform a thorough history and physical examination to define dysfunction of adjacent structures and to uncover any relevant history of eye surgery or trauma. It is especially important to exclude the possibility of a compressive lesion of the third nerve – because an aneurysm of the posterior communicating artery cannot be missed, considering a magnetic resonance angiography (MRA) or even a conventional angiogram in all patients with isolated oculoparasympathetic dysfunction is worthwhile.

In patients with isolated pupilloconstriction defects that remain undiagnosed after history and physical examination, use dilute pilocarpine drops to investigate for the possibility of an Adie's tonic pupil. If denervation supersensitivity is absent, then use concentrated pilocarpine drops to investigate for pharmacological blockade. One final consideration is benign episodic unilateral mydriasis, a diagnosis of exclusion that may be associated with migraine.[5]

Oculoparasympathetic dysfunction that remains undiagnosed after comprehensive investigation may require referral to an ophthalmologist.

Anisocoria worse in the dark (sympathetic dysfunction)

Damage to the oculosympathetic pathway is known as Horner's syndrome, and when complete, is characterized by ipsilateral miosis, ptosis, and facial anhidrosis. The oculosympathetic fibers follow a three-neuron pathway (Figure 7.2):

First-order neuron

The first-order neuron is found in the hypothalamus. Its axons descend through the lateral brainstem and cervical spinal cord. Anisocoria is unlikely to be the major finding of a lateral brainstem lesion, as nearby structures are also likely to be affected, producing Wallenberg's syndrome (Chapter 21). Spinal cord lesions are similarly unlikely to produce anisocoria as the major complaint.

Second-order neuron

The first synapse in the oculosympathetic pathway occurs at the C8–T1 level of the spinal cord in the ciliospinal center of Budge. Axons that arise from the second-order neuron pass through the mediastinum, traveling superior to the apex of the lung and inferior to the subclavian artery. This is a common site for the oculosympathetic tract to be compressed by an apical lung cancer (Pancoast tumor), usually in association with a painful ipsilateral brachial plexopathy (Chapter 16). The second-order neuron is also vulnerable to injury from attempted subclavian venous catheter placement.

Third-order neuron

The axons of the second-order neuron synapse in the superior cervical ganglion. Axons to the eyelid and pupil travel with the internal carotid artery, while those that control facial perspiration follow the external carotid artery. Lesions of the first- and second-order neurons therefore produce the complete triad of Horner's syndrome, whereas a lesion of the third-order neuron leads to anisocoria and ptosis without facial anhidrosis. Carotid artery dissection is the most serious cause of Horner's syndrome affecting the third-order neuron and is associated with severe ipsilateral headache and facial pain (Chapter 19). Cluster headache and the indomethacin-responsive headaches may present identically. Intracranial oculosympathetic fibers travel with the ophthalmic nerve through the cavernous sinus and into the orbit with the long ciliary nerves to reach the pupillodilators.

Clinical approach

Although eye drops containing cocaine and hydroxyamphetamine help to localize the site of Horner's syndrome, using them is too time-consuming to be employed effectively in the emergency setting. The diagnosis of Horner's syndrome is largely made by the company it keeps: Wallenberg's syndrome in a patient with a lateral brainstem lesion, painful ipsilateral brachial plexopathy in a patient with a Pancoast tumor, ipsilateral headache in a patient with carotid artery dissection, and ipsilateral ocular motor abnormalities in a patient with a cavernous sinus lesion. Patients in whom none of these neighboring signs is present require imaging studies to help localize the dysfunction, including MRI of the brain (paying particular attention to the lateral brainstem and cavernous sinus), MR or CT angiography of the cervical vessels, and CT scan of the chest.

Physiological anisocoria

Anisocoria of up to 1 mm, usually worse in the dark, may be observed in the absence of any recognizable sympathetic or parasympathetic pathology. Physiological anisocoria is usually longstanding and is best diagnosed by examining old photographs. In many cases, however, it remains a diagnosis of exclusion, and careful evaluation for other sources of anisocoria should be conducted first.

References

1. Caplan LR. Ptosis. *J Neurol Neurosurg Psychiatry* 1974;**37**:1–7.

2. Grandas F, Elston J, Quinn N, Marsden CD. Blepharospasm: a review. *J Neurol Neurosurg Psychiatry* 1988;**51**:767–772.

3. Lepore FE, Duvoisin RC. "Apraxia" of eyelid opening: an involuntary levator inhibition. *Neurology* 1985;**35**:423–427.

4. Defazio G, Livrea P, Lamberti P, et al. Isolated so-called apraxia of eyelid opening: report of 10 cases and a review of the literature. *Eur Neurol* 1998;**39**:204–210.

5. Jacobson DM. Benign episodic unilateral mydriasis. *Ophthalmology* 1995;**102**:1623–1627.

Facial weakness, dysarthria, and dysphagia

Lower brainstem (bulbar) symptoms

The unifying feature of facial movement, speech, and swallowing is that the lower motor neurons that control them all lie within the pons and medulla. Because these motor neurons occupy a small volume within the brainstem, a tiny focus of ischemia, inflammation, or neoplasia often leads to simultaneous facial weakness, dysarthria, and dysphagia.

Facial weakness

Anatomy

Figures 8.1 and 8.2 are rough schematics of the innervation of the muscles of facial expression and associated structures. Fibers derived from the motor cortex descend through the corona radiata, the internal capsule, and the cerebral peduncle to reach the contralateral facial nucleus. Most of the fibers from the lower one-third of the motor cortex project to neurons within the contralateral facial nucleus, while direct cortical projections to the components of the facial nucleus that control the upper part of the face are less robust.[1] The facial nerve fascicles travel medially through the pons, curving around the abducens nucleus. They then turn laterally to emerge from the ventrolateral pons as the facial nerve. The nerve courses through the cerebellopontine angle and enters the internal auditory meatus. In both locations, the facial nerve lies in proximity to the vestibulocochlear nerve. The facial nerve then passes from the internal auditory meatus to the facial canal. There are two clinically important branches that arise from the nerve within the facial canal: the nerve to the stapedius, which helps to dampen the vibration of the stapes, and the chorda tympani, which contains taste fibers from the anterior two-thirds of the tongue. It is important to note that the neurons for these taste fibers are actually in the nucleus of the solitary tract, not the facial nucleus. The facial nerve emerges from the facial canal via the stylomastoid foramen to innervate the muscles of facial expression.

Examination of the functions of the facial nerve

Accurate localization of facial weakness requires comprehensive neurological examination of the four clinically important functions of the facial nerve:

1. Examine the upper half of the face by asking the patient to lift their eyebrows, wrinkle their forehead, and close their eyes tightly. In patients with severe upper facial weakness, the sclera will be visible when the patient attempts to close the eye (Bell's phenomenon).
2. Examine the lower half of the face by asking the patient to show their teeth and hold air in their cheeks.
3. Although the stapedius cannot be tested at the bedside, ask the patient whether loud or high-pitched noises are particularly irritating.
4. Finally, check taste on the anterior two-thirds of the tongue by using a sweetened fruit drink. This works much more effectively than sugar. Pipette a very small volume of the fruit drink into a straw and have the patient close their eyes. Place one drop on the affected side of the tongue first and ask the patient whether they can taste the sweetness. It is important that the patient keeps their mouth open during this study to prevent spread of the fruit drink to the other side of the tongue or to the posterior taste buds. If they do not taste anything on the affected side, place one drop of fruit drink on the normal side of the tongue to verify that taste is intact on that side.

Differentiating between central and peripheral facial weakness

Acute-onset, unilateral facial weakness is a common problem for which emergency room physicians often request neurological consultation. The principal question is whether the facial weakness is due to stroke and requires inpatient evaluation, or to Bell's palsy,

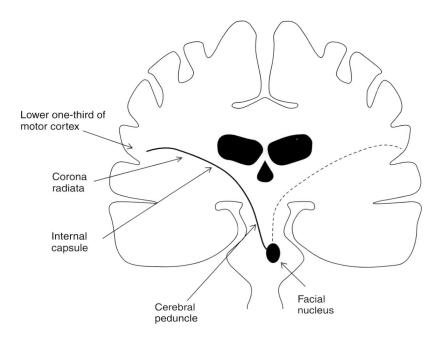

Figure 8.1 Schematic showing upper motor neuron control of facial movement. The portion of the facial nucleus that innervates the lower half of the face receives predominantly contralateral (solid line) but also some ipsilateral (dashed line) innervation from the lower one-third of the motor cortex. The portion of the facial nucleus that innervates the upper half of the face receives little cortical input.

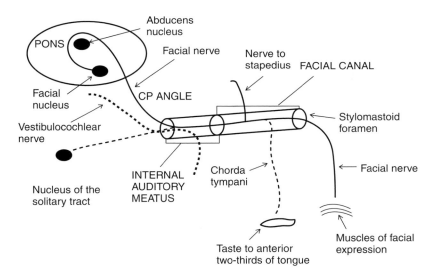

Figure 8.2 Simplified schematic of the facial nerve. CP angle = cerebellopontine angle. See text for details.

which may be managed on an outpatient basis. For clinical purposes, the most reliable way to differentiate between central and peripheral lesions is by examining the upper half of the face: cortical lesions do not tend to affect the upper half of the face, as the motor neurons that innervate the upper half of the face receive scant cortical input. Keep in mind, however, that stroke within the pons (a lesion of the CNS that affects the facial nerve fascicles) may produce facial weakness that appears to be peripheral in origin. Neighborhood signs

and symptoms, therefore, are often necessary to localize the source of facial weakness:

1. Hand weakness ipsilateral to facial weakness strongly suggests pathology involving the contralateral motor cortex, as the face and hand areas are adjacent to each other on the motor homunculus.
2. Paralysis of ipsilateral conjugate gaze or of ipsilateral eye abduction places the lesion in the pons where the facial nerve fascicles cross

63

the abducens nucleus and nerve. Contralateral limb weakness due to a lesion of the adjacent corticospinal tract is often present.

3. The combination of facial weakness and dysphagia point to a lesion involving both the pons and medulla.

4. Ipsilateral hearing loss points to a lesion involving the facial nerve in combination with the vestibulocochlear nerve in the cerebellopontine angle (Chapter 23) or internal auditory meatus.

5. Ipsilateral hyperacusis (intolerance of high-pitched sounds) accompanies facial nerve lesions proximal to the departure of the nerve to the stapedius, provided that the vestibulocochlear nerve is spared.

6. Loss of taste to the anterior two-thirds of the tongue accompanies lesions within the cerebellopontine angle, internal auditory meatus, or facial canal proximal to the takeoff of the chorda tympani. This is the most common pattern of deficits in Bell's palsy.

7. Isolated weakness of the muscles of facial expression of both the upper and lower halves of the face points to a lesion of the nerve in the facial canal distal to the takeoff of the chorda tympani.

Causes of facial weakness

Supranuclear lesions

Cortical lesions, because of the organization of the motor homunculus, usually produce contralateral facial weakness accompanied by hand weakness. Lesions within the corona radiata or internal capsule are usually accompanied by arm and leg weakness. In both cases, the upper half of the face should be spared. Strokes are the most common cause of supranuclear facial lesions.

Pontine lesions

Pontine lesions (most commonly strokes, tumors, or demyelinating diseases) cause flaccid facial palsy that mimics Bell's palsy. Although the lesion is in the brainstem, fascicular lesions within the pons are technically peripheral in nature. As noted above, the facial nerve fascicles first run in proximity to the abducens nucleus and then the corticospinal tract. Clues suggesting that pontine stroke is the source of facial weakness therefore include deviation of the eyes to the opposite side, ipsilateral lateral rectus palsy, or contralateral hemiparesis.

Because the fascicles of the facial nerve in the pons do not contain taste fibers (which run in the chorda tympani), finding preserved taste in patients with fascicular lesions and impaired taste in those with peripheral nerve lesions is an important clinical tool to differentiate between the two lesion sites.

Bell's palsy and other lesions of the facial nerve proper

Bell's palsy is a facial nerve disorder characterized by profound unilateral facial weakness that develops over the course of several hours. A patient with Bell's palsy may note difficulty with closing their eye and may slur their speech or lose food from the corner of their mouth. They may also note reduced taste, or feel that loud noises are particularly intense. Although the patient may report that their face feels numb, this abnormal sensation is actually caused by difficulty moving the face rather than by specific involvement of sensory fibers in the trigeminal nerve. Bell's palsy is considered an idiopathic disease, but most cases are likely caused by herpes zoster or herpes simplex virus infections of the facial nerve. Indicators of "nonidiopathic" Bell's palsy include headache, fever, involvement of other cranial nerves, and bilateral facial palsies, all of which should prompt further investigation including lumbar puncture and testing for Lyme disease, sarcoidosis, HIV, and Sjögren's syndrome.

The mainstays of treatment of Bell's palsy are steroids and antiviral agents such as acyclovir. The most recently published large study, however, suggests that steroids improve recovery in patients with Bell's palsy, but that the addition of valacyclovir does not offer an additional benefit.[2] Treat patients diagnosed within 3 days of symptom onset, therefore, with prednisone 60–80 mg for 1 week. Provide artificial tears and an eye patch to prevent corneal abrasions for patients who have difficulty with closing the eye. Prognosis of Bell's palsy depends on the initial degree of deficits: approximately 60% of patients with complete paralysis make a full recovery, compared with 95% with incomplete paralysis at diagnosis.[3] Younger patients and those whose recovery begins within 3 weeks of onset also have better outcomes.

Incidental facial weakness

Incidental mild facial asymmetry is a frequent finding on neurological examination. The question arises as to whether this facial weakness is a component of the process that brings the patient to neurological attention (which becomes especially relevant in patients with suspected multifocal disease such as multiple sclerosis) or whether it is a preexisting, incidental finding. Asking the patient or available family members whether the facial weakness is old is frequently unhelpful. The first way to determine whether facial asymmetry is new or old is to examine old pictures such as a driver's license photo or family portrait. The second is to take advantage of synkinesis: axon sprouts that form during healing of facial nerve injuries often innervate both the orbicularis oculi and orbicularis oris, so that when a patient with an old facial nerve palsy blinks, the ipsilateral corner of the mouth rises.

Dysarthria

Dysarthria is defined as a disorder of the mechanical production of speech. Although it is distinct from aphasia, it is common in patients with nonfluent aphasias such as Broca's aphasia and transcortical motor aphasia (Chapter 3). The following are the most important subtypes of dysarthria[4]:

Spastic (upper motor neuron) dysarthria

The upper motor neurons for speech are found in the mouth area of the motor cortex in the precentral gyrus. Fibers descend through the subcortical white matter and internal capsule to reach the lower motor neurons in the pons and medulla. Spastic dysarthria has a harsh, strained, mechanical quality. Words are spoken slowly and with great effort. On examination, the jaw jerk and gag reflex may be brisk. The three main causes of spastic dysarthria are amyotrophic lateral sclerosis (Chapter 10), progressive supranuclear palsy (Chapter 13), and the pseudobulbar state caused by chronic ischemic disease of the subcortical white matter (see below).

Flaccid (lower motor neuron) dysarthria

Patients with flaccid dysarthria have thick, muddy speech, usually secondary to generalized disorders of the motor neuron, neuromuscular junction, or muscle. Common causes include amyotrophic lateral sclerosis, bulbar myasthenia gravis, oculopharyngeal muscular dystrophy, and inflammatory myopathy. Individual neuropathies of the facial, hypoglossal, and vagus nerves may also cause flaccid dysarthria, but are less common than these generalized disorders. The standard technique to differentiate among the mononeuropathies that lead to dysarthria is to test labial, lingual, and guttural sounds:

- The facial nerve innervates the lips and other muscles of facial expression. Facial nerve lesions cause the greatest difficulties producing labial sounds such as "puh."
- The hypoglossal nerve innervates the tongue. Hypoglossal nerve lesions lead to difficulties producing lingual sounds such as "tuh."
- The vagus nerve innervates the laryngeal muscles. Lesions of this nerve produce difficulties with making guttural sounds such as "kuh" or "guh." Injury to the vagus nerve, and more specifically its recurrent laryngeal branch, however, more often leads to hoarseness.

Extrapyramidal dysarthrias

Tremor, myoclonus, chorea, and tics are manifestations of extrapyramidal disease that may affect speech in fairly predictable ways. Moderate to severe Parkinson's disease is usually accompanied by slow, hypophonic (reduced in volume), and monotonous speech. Spasmodic dysphonia is a dystonic disorder of the laryngeal muscles: in adductor spasmodic dysphonia, speech is cut off and choppy, while in abductor spasmodic dysphonia, speech is breathy and whispery. Spasmodic dysphonia, similar to the other focal dystonias, may be treated with botulinum toxin injections. Multisystem atrophy may produce a fairly unique, high-pitched quivering dysarthria.

Scanning (cerebellar) dysarthria

This is the classic speech pattern in patients with disease of the cerebellum and its connections. The speech has a halting, uncoordinated pattern with awkward volume modulations and separations between words and phrases. The best-known cause of scanning speech is advanced multiple sclerosis.

"Slurred" speech

Unfortunately, many patients with acute dysarthria do not fit neatly into one of the four common subtypes described in this section, and are most appropriately labeled as having "slurred speech." This is common in patients with substance intoxication or metabolic disturbances. Although many patients with stroke have slurred speech, it is rarely an isolated problem, as it is usually accompanied by facial or hand weakness or by a language disturbance.

Dysphagia

Swallowing is divided into oral, pharyngeal, and esophageal phases. The first important task in evaluating dysphagia, therefore, is to determine which phase is dysfunctional by asking the patient where the food gets stuck. If they point to the mouth (oral phase) or back of the throat (pharyngeal phase), the dysphagia may be due to neurological dysfunction. If they point instead to the sternum, they have an esophageal problem and should be referred to a gastroenterologist. The other piece of important information that must be determined from the history is which consistencies are difficult for the patient to swallow: dysphagia for liquids or nasal regurgitation during swallowing strongly suggests neurological disease. In some cases, it may be difficult to determine whether dysphagia is caused by oral or pharyngeal phase dysfunction, and video swallowing studies are needed to localize the problem. Many of the causes of dysphagia discussed below are irreversible, and patients must be treated with dietary restrictions or, when dysphagia is severe, feeding tubes.

Oral phase dysphagia

Trigeminal nerve lesions

The muscles of mastication are innervated by the trigeminal nerve. Because trigeminal nerve lesions rarely produce dysphagia, they will not be discussed further.

Hypoglossal nerve lesions

Supranuclear control of tongue movement is derived from the lower one-third of the precentral gyrus. The lower motor neurons are located in the dorsomedial medulla (Chapter 21, Figure 21.2). These motor neurons give rise to the hypoglossal nerve fascicles, which course anteriorly through the medulla, passing through the corticospinal tracts to emerge from the medulla. After emerging from the hypoglossal canal, the nerve takes a long course through the neck, looping around the internal carotid artery, external carotid artery, and internal jugular vein before supplying the muscles of the tongue. Most tongue muscles have bilateral cortical innervation, while the genioglossus has predominantly contralateral innervation.

When examining a patient with suspected tongue weakness or oral phase dysphagia, first observe the tongue as it rests in the floor of the mouth. Look for atrophy, particularly scalloping at the edges. Also look for fasciculations or wriggling movements of the tongue. Both atrophy and fasciculations may suggest motor neuron disease. Next, ask the patient to stick their tongue out straight. Deviation to one side suggests either an ipsilateral hypoglossal nuclear or nerve lesion or a contralateral hemispheric lesion. Finally, ask the patient to push their tongue into their cheek. Look for asymmetries in resistance as you press the tongue inwards through the cheek.

The first common localization of tongue weakness is the hypoglossal motor neurons themselves, as in amyotrophic lateral sclerosis. Although tongue weakness is common in this disorder, it is almost always accompanied by other signs, as discussed in Chapter 10. Infarction of the hypoglossal nerve fascicles within the medial medulla is the next common cause of tongue weakness. Because the fascicles cross through the corticospinal tract, patients with fascicular lesions usually have contralateral hemiparesis (medial medullary syndrome of Dejerine). Hypoglossal nerve lesions within the posterior fossa are often due to trauma or to mass lesions, and affect the glossopharyngeal, vagus, and accessory nerves simultaneously. Finally, lesions of the hypoglossal nerve within the neck may occur as a result of carotid endarterectomy or retropharyngeal mass.

Pharyngeal phase dysphagia

Supranuclear lesions (the pseudobulbar state)

Because the motor neurons of the nucleus ambiguus (see below) receive supranuclear inputs from both hemispheres, unilateral lesions do not produce dysphagia. Bilateral lesions, however, are quite common in patients with the "pseudobulbar state" characterized by dysphagia, spastic dysarthria, and emotional incontinence. A patient with emotional incontinence laughs or cries in situations that are not congruent with their actual emotional state, so-called pathological laughter and crying. For example, they may burst out laughing when given devastating news or start to cry unexpectedly when they are told the time. Attacks are frequent and spontaneous. Although the patient is not emotionally bothered by the symptoms, attacks may pose challenges in social settings. One examination clue to the diagnosis of the pseudobulbar state is the presence of a hyperactive gag reflex. The pseudobulbar state has two basic causes. The first is bilateral subcortical white matter disease caused by ischemia or demyelination. The second is upper motor neuron degeneration secondary to amyotrophic lateral sclerosis or primary lateral sclerosis. Unfortunately, treatments for dysphagia related to supranuclear lesions are limited. Pathological laughter and crying, however, may improve with antidepressants.

Nuclear lesions

The nucleus ambiguus within the lateral medulla contains the motor neurons that mediate swallowing. Isolated lesions at this level are rare, and adjacent brainstem structures including the vestibular nuclei, Horner's tract, the spinal trigeminal tract and nucleus, and the spinothalamic tract are often involved simultaneously. The classic lesion of the lateral medulla is Wallenberg's syndrome (Chapter 21). Other causes of nuclear lesions include amyotrophic lateral sclerosis, tumors, demyelinating disease, and syringobulbia.

Glossopharyngeal and vagus nerve lesions

The glossopharyngeal and vagus nerves contain motor, sensory, and parasympathetic fibers. They are often discussed together because they arise from shared brainstem structures, lie in proximity to each other as they exit the brainstem, and perform similar functions. The swallowing fibers that contribute to both nerves are derived from the nucleus ambiguus. The nerves may be affected in isolation or in combination:

- Because the stylopharyngeus is the only pharyngeal muscle innervated by the glossopharyngeal nerve, isolated nerve lesions produce only mild, if any, dysphagia. Clinical signs of glossopharyngeal nerve lesions include loss of taste on the posterior one-third of the tongue and a decreased gag reflex.
- Isolated vagus nerve lesions lead to severe dysphagia, as the vagus nerve innervates all of the pharyngeal muscles with the exception of the stylopharyngeus. Because the vagus nerve also innervates the laryngeal muscles, the patient also develops a hoarse dysarthria. Clinical signs of vagus nerve lesions include decreased ipsilateral palate elevation and a decreased gag reflex.
- After emerging from the lateral medulla, the glossopharyngeal and vagus nerves exit the skull with the accessory nerve through the jugular foramen. In addition to the signs and symptoms of glossopharyngeal and vagus nerve lesions, jugular foramen processes lead to signs of

accessory nerve dysfunction including weakness of the ipsilateral sternocleidomastoid (weakness of head turning in the contralateral direction) and trapezius (weakness of ipsilateral shoulder shrug).

Neuromuscular junction lesions

Bulbar myasthenia gravis is an important, treatable cause of dysphagia that often leads to urgent hospitalization. While the classic temporal profile of myasthenia gravis is one of fluctuating deficits, patients with severe bulbar myasthenia gravis usually progress rapidly over hours to days. Agents such as oral pyridostigmine are obviously ineffective for bulbar myasthenia gravis, as the patient cannot swallow their medications. Intravenous pyridostigmine (1–2 mg) may be used as a temporizing measure, but almost all patients with severe bulbar myasthenia gravis should be treated with intravenous immunoglobulin or plasmapheresis as if they were in myasthenic crisis (Chapter 12). The other important cause of pharyngeal dysphagia secondary to neuromuscular junction dysfunction is botulism (Chapter 12). Lambert–Eaton myasthenic syndrome does not usually impair swallowing.

Myopathic lesions

Oculopharyngeal muscular dystrophy (OPMD) is an autosomal dominantly inherited disorder characterized by dysphagia and extraocular movement weakness. It is most common in people of French–Canadian background. Unlike most muscular dystrophies, it typically begins in middle age. The diagnosis is straightforward when there is a positive family history. If this is not available, muscle biopsy showing distinctive rimmed vacuoles or genetic testing may help to establish the diagnosis. Although cricopharyngeal myotomy may help some patients with OPMD, the treatment of this condition is largely supportive.

Inflammatory myopathies and mitochondrial myopathies may on occasion present with dysphagia as the first symptom.

Extrapyramidal lesions

Bradykinesia of swallowing is often a later feature of extrapyramidal disorders such as Parkinson's disease. It may be present earlier in the course of atypical parkinsonian syndromes such as multisystem atrophy and progressive supranuclear palsy.

References

1. Jenny AB, Saper CB. Organization of the facial nucleus and corticofacial projection in the monkey: a reconsideration of the upper motor neuron facial palsy. *Neurology* 1987;**37**:930–939.

2. Engstrom M, Berg T, Stjernquist-Desatnik A, et al. Prednisolone and valaciclovir in Bell's palsy: a randomised, double-blind, placebo-controlled, multicentre trial. *Lancet Neurol* 2008;**7**:993–1000.

3. Peitersen E. Bell's palsy: the spontaneous course of 2,500 peripheral facial nerve palsies of different etiologies. *Acta Otolaryngol* 2002;**S549**:4–30.

4. Darley FL, Aronson AE, Brown JR. *Motor Speech Disorders*. Philadelphia: W. B. Saunders Company; 1975.

Dizziness and vertigo

"What do you mean by dizziness?"

The first step in evaluating the patient with acute dizziness is to determine precisely what they mean when they tell you they are dizzy. The three sensations that patients describe most commonly when they use the term dizziness are lightheadedness, imbalance, and vertigo. While all three are of potential interest to the neurologist, it is vertigo that is most specific for neurological disease. Lightheadedness and imbalance will therefore be discussed only briefly.

Lightheadedness

Although lightheadedness or presyncope is usually the province of internists and cardiologists, many patients with frequent, intolerable symptoms are referred to neurologists for evaluation and treatment. After performing a careful history, it is necessary to review the basic assessment, especially electrocardiograms, echocardiograms, and telemetry data, to make sure that there is no medical explanation for the symptoms. Ensure that the patient is not volume depleted and check for any recent changes in antihypertensive medications or sedatives. For patients in whom the cause of lightheadedness is still in question, tilt-table testing and extended cardiac telemetry (i.e. a Holter monitor) may help to distinguish among cardiogenic syncope, orthostatic hypotension, neurally mediated syncope, and paroxysmal tachycardia syndrome.

Cardiogenic syncope

Arrhythmias, aortic stenosis, and hypertrophic obstructive cardiomyopathy are common and serious cardiogenic causes of presyncope and syncope, which require the attention of a cardiologist.

Orthostatic hypotension

Orthostatic hypotension is defined as a drop in systolic blood pressure of >20 mmHg or diastolic blood pressure of >10 mmHg that occurs within 3 minutes of standing.[1] Orthostatic hypotension is often secondary to antihypertensive medications or volume depletion. Primary neurological conditions that predispose to orthostatic hypotension include multisystem atrophy, pure autonomic failure, and Parkinson's disease. Conservative measures to treat orthostatic hypotension include adjusting any contributory medications, encouraging adequate hydration, increasing salt intake, and raising the head of the bed at night. Elastic stockings to reduce peripheral venous pooling are another nonpharmacological option, but are poorly tolerated by most patients, especially in the summer. If conservative measures fail, the two main medical options are the mineralocorticoid fludrocortisone (initiated at 0.1 mg qd and titrated to 0.5 mg qd as needed) and the α-adrenergic agonist midodrine (initiated at 2.5 mg tid and increased to 10 mg tid as tolerated). Do not give either agent in the evening, as doing so may produce nocturnal hypertension and worsen daytime hypotension. Both agents may produce supine hypertension as a side effect.

Neurally mediated syncope

Neurally-mediated syncope (the vasovagal response) is a complex and incompletely understood phenomenon. It occurs as a result of peripheral vasodilation and bradycardia secondary to increased vagal output to the sinus node of the heart. Neurally mediated syncope is most often provoked by a painful, stressful, or emotional stimulus. Other common precipitants include urination, defecation, and the Valsalva maneuver. Carotid sinus syncope is a rare form of neurally mediated syncope, which results from pressure in the area of the carotid artery or sudden head turning. Lightheadedness in neurally mediated syncope is often accompanied by weakness, tremulousness, blurred vision, diaphoresis, and nausea. If the diagnosis is not obvious from the history, it may be made with the help of tilt-table testing. Patients with neurally mediated syncope should be educated on how to identify and avoid precipitants of their attacks. Volume expansion and fludrocortisone may be helpful.

Postural tachycardia syndrome

Postural tachycardia syndrome (POTS) is a poorly understood disorder characterized by lightheadedness or fainting that occurs upon standing and is accompanied by tachycardia but not hypotension. Most patients with POTS are young women and, because the symptoms that accompany POTS may resemble panic attacks, patients are often misdiagnosed with anxiety disorders long before the correct diagnosis is contemplated. Postural tachycardia syndrome is diagnosed by finding a symptomatic increase in heart rate of >30 beats/minute without a drop in blood pressure upon assuming an upright position, either by standing in the office or by a tilt table test.[2] Unfortunately, treatments such as volume repletion, fludrocortisone, and midodrine usually do not lead to substantial improvement.

Dizziness of psychological origin

Patients with anxiety and panic disorders may describe a sensation of dizziness that has features distinct from vertigo, including a sensation of floating, lightheadedness, or depersonalization. These patients often come to neurological attention when other symptoms of a panic attack are absent. Careful psychiatric assessment and exclusion of syncope and neurological disorders help to make the diagnosis. Pharmacological and behavioral management of the responsible anxiety or panic disorder may reduce or cure symptoms.

Imbalance

Imbalance is a sensation that is often difficult to describe more specifically than "dizziness." Some patients will use the term "off balance" or may tell you that they feel as if they are on a ship at sea. Imbalance has a wide variety of etiologies, but, in general, they all have some component of proprioceptive loss secondary to cervical myelopathy, polyneuropathy, or orthopedic conditions. Evaluation and treatment of imbalance is discussed further in Chapter 18.

Evaluation of vertigo

History

Vertigo is the sensation of environmental movement or rotation produced by dysfunction of the vestibular labyrinth, vestibular nerve, brainstem, or cerebellum. As a general rule, peripheral (labyrinthine and vestibular nerve) dysfunction is benign, while central (brainstem and cerebellar) dysfunction is serious and possibly life-threatening. Distinction between central and peripheral localizations is therefore crucial to determine which patients require further evaluation and monitoring. *The most reliable indicator of central vertigo is the presence of accompanying CNS dysfunction such as diplopia, facial numbness, dysarthria, and dysphagia.* Features that are more consistent with (but not pathognomonic for) peripheral nervous system pathology include hearing loss, aural fullness, and tinnitus. Several other symptoms may also help to distinguish between central and peripheral nervous system dysfunction, but are less reliable. For example, symptom duration of several minutes is more likely to reflect a central process, whereas symptoms that last for seconds at a time are more consistent with peripheral disease. Occipital or nuchal headaches are more typical of CNS processes such as cerebellar or brainstem hemorrhages. Changes in symptoms with head position are more characteristic of peripheral nervous system disorders. Older patients and those with risk factors for vascular disease are more likely to have central vestibular dysfunction than are younger, otherwise healthy people.

Neurological examination

Neurological examination is often more helpful than the history in distinguishing between central and peripheral causes of vertigo. Cranial nerve findings including anisocoria, ocular misalignment, facial numbness, facial weakness, asymmetric hypoactive gag reflex, and tongue deviation favor brainstem pathology (Chapters 7 and 8). Any weakness or sensory deficits in the limbs also point to a brainstem process. Hearing loss more commonly accompanies peripheral causes of vertigo. The following examination techniques are helpful in assessing the vertiginous patient.

"Cerebellar" signs

For clinical purposes, the cerebellum may be divided roughly into the midline, which coordinates truncal movements, and the hemispheres, which coordinate appendicular movements. A number of examination findings reflect pathology in the cerebellum or its connections within the brainstem and cerebral hemispheres.

Finger-to-nose test

Limb dysmetria may be elicited by asking the patient to move their finger rapidly back and forth between their nose and your finger. In order to maximize the yield of this task, instruct the patient to abduct their arm so that the elbow is at shoulder height and place the target an entire arm's length away from them. A patient with ipsilateral cerebellar hemispheric dysfunction will miss or overshoot the target and may also miss their nose or strike it with excessive force. In some patients with cerebellar system dysfunction, finger-to-nose testing will uncover intention tremor, which is a tremor manifest near the end of a directed movement (Chapter 14).

Overshoot

The overshoot phenomenon is elicited by having the patient attempt to perform mirror movements. Instruct them to align their hand opposite yours and then mirror your hand as you move it rapidly in the vertical or horizontal plane and then stop it abruptly. A patient with an ipsilateral cerebellar hemispheric lesion will not be able to stop in time, terminating their movements several inches past the target.

Rebound

Ask the patient to extend their arms in front of them with their wrists pronated. Tap the dorsal surfaces of each forearm briskly, observing for abnormal, large amplitude oscillations as the arm returns to its resting position. Rebound also points to an ipsilateral cerebellar hemispheric lesion

Heel–knee–shin test

Instruct the patient to tap the knee with the opposite heel and then run it up and down the surface of the shin. Clumsiness or an inability to complete this kind of movement points to an ipsilateral cerebellar hemispheric lesion.

Truncal ataxia

Patients with midline cerebellar lesions are unable to sit upright, tending to fall to the side with any perturbation of the trunk. Patients with hemispheric lesions tend to fall to the side of the lesion.

Nystagmus

Nystagmus is an abnormal ocular oscillation. Jerk nystagmus is characterized by an abnormal slow movement in one direction followed by a fast corrective movement in the opposite direction. By convention, it is named for the direction of the fast phase. Pendular nystagmus is characterized by eye movements of similar velocity in both directions. Examine for nystagmus in the primary position (with the eyes looking straight ahead) and in all directions of gaze, noting the direction, amplitude, and velocity of nystagmus in each position. Subtle nystagmus is often only observable when visual fixation is removed. The best way to do this at the bedside is to have the patient close one eye while you look into the other eye with an ophthalmoscope. When examining for nystagmus using this method, keep in mind that the fundus moves in the direction opposite to the direction that the eye moves when it is opened. A detailed discussion of the neuroanatomy of nystagmus is beyond the scope of this text. For clinical purposes, the following are several rules of thumb that allow nystagmus to be used in localizing vertigo[3]:

- Endpoint nystagmus is a low-amplitude, low-frequency nystagmus that occurs with ocular fixation. It fatigues after two to three beats and is usually a normal variant.
- Horizontal and horizontal–torsional nystagmus suggests contralateral peripheral vestibular dysfunction, often vestibular neuritis. This nystagmus may be present in the primary position, but is usually more prominent when looking in the direction of the fast phase of nystagmus.
- Horizontal nystagmus that reverses direction every 2 minutes is called periodic alternating nystagmus and points to dysfunction of the cerebellar midline.
- Horizontal nystagmus that is relatively symmetric in all directions of gaze is usually congenital. People with this form of nystagmus do not actually have oscillopsia (the sensation that objects are moving back and forth). It is important to recognize this form of nystagmus, as it may lead to unnecessary evaluation for serious brainstem pathology if it is misinterpreted.
- Bruns nystagmus suggests a cerebellopontine angle tumor: when gaze is directed towards the side of the tumor, there is a large-amplitude horizontal nystagmus due to brainstem compression, and when the gaze is directed to the contralateral side, there is a small-amplitude horizontal nystagmus away from the tumor due to vestibular paralysis.[4]

- Downbeating nystagmus in the primary position or with lateral gaze suggests vestibulocerebellar dysfunction, medication toxicity, or a cervicomedullary junction lesion such as a Chiari malformation.[5]
- Purely upbeating nystagmus also points to drug intoxication or to medullary dysfunction. Unless there is a clear history of intoxication with a medication or drug of abuse, purely vertical nystagmus should prompt imaging of the brainstem.
- Upbeating nystagmus with a torsional component, when it is elicited by the Dix–Hallpike maneuver, is classical for benign paroxysmal positional vertigo.
- Purely torsional nystagmus is uncommon and points to brainstem rather than peripheral vestibular dysfunction.
- Pendular nystagmus also reflects brainstem dysfunction. In some cases, benign congenital nystagmus has a pendular appearance.
- Almost all nystagmus involves both eyes. Causes of true or apparent monocular nystagmus include:
  - myasthenia gravis
  - internuclear ophthalmoplegia
  - congenital monocular blindness
  - superior oblique myokymia

The following abnormal eye movements may be misinterpreted as nystagmus:
- Ocular bobbing and dipping are seen in comatose patients with brainstem dysfunction and are discussed further in Chapter 2.
- Square-wave jerks are binocular saccadic movements that occur in the direction opposite to visual fixation and last for a fraction of a second before the eyes return to the primary position. They are frequent in normal subjects, but may also occur in patients with parkinsonian syndromes, especially progressive supranuclear palsy and multisystem atrophy.[6]
- Opsoclonus is characterized by irregular, sometimes chaotic, horizontal and vertical eye movements. It is often present in conjunction with myoclonus (Chapter 14), and in this setting is associated with a paraneoplastic syndrome or autoimmune disease.

Head-thrust test

A positive head-thrust test is useful in establishing a unilateral peripheral vestibular lesion.[7] To perform the test, instruct the patient to fix their gaze on a target approximately 10 feet away. Next, grasp the head by the vertex and chin, and rotate it horizontally by about 20°. The rotation must be done fairly quickly. In a patient with a unilateral vestibular lesion, rotation of the head *towards* the affected side will lead to a catch-up saccade opposite to the direction of head rotation. Rotation of the head *away* from the affected side will be accompanied by normal eye movements without any refixation.

Dix–Hallpike maneuver

The Dix–Hallpike maneuver is used to elicit nystagmus or reproduce vertigo in patients with benign paroxysmal positional vertigo (BPPV).[8] To perform the Dix–Hallpike maneuver, the patient should be seated upright (Figure 9.1A). Warn the patient that the maneuver may lead to intense vertigo. Grasp the head on both sides and quickly turn the head to the side while bringing the patient backwards so that the head lies over the edge of the bed (Figure 9.1B). When the Dix–Hallpike maneuver is performed for patients with the posterior canal variant of BPPV, it produces a torsional upbeat nystagmus beating towards the side of the involved ear. Characteristically, this maneuver

A

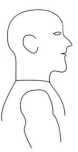

B

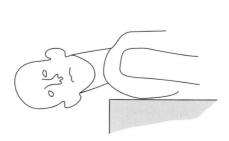

Figure 9.1 The Dix–Hallpike maneuver for right-sided benign paroxysmal positional vertigo. See text for details.

fatigues when it is repeated. A less common variant of BPPV involves the horizontal semicircular canal, in which case the nystagmus beats horizontally towards the involved ear. It is important to keep the head turned and hanging over the side of the bed after performing the maneuver, as nystagmus secondary to BPPV is usually associated with a latency of up to 30–45 seconds. If the Dix–Hallpike maneuver is negative when the head is turned to the right, sit the patient upright and repeat the maneuver in the opposite direction.

Imaging of the patient with vertigo

The need for neuroimaging in patients with signs and symptoms of central vertigo is clear cut. The studies of choice are MRI of the brain with magnetic resonance angiography (MRA) of the posterior circulation. CT scans do not provide adequate images of the posterior fossa and are therefore of limited value in evaluating patients with suspected central vertigo. Patients with brief episodes of vertigo and an examination that is normal or shows only horizontal nystagmus and possibly mild gait instability generally do not require neuroimaging. With the rare exception of patients with posterior inferior cerebellar artery infarction, most such patients have peripheral vestibulopathy.[9] It is prudent to image older patients and those who have risk factors for vascular disease if any uncertainty remains about the localization after the history and physical examination.

Causes of vertigo

Vertebrobasilar ischemia and infarction

Vertebrobasilar vascular disease is the most dangerous cause of acute-onset vertigo. Symptoms begin suddenly, and some patients have transient ischemic attacks before stroke occurs. Because the blood vessels of the posterior circulation are usually affected in a patchy, irregular manner, there is considerable variability in the presentation of vertebrobasilar strokes. More precisely localizable vertebrobasilar syndromes that are exceptions to this rule include Wallenberg's syndrome and cerebellar infarction (Chapter 21). Signs and symptoms that accompany vertigo are highly variable and include diplopia, facial pain and numbness, dysarthria, dysphagia, and sensorimotor signs and symptoms in the limbs. The diagnosis of vertebrobasilar infarction is confirmed by MRI. In some cases, MRA may help to identify the responsible vessel. Consider the diagnosis of vertebral artery dissection in patients with posterior circulation strokes accompanied by neck pain, and confirm the diagnosis with MRA or computed tomography angiography (CTA) of the cervical vasculature.

Vestibular neuritis

Presumed viral infection of the vestibular nerve is among the most common causes of acute vertigo. A viral prodrome may or may not precede vestibular neuritis. Symptoms usually develop over several hours to days and last for up to a few weeks at a time. Vertigo is typically quite severe and is associated with nausea and vomiting. Some patients have a combination of vestibular neuritis and hearing loss known as neurolabyrinthitis. The nystagmus due to vestibular neuritis is either horizontal or horizontal with a torsional component and directed away from the involved ear. A positive head-thrust test helps to establish the diagnosis in some cases. There is no specific treatment for the underlying cause of vestibular neuritis. Supportive care includes vestibular suppressants such as the antihistamine meclizine (25–50 mg q6h) or the benzodiazepine lorazepam (0.5–1 mg q6h). Patients with severe or persistent symptoms may require vestibular rehabilitation.

Benign paroxysmal positional vertigo

This is characterized by brief (<30–60 seconds), episodic vertigo, which occurs with changes in head position, often when turning over in bed or bending the head backwards while reaching for something on a high shelf. Because of the intensity of the episodes, patients may report that symptoms last for up to a few minutes at a time. Precipitating factors include head trauma, vestibular neuritis, and a perilymph fistula. The pathophysiology of BPPV involves excessive stimulation of the cupula by otoconial debris in the semicircular canal, which in turn leads to increased firing of the ampullary nerve, resulting in the characteristic vertigo and nystagmus. The diagnosis is established via the Dix–Hallpike maneuver (see above). In patients with the posterior semicircular canal variant, this maneuver produces nystagmus that is upbeating and torsional towards the lower ear. In patients with the less common horizontal canal variant, the nystagmus is horizontal and also beats towards the lower ear. Nystagmus may occur in the opposite direction in patients recovering from acute BPPV, or may be absent entirely.

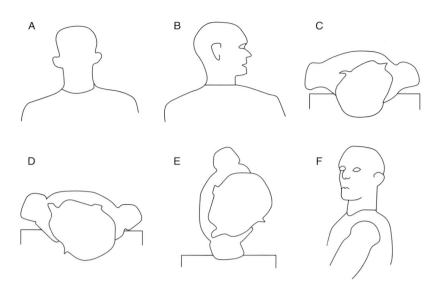

Figure 9.2 The Epley maneuver for right posterior canal variant benign paroxysmal positional vertigo. See text for details.

The Epley or particle-repositioning maneuver is an effective treatment for patients with the posterior semicircular canal variant of BPPV (Figure 9.2):[10]

1. The patient should be seated upright (Figure 9.2A).
2. Instruct them to turn their head 45° towards the symptomatic side (Figure 9.2B).
3. Next, the patient should bring their head backwards so that they are lying over the edge of the bed (Figure 9.2C). They should wait 30 seconds in this position.
4. Next, they should rotate their head 90° so that they are facing in the opposite direction (Figure 9.2D). Wait 30 seconds in this position.
5. Instruct the patient to rotate the entire head and body 90° toward the unaffected side and wait for 30 seconds in this position (Figure 9.2E).
6. Finally, instruct the patient to sit up while keeping the head rotated 45° with respect to the body. Wait 30 seconds in this position (Figure 9.2F).

In some patients with BPPV, the vertigo may be so severe that the Epley maneuver is poorly tolerated. These patients may benefit from pretreatment with vestibular suppressants such as meclizine. Because symptoms tend to recur over time, give patients written instructions or pictures on how to perform the Epley maneuver so that they may treat themselves at home without delay.

Treat the horizontal variant of BPPV with the barbecue-spit maneuver (Figure 9.3).[11] The patient lies supine (Figure 9.3A) and then rotates 90° so that the affected ear is facing downwards (Figure 9.3B). Instruct them to wait for 30 seconds in this position. The patient then completes three successive 90° rotations, waiting for 30 seconds in between each rotation (Figures 9.3C–E).

Ménière's disease

Ménière's disease is thought to occur as a consequence of endolymphatic fluid buildup in the inner ear. The classical symptom cluster of Ménière's disease is recurrent, spontaneous vertigo, sensorineural hearing loss, aural fullness, and tinnitus.[12] The diagnosis may be missed in its early stages when vertigo is the sole symptom. Episodes of vertigo last for between 20 minutes and a few hours. Several days of milder imbalance may follow the intense vertiginous spells. During attacks, low-frequency hearing loss may be detected with a 256 Hz tuning fork, although formal audiometric testing is usually required. Hearing loss progresses with recurrent attacks. Prophylaxis for Ménière's disease includes salt restriction and diuretics such as hydrochlorthiazide (50 mg qd) or acetazolamide (500 mg bid). Acute attacks respond to vestibular suppressants. Patients with symptoms that are refractory to medical treatment should be referred to an otorhinolaryngologist for consideration of endolymphatic sac surgery, transtympanic gentamicin, or labyrinthectomy.[13]

Migraine

When vertigo occurs as a migraine aura (Chapter 19), the diagnosis is straightforward. More difficult from a

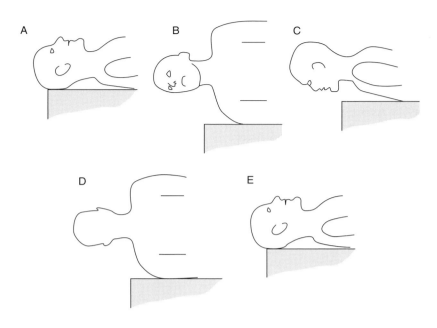

Figure 9.3 The barbecue-spit maneuver for right horizontal canal variant benign paroxysmal positional vertigo. See text for details.

diagnostic perspective, however, are attacks of vertigo in migraineurs that last for hours to days and occur independently of the headaches. Patients with such episodes are often diagnosed with Ménière's disease or chronic undifferentiated dizziness. Overall, migraine-associated dizziness accounts for only 2% of episodic dizziness, and other more common conditions should be excluded prior to committing to this diagnosis.[14] Migraine abortive and prophylactic agents may help stop these attacks and reduce the frequency with which they recur.

Medication toxicity

Vestibulotoxic medications that commonly produce vertigo include aminoglycosides, anticonvulsants, sedatives, and cisplatin. In some but not all cases, discontinuing the responsible medication may reverse the symptoms.

Perilymph fistula

This condition results from a leakage of perilymph fluid through the labyrinthine membrane. The classic constellation of symptoms is a popping sound in the ear accompanied by a combination of sudden hearing loss, tinnitus, and vertigo. Symptoms are precipitated by sneezing, straining, and coughing. The diagnosis is established by finding a positive fistula sign: symptoms are reproduced when the patient attempts to "pop" his or her ears while squeezing the nose closed. Instruct

patients with perilymph fistula to avoid precipitating activities and to take vestibular suppressants such as meclizine during acute attacks. Refer patients with refractory symptoms to an otorhinolaryngologist for definitive treatment.

Epileptic dizziness

In rare circumstances, a sudden brief feeling of instability or frank vertigo may be a seizure manifestation, usually pointing to a focus in the posterior–superior temporal lobe.[15] Epileptic dizziness or vertigo should be considered only after more common conditions are thoroughly excluded. Because it so uncommon, epileptic dizziness must be confirmed with an EEG demonstrating epileptiform discharges during an episode.

Cerebellopontine angle tumors

Acoustic neuromas and meningiomas are the most common tumors of the cerebellopontine angle (CPA) (Chapter 23). These tumors generally grow slowly, and compensation from the contralateral vestibular system makes acute vertigo uncommon.[16] Other signs and symptoms of CPA tumors include facial numbness, facial weakness, hearing loss, and disequilibrium. Surgical intervention should be considered for patients with progressive symptoms or evidence of tumor expansion on serial neuroimaging studies.[16]

Chronic undifferentiated dizziness

This diagnosis may represent a *forme fruste* of migraine, Ménière's disease, or vestibular neuritis. Many patients with this condition are dismissed as having psychiatric disorders. A viral prodrome or mild head trauma frequently precedes symptom onset by several weeks, but it is hard to prove that either process is really responsible for the symptoms. Most patients describe a sense of being off balance rather than frank vertigo. They do not usually have hearing problems, ocular motility disorders, or falls. Examination is normal with the possible exception of subtle horizontal nystagmus. Chronic undifferentiated dizziness is ultimately a diagnosis of exclusion. A thorough evaluation should include electronystagmography, caloric testing, neuroimaging studies, and lumbar puncture. Some patients respond to vestibular rehabilitation and vestibular suppressant medications. I have found that agents used for migraine prophylaxis are helpful to a small minority.

Postconcussion syndrome and posttraumatic dizziness

Post concussion syndrome includes headache, irritability, forgetfulness, poor concentration, and dizziness (Chapter 4). The dizziness is often due to labyrinthine trauma or BPPV. In many cases, however, the dizziness of postconcussion syndrome is a vague sense of imbalance rather than true vertigo.

Multiple sclerosis

Demyelinating lesions involving the cerebellum or its connections within the brainstem may lead to vertigo (Chapter 22). As a presenting complaint of MS, however, vertigo is uncommon.

Paraneoplastic cerebellar degeneration

The most common antibodies that lead to paraneoplastic cerebellar degeneration are anti-Yo (breast and ovarian cancers), anti-Hu (small-cell lung cancer), anti-Tr (Hodgkin's lymphoma), and anti-Ri (breast and ovarian cancers).[17] Treatment should focus on the underlying cancer. Unfortunately, the cerebellar degeneration associated with these syndromes is progressive, and most patients lose the ability to ambulate.

Episodic ataxia

The episodic ataxias are a group of uncommon channelopathies characterized (as their name suggests) by recurrent bouts of ataxia.[18] Episodic ataxia type 2 in particular may cause episodic vertigo and headaches that are precipitated by stress and fatigue and which may last for hours or days at a time. Acetazolamide (500–1000 mg) reverses the symptoms of an acute attack.

References

1. The Consensus Committee of the American Autonomic Society and the American Academy of Neurology. Consensus statement on the definition of orthostatic hypotension, pure autonomic failure, and multiple system atrophy. *Neurology* 1996;**46**:1470.

2. Jacob G, Costa F, Shannon JR, et al. The neuropathic postural tachycardia syndrome. *N Engl J Med* 2000;**343**:1008–1014.

3. Serra A, Leigh RJ. Diagnostic value of nystagmus: spontaneous and induced ocular oscillations. *J Neurol Neurosurg Psychiatry* 2002;**73**:615–618.

4. Baloh RW, Konrad HR, Dirks D, Honrubia V. Cerebellar-pontine angle tumors. Results of quantitative vestibulo-ocular testing. *Arch Neurol* 1976;**33**:507–512.

5. Baloh RW, Spooner JW. Downbeat nystagmus: a type of central vestibular nystagmus. *Neurology* 1981;**31**:304–310.

6. Rascol O, Sabatini U, Simonetta-Moreau M, et al. Square wave jerks in parkinsonian syndromes. *J Neurol Neurosurg Psychiatry* 1991;**54**:599–602.

7. Halmagyi GM, Curthoys IS. A clinical sign of canal paresis. *Arch Neurol* 1988;**45**:737–739.

8. Dix MR, Hallpike CS. The pathology, symptomatology and diagnosis of certain common disorders of the vestibular system. *Proc R Soc Med* 1952;**45**:341–354.

9. Norrving B, Magnusson M, Holtas S. Isolated acute vertigo in the elderly; vestibular or vascular disease. *Acta Neurol Scand* 1995;**91**:43–48.

10. Epley JM. The canalith repositioning procedure: for treatment of benign paroxysmal positional vertigo. *Otolaryngol Head Neck Surg* 1992;**107**:399–404.

11. Lempert T, Tiel-Wick K. A positional maneuver for treatment of horizontal-canal benign positional vertigo. *Laryngoscope* 1996;**106**:476–478.

12. American Academy of Otolaryngology-Head and Neck Foundation. Committee on Hearing and Equilibrium guidelines for the diagnosis and evaluation of therapy in Ménière's disease. *Otolaryngol Head Neck Surg* 1995;**113**:181–185.

13. Sajjadi H, Paparella MM. Meniere's disease. *Lancet* 2008;**372**:406–414.

14. Cutrer FM, Baloh RW. Migraine-associated dizziness. *Headache* 1992;**32**:300–304.

15. Kogeorgos J, Scott DF, Swash M. Epileptic dizziness. *BMJ* 1981;**282**:687–689.

16. Selesnick SH, Jackler RK, Pitts LW. The changing clinical presentation of acoustic tumors in the MRI era. *Laryngoscope* 1993;**103**:431–436.

17. Shams' ili S, Grefkens J, de Leeuw B, et al. Paraneoplastic cerebellar degeneration associated with antineuronal antibodies: analysis of 50 patients. *Brain* 2003;**126**:1409–1418.

18. Jen J, Yue Q, Nelson SF, et al. A novel nonsense mutation in CACNA1A causes episodic ataxia and hemiplegia. *Neurology* 1999;**53**:34–37.

Proximal and generalized weakness

Weakness and its mimics

Weakness is both a sign and symptom of motor dysfunction characterized by the failure of a movement to generate an appropriate force. Careful questioning of many patients referred for weakness reveals that the problem is not actually weakness, but rather a condition that mimics it:

- Fatigue is the common sensation of tiredness or physical exhaustion that accompanies medical conditions such as hypothyroidism and anemia, sleep disorders, and depression. Although fatigued patients often describe themselves as weak, formal motor testing shows that they actually possess full strength.
- Bradykinesia is slowness of movement. It is a core feature of parkinsonism, and is discussed in greater detail in Chapter 13.
- Musculoskeletal system dysfunction may reduce the range of motion of a joint but does not produce actual weakness.
- Pain from any source may restrict movement and be erroneously interpreted as weakness.
- Sensory loss that impairs joint position sensation may lead to the impression of weakness. The telltale sign that sensory loss is the cause of impaired movement is that the joint moves normally when the patient looks directly at it, but fails to move appropriately when they look away.

The evaluation of weakness

The key step in diagnosing the weak patient is to define the distribution and speed of onset of weakness by history and physical examination. The most common gradual-onset patterns of weakness are:

- proximal (this chapter)
- distal (Chapter 15)
- extraocular muscle (Chapter 6)
- focal limb (Chapter 11)

- bulbar (Chapter 8)
- facial (Chapter 8)
- myelopathic (Chapter 17)

Rapidly developing weakness is discussed further in Chapters 12 and 21.

Even if the history strongly suggests one of these patterns, it is imperative to perform a comprehensive neurological examination. Patients are frequently unaware of or adapt to minor weakness, and you will miss subtle signs of more widespread motor system dysfunction if you focus only on the weakness that the patient describes. This is often true for patients with amyotrophic lateral sclerosis, in whom the diagnosis is routinely overlooked for several months due to exclusive focus on a single weak muscle group.

While it is tempting to proceed directly to power testing when evaluating a weak patient, you will miss important diagnostic clues if you fail to examine muscle bulk. Look for muscle atrophy in both proximal and distal muscles, around the temples, and in the tongue. Muscles in which atrophy is obvious include the deltoid, periscapular muscles, abductor pollicis brevis, first dorsal interosseous, quadriceps, and extensor digitorum brevis.

After examining muscle bulk, examine muscle tone in the upper and lower extremities. Instruct the patient to lie still and relax. Move the arms at the elbows and wrists, looking for an increase in resistance. Check tone in the legs while the patient lies flat. Grasp the thigh and lower leg from above and shake the leg, looking for movement at the foot: normally, the foot moves back and forth loosely, but in patients with hypertonicity, the foot remains stiff at the ankle. Abnormalities of tone include:

- Flaccidity: a floppy decrease in tone, which points to a peripheral nervous system lesion or to a hyperacute CNS lesion (e.g. acute stroke or spinal shock).
- Spasticity: the form of hypertonicity caused by disease of the pyramidal system. The initial

limb movement is met with the greatest amount of resistance, which then dissipates as joint displacement increases. Spasticity is most obvious when attempting to extend the flexed arm or wrist, or attempting to flex the extended leg.

- Rigidity: the increase in tone caused by extrapyramidal disease. It is independent of the velocity and direction of movement.
- Paratonia: caused by frontal lobe degeneration and characterized by an increase in tone that varies with the amount of resistance applied by the examiner.

When examining power, oppose the muscle being tested with a muscle of approximately equal strength. Use extra effort for large, physically fit patients. You will often need to exercise a mechanical advantage to find subtle weakness in muscles such as the quadriceps, tibialis anterior, and gastrocnemius, as these muscles tend to be strong when using conventional muscle strength testing techniques. Subtle weakness of the gastrocnemius, in fact, may be detected only by an inability of the patient to stand on their toes. The genioglossus, abductor digiti minimi, and iliopsoas lie at the other extreme, and you should give these muscles a mechanical advantage to avoid incorrectly labeling them as weak. Be aware of "giveway" weakness caused by pain or poor effort: encourage the patient to push as hard as they can for even as little as 1 second if it appears that they are not giving maximal effort.

While there is no substitute for detailed knowledge of the nerve roots, nerves, and muscles that control joint movement, relearning all the details of first-year medical school anatomy is often not necessary to localize the source of weakness in a given patient. Table 10.1 distills this information to a high-yield format of the 20 most commonly tested movements for use on the ward and in the clinic. The muscles are organized into proximal and distal groups, whether they are weak in pyramidal (corticospinal) lesions, and by the nerve root and nerves that innervate them. *Aids to the Examination of the Peripheral Nervous System*[1] is an additional, invaluable guide to the sensorimotor examination.

Proximal weakness

History

The proximal muscles are those that are close to the trunk. Complaints of proximal muscle weakness include difficulty when reaching overhead, combing or brushing the hair, rising from a seated position, or ascending stairs. The patient may describe themselves as "walking like a cowboy" with bowed legs and side-to-side waddling. Contrary to popular belief, proximal weakness is not pathognomonic for myopathic disease. Other localizations that commonly produce proximal weakness include the motor neuron, nerve root, nerve plexus, neuromuscular junction, and, in some cases, the peripheral nerves.

Associated features

Although mild muscle tenderness is a feature of many myopathic disorders, severe pain is uncommon in myopathy. In the absence of trauma, rhabdomyolysis and myoglobinuria suggest the possibility of a metabolic myopathy. Rash points to dermatomyositis or to an overlap myopathy. Diplopia, ptosis, and dysphagia are seen in patients with myasthenia gravis or oculopharyngeal muscular dystrophy. Dry eyes and dry mouth often accompany Lambert–Eaton myasthenic syndrome (LEMS). Cramps, fasciculations, and muscle atrophy are features of amyotrophic lateral sclerosis.

Examination

Muscle bulk

Proximal weakness with prominent muscle atrophy suggests muscular dystrophy, a cachectic myopathy, or motor neuron disease. Most patients with inflammatory myopathies do not have muscle wasting in the early stages. Neuromuscular junction disorders do not affect muscle bulk.

Muscle strength

Muscle strength testing should always begin with an examination of neck flexion and extension, especially for patients with proximal muscle weakness. In most patients, neck flexors become weak before neck extensors. The proximal muscles of the arms include the deltoids, biceps, and triceps. In the legs, the proximal muscles are the iliopsoas, quadriceps, gluteal muscles, and hip adductors.

Exercise testing

Muscle fatigability is the defining feature of myasthenia gravis. This is most easily assessed at the deltoid. First, test the maximal strength of shoulder abduction. Next, instruct the patient to abduct the arm 20–30 times in succession at a frequency of approximately twice per

Table 10.1 Commonly tested movements in localizing weakness

Action	Principal muscle or muscles	Proximal or distal	Weak in pyramidal lesion?	Nerve roots	Nerve
Neck flexion	Multiple	Proximal	No		
Neck extension	Multiple	Proximal	No		
Shoulder abduction	Deltoids	Proximal	Yes	C5–6	Axillary
Elbow flexion	Biceps	Proximal	No	C5–6	Musculocutaneous
Elbow extension	Triceps	Proximal	Yes	C6–8	Radial
Wrist flexion	Flexor carpi radialis, flexor carpi ulnaris	Distal	No	C6–7, C8–T1	Median (FCR) and ulnar (FCU)
Wrist extension	Extensor carpi radialis brevis, extensor carpi radialis longus, extensor carpi ulnaris	Distal	Yes	C7	Radial
Extension of fingers at MCP joints	Extensor digitorum communis and extensor indicis	Distal	Yes	C7–8	Radial
Extension of fingers at PIP and DIP joints	Lumbricals	Distal	Yes	C8–T1	Median and ulnar
Finger abduction	Abductor digiti minimi, dorsal interossei	Distal	Yes	C8–T1	Ulnar
Thumb abduction	Abductor pollicis brevis	Distal	No	C8–T1	Median
Hip flexion	Iliopsoas	Proximal	Yes	L2–3	Femoral/L2–3 roots
Hip abduction	Gluteus medius and minimus	Proximal	Yes	L5–S1	Superior gluteal
Hip adduction	Adductor longus and magnus	Proximal	No	L2–3	Obturator
Knee flexion	Hamstrings	Proximal	Yes	L5–S1	Sciatic
Knee extension	Quadriceps	Proximal	No	L2–4	Femoral
Foot dorsiflexion	Tibialis anterior	Distal	Yes	L4–5	Peroneal
Foot plantarflexion	Gastrocnemius	Distal	No	S1	Tibial
Toe extension	Extensor hallucis, extensor digitorum	Distal	Yes	L5	Peroneal
Toe flexion	Flexor digitorum	Distal	No	S1	Tibial

DIP = distal interphalangeal, FCR = flexor carpi radialis, FCU = flexor carpi ulnaris, MCP = metacarpophalangeal, PIP = proximal interphalangeal.

second. Observe for either a failure to complete the series of contractions or a decrease in strength when testing the patient after the final contraction. If necessary, use contralateral shoulder abduction as a control for patients with subtle weakness.

All patients with proximal weakness should also undergo testing for postexercise facilitation, the characteristic finding of the presynaptic neuromuscular junction LEMS. To test for postexercise facilitation, instruct the patient to contract a weak muscle maximally against resistance for 10 seconds. Postexercise facilitation is present if there is a clear improvement in muscle strength after brief exercise.

Reflexes

Patients with myopathies usually have normal deep tendon reflexes unless there is substantial weakness or muscle atrophy. Lambert–Eaton myasthenic syndrome classically causes diminished or absent reflexes that reappear when the reflex is checked after 10 seconds of sustained exercise. Neuropathic and radiculopathic conditions should produce hyporeflexia or areflexia. Upper motor neuron dysfunction in amyotrophic lateral sclerosis (ALS) may produce hyperreflexia, but because ALS is a disease of both the upper and lower motor neurons, it may cause either an increase or decrease in reflexes.

Sensation

Sensory examination is usually normal in patients with proximal weakness. Exceptions include LEMS and neuropathic conditions such as chronic inflammatory demyelinating polyneuropathy. Do not assign too much weight to mild distal pinprick loss, as this is often secondary to a preexisting but trivial polyneuropathy.

Gait

Patients with proximal muscle weakness waddle from side to side, the so-called Trendelenburg gait (Chapter 18). To elicit Trendelenburg's sign, observe the patient from behind and instruct them to stand on one foot. The sign is present when the trunk droops towards the side of the elevated leg. Patients with proximal muscle weakness require several attempts to rise from a seated position, and may be unable to do it at all. This test is even more difficult if the patient attempts to do it when their arms are folded across their chest.

Other signs and symptoms

Bulbar weakness accompanies amyotrophic lateral sclerosis and myasthenia gravis but is not universal in either condition, especially in their early stages. Dysphagia is prominent in oculopharyngeal muscular dystrophy and may also occur in patients with advanced inflammatory myopathies. Diplopia and ptosis in patients with proximal weakness strongly suggest myasthenia gravis, a mitochondrial myopathy, or oculopharyngeal muscular dystrophy, and essentially exclude the possibility of amyotrophic lateral sclerosis. Myotonia is impaired relaxation of a muscle, and is the characteristic finding of myotonic dystrophy and myotonia congenita. If myotonia is not immediately obvious when the patient fails to loosen their grip after shaking your hand, test for percussion myotonia by briskly tapping the tongue, deltoid, or thenar eminence with a reflex hammer (Chapter 14). Myoedema is a mounding of the muscles upon percussion, seen in patients with hypothyroidism.

Laboratory testing in the patient with proximal weakness

Creatine kinase

Creatine kinase (CK) catalyzes the conversion of creatine and ATP to phosphocreatine and ADP. Phosphocreatine is the largest phosphate reserve for regenerating ATP during active muscle contraction. When muscle cells are damaged by a myopathic process, the serum CK level increases. Although CK is the most sensitive and specific laboratory marker for myopathy, as many as one-third of otherwise normal subjects have CK levels greater than the upper limit of normal of approximately 150 U/liter.[2] This leads to a large number of referrals for patients with asymptomatic or minimally symptomatic hyperCKemia (see Box 10.1). The CK level should be elevated in patients with inflammatory myopathy, dystrophinopathy, limb-girdle dystrophy, and hypothyroidism – question these diagnoses if CK is normal. The CK level may be normal in patients with cachectic myopathy, steroid myopathy, and hyperthyroidism. While an elevated CK level is considered synonymous with myopathy, neuromuscular diseases including ALS, Guillain–Barré syndrome, and even benign cramps may all cause modest CK elevations. Heavy exercise, large muscle bulk, and African ancestry may also increase the CK level in the absence of muscle disease.

> **Box 10.1 HyperCKemia**
>
> The CK level is often checked by primary care physicians in patients with nonspecific complaints including myalgias and fatigue. This is especially true in patients who take statins. Because most patients with mildly elevated CK levels do not actually have a myopathic disorder, this finding must be interpreted cautiously. The largest study of patients with so-called "idiopathic hyperCKemia" found relevant neuromuscular disorders in only 18% of 114 patients with persistently elevated CK levels.[3] Careful reading of this study shows, however, that none of these patients had a treatable neuromuscular disorder. Although there are no firm guidelines, it is difficult to rationalize further evaluation of otherwise strong, minimally symptomatic patients with hyperCKemia of <1000 U/liter.

Aldolase

Aldolase is an important glycolytic enzyme found in muscle and the liver. It may be elevated in patients with muscle disease, but usually adds little to the diagnostic evaluation of a patient with suspected myopathy.

Nerve conduction studies and electromyography

Nerve conduction studies (NCS) and electromyography (EMG) are often helpful diagnostic studies for patients with weakness secondary to peripheral nervous system dysfunction (Figure 10.1).[4] In brief, for patients with proximal and generalized weakness, nerve conduction studies are useful in pinpointing sites of focal nerve compression and differentiating between axonal and demyelinating polyneuropathies. Needle EMG helps to localize radiculopathy, detect myopathic processes, and confirm the diagnosis of motor neuron disease. Repetitive nerve stimulation and single-fiber EMG establish the presence of neuromuscular junction disorders. It is important to recognize the limitations of neurophysiological testing: as Preston and Shapiro note in their essential textbook on electrodiagnosis, EMG is an extension of the clinical examination, and is

unlikely to establish a specific diagnosis if the diagnosis is not considered prior to performing the test.[5]

Muscle biopsy

Muscle biopsy is routinely performed when a myopathic process is suspected. While a muscle biopsy may help to diagnose many exotic varieties of muscle and nerve disease, it is most important for patients with inflammatory, toxic, or endocrine myopathies, because these are potentially treatable conditions. Special histochemical stains and electron microscopy may aid in diagnosis, but rarely do these studies increase the likelihood of finding a treatable condition.

Forearm exercise testing

The basis of the forearm exercise test is that muscle contraction leads to increases in the metabolic by-products lactate and ammonia. To perform forearm exercise testing, draw lactate and ammonia levels from the antecubital vein. Next, have the patient contract the forearm and hand muscles for 1 minute using a dynamometer. Draw lactate and ammonia levels at 1, 3, and 5 minutes following exercise. In normal subjects, there is a rise in both lactate and ammonia after exercise, usually to at least twice the resting value. In patients with myopathies due to glycolytic enzyme deficiencies, lactate does not rise but ammonia does. In patients with myoadenylate deaminase deficiency, ammonia rises but lactate does not. A frustratingly common finding in forearm exercise testing is that both the ammonia and lactate fail to rise sufficiently, suggesting inadequate exercise quality. Because forearm exercise testing is rarely helpful in establishing a diagnosis in adult patients and never uncovers a treatable condition, I rarely perform it.

Causes of proximal weakness

Inflammatory myopathies

The shared features of the inflammatory myopathies are proximal muscle weakness, CK elevation, myopathic EMG changes, and inflammatory infiltrates on muscle biopsy. Severe cases are associated with dysarthria, dysphagia, and diaphragmatic weakness. Muscle aches and pains, if present, are not prominent. In adults, inflammatory myopathies are among the most important causes of proximal weakness, as they are often treatable. The four common inflammatory myopathies may be distinguished on clinical as well as pathological grounds.

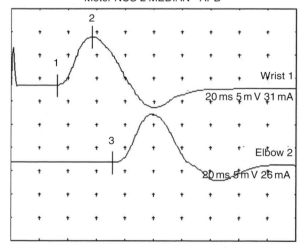

Figure 10.1 Motor nerve conduction study (NCS) of the left median nerve recording from the abductor pollicis brevis (APB). The median nerve is stimulated at the wrist (top trace) and at the elbow (bottom trace). Parameters of interest are the distal latency (the time elapsed between stimulation and the onset of the first motor response at point 1, the response amplitude (the difference in heights between points 1 and 2), and the conduction velocity (obtained by subtracting the time elapsed between points 3 and 1 and dividing by the distance between the stimulation sites). Axonal neuropathies are characterized by low amplitudes and mildly reduced conduction velocities. Demyelinating neuropathies are characterized by mildly reduced amplitudes and markedly reduced conduction velocities.

Polymyositis

Polymyositis is the least common of the three primary inflammatory myopathies. Patients with polymyositis have proximal muscle weakness and elevated CK levels. Muscle biopsy shows endomysial lymphocytic infiltrates that invade nonnecrotic muscle fibers. Corticosteroids are the first-line treatment for polymyositis. Prednisone should be initiated at 60–80 mg qd for 2–3 months. The daily dose is tapered subsequently by 5–10 mg each week. A steroid-sparing agent should be added for patients who respond incompletely. Methotrexate is usually the agent of first choice. This should be started at 2.5 mg qwk and increased by 2.5 mg qwk to reach a goal of 15–20 mg qwk. Obtain a chest X-ray and pulmonary function tests before starting methotrexate and at least every 6 months to screen for pulmonary fibrosis. Because methotrexate may also be hepatotoxic, check liver function tests at least every 2 months. Persistently elevated liver function tests should prompt referral for liver biopsy. For patients who do not respond to methotrexate, azathioprine is usually the next choice among the steroid-sparing agents. Start azathioprine at 50 mg/day and titrate up by 50 mg each week to a dose of 1–2 mg/kg over 2–3 weeks. Monitor complete blood counts weekly for the first month, then biweekly for the next month, then every month for the entire course of therapy. Check liver function tests every 3 months in patients who take azathioprine.

Dermatomyositis

Dermatomyositis is the most common of the idiopathic inflammatory myopathies. In addition to proximal muscle weakness, patients with dermatomyositis have several characteristic skin changes.[6] The heliotrope rash is a symmetric violaceous mask around the upper and lower borders of the eyes. Gottron's papules are elevated violaceous plaques that involve bony prominences, most typically the metacarpophalangeal and interphalangeal joints. Two other typical skin changes are the V sign (erythema over the anterior neck and chest) and the shawl sign (erythema over the posterior neck and shoulders). Unlike polymyositis and inclusion body myositis, dermatomyositis is a multisystem disorder that often involves the gastrointestinal and pulmonary systems in addition to the skin and skeletal muscle. The CK level is elevated in the overwhelming majority of patients with dermatomyositis. Muscle biopsy shows perimysial inflammation of lymphocytes and perifascicular atrophy.

Approximately 25% of patients with dermatomyositis have an underlying malignancy and are at greater risk of developing a malignancy both before and after the diagnosis.[6] Patients with dermatomyositis should therefore undergo annual screening for age- and gender-appropriate cancers. When the diagnosis of dermatomyositis is established, it is important to test for antibodies to Jo-1, a tRNA synthetase (also seen in patients with polymyositis, but less frequently), which is associated with a greater likelihood of pulmonary disease, and therefore warrants more caution when considering treatment with methotrexate. Treat dermatomyositis using an approach similar to that described for polymyositis.

Inclusion body myositis

Inclusion body myositis (IBM) is distinguished from the other inflammatory myopathies by early involvement of wrist flexors and finger flexors in addition to proximal muscles. The CK level may be elevated more modestly in IBM than in the other inflammatory myopathies. Diagnostic muscle biopsy abnormalities include inflammatory infiltrates and inclusions within muscle fibers. Unfortunately, IBM does not respond to treatment with corticosteroids or other immunosuppressants.

Overlap myopathies

Overlap myopathies are inflammatory myopathies that occur in the context of a rheumatological disorder such as systemic lupus erythematosus, scleroderma, or rheumatoid arthritis. Like polymyositis and dermatomyositis, overlap myopathies are usually steroid responsive.

Muscular dystrophies

Dystrophinopathies

Duchenne's muscular dystrophy is an X-linked disorder produced by an out-of-frame shift in the gene that encodes the muscle membrane protein dystrophin. Duchenne's muscular dystrophy is always diagnosed in childhood, and survival past early adulthood is not typical. Milder dystrophinopathies, however, may present for the first time in one of several ways in adulthood. Becker's muscular dystrophy is produced by an in-frame shift in the dystrophin gene, and leads to proximal weakness, sometimes affecting the quadriceps in isolation.[7] Female carriers of the dystrophin mutation may also present with proximal weakness in adulthood.[8] Molecular diagnosis is available for patients with suspected dystrophinopathies. Treatment of dystrophinopathies in adults is generally supportive.

Limb-girdle muscular dystrophies

The limb-girdle muscular dystrophies are a heterogeneous group of disorders that produce hip and shoulder muscle weakness. They may be inherited in any fashion, and may not become clinically obvious until adulthood. Although many patients choose to pursue genetic testing for the peace of mind of having a diagnosis, there are no medications that reverse limb-girdle muscular dystrophy symptoms.

Thyroid myopathies

Both hypothyroidism and hyperthyroidism may result in myopathy. While thyroid myopathies are among the more common of the endocrine myopathies, they are often recognized and treated by primary care physicians or endocrinologists without coming to the attention of neurologists. Levels of CK are usually elevated in patients with hypothyroid myopathy and normal or mildly elevated in patients with hyperthyroid myopathy. In patients with no other explanation, checking thyroid function studies may help to establish the diagnosis in a patient who presents with a suspected myopathy.

Toxic and iatrogenic myopathies

The most important medications and toxins that lead to myopathy are statins, ethanol, and corticosteroids. Other important causes are chloroquine, colchicine, hydroxychloroquine, penicillamine, and zidovudine.

Statin-induced myopathy

3-Hydroxy-3-methylglutaryl-coenzyme A (HMG-CoA) reductase inhibitors (statins) are commonly prescribed cholesterol-lowering agents that produce a wide variety of muscle pathology ranging from asymptomatic CK elevation, to mild muscle aches and cramps, to frank myopathy, to rhabdomyolysis.[9] Despite popular opinion that suggests otherwise, atorvastatin, fluvastatin, pravastatin, and simvastatin are all equally likely to lead to myopathy.[10] It should not be assumed that a statin is the cause of proximal weakness in a patient who happens to be taking one of these medications: thorough evaluation for other causes of proximal weakness should be conducted before assigning responsibility to the statin. The best treatment for muscle problems in patients taking statins is not entirely clear. For patients with tolerable muscle aches or asymptomatic CK elevations, it is usually safe to continue the statin. For patients with rhabdomyolysis or frank myopathy, discontinue the statin immediately and avoid prescribing statins in the future. Alternative lipid-lowering agents including ezetimibe, gemfibrozil, or niacin may also produce myopathic side effects similar to those produced by the statins. Among the lipid-lowering agents, cholestyramine is likely associated with the smallest risk for muscle pathology.

Alcohol-related myopathies

Excessive alcohol use causes two types of myopathy. The first type is an acute-onset necrotizing myopathy with severe muscle weakness, cramps, and myalgias. More commonly, many years of heavy alcohol use leads to a painless proximal myopathy that develops over weeks to months. The exact lifetime dose of alcohol necessary to produce this myopathy and the role of nutritional deficiencies are unclear. Moderate alcohol use (one or two drinks per day) is likely not sufficient to cause a myopathy. Discontinuing alcohol use may improve symptoms.

Steroid myopathy

Chronic corticosteroid use may lead to a myopathy. Although the exact duration of therapy required before the myopathy develops is not clear, 4 weeks is a probable minimum. The typical clinical picture is painless proximal muscle weakness greater in the legs than in the arms, mild or no CK elevation, and normal EMG. Other features of chronic steroid use are usually present. In most patients, the chronology of steroid administration and symptom development makes diagnosis straightforward. For patients who receive steroids for inflammatory myopathy or myasthenia gravis, establishing whether the problem is steroid myopathy or the condition for which the steroids are being prescribed may be more challenging. In these cases, muscle biopsy demonstrating type II muscle fiber atrophy may be necessary to make the diagnosis. Symptoms usually improve several weeks to months after steroid discontinuation. Physical activity may help to prevent steroid myopathy.

Other myopathies

Almost all treatable myopathies are due to inflammatory, iatrogenic, toxic, or endocrine processes. Two uncommon myopathies deserve mention because they may be treatable. Acid maltase deficiency is a metabolic myopathy characterized by proximal weakness and respiratory failure due to diaphragmatic dysfunction, which may respond to weekly infusions of α-glucosidase.[11] Mitochondrial myopathy is often part of a multisystem disorder, and is usually treated with a cocktail containing vitamin E, creatine monohydrate, and coenzyme Q10 with variable results. Other dystrophic and metabolic myopathies are usually not treatable, and the length to which a diagnosis is pursued is largely determined by the patient's curiosity and interest in genetic counselling.

Generalized myasthenia gravis

Myasthenia gravis is an autoimmune disease produced by antibodies that disrupt the function of the postsynaptic neuromuscular junction. Although many patients develop fixed weakness, fatigability with exercise is the distinguishing feature of myasthenia gravis. Other common forms of myasthenia gravis include ocular myasthenia (Chapter 6), myasthenic crisis (Chapter 12), and bulbar myasthenia (Chapter 8). Patients with generalized myasthenia usually, but not always, have preceding or accompanying ocular signs and symptoms. In their absence, the diagnosis may be challenging.

The two bedside tests that may be used to confirm a diagnosis of myasthenia gravis are the ice test and the edrophonium or tensilon test, both of which are described in more detail in Chapter 6, as they are more reliable in patients with ocular symptoms than in patients with isolated proximal weakness.

Beyond history and physical examination, a wide variety of diagnostic tests is available for patients with suspected myasthenia gravis. The diagnosis is most often established by finding acetylcholine receptor (AChR)-binding antibodies in the blood. A very small minority of patients without AChR-binding antibodies have blocking or modulating antibodies. Of the 20% of myasthenics without AChR antibodies, half possess antibodies to muscle-specific tyrosine kinase (MuSK). Patients with no detectable AChR or MuSK antibodies are called seronegative myasthenics, and require electrophysiological testing to establish the diagnosis. The characteristic finding is the electrodecremental response to 3 Hz repetitive nerve stimulation (Figure 10.2). If repetitive nerve stimulation is normal, single-fiber EMG showing abnormal jitter and blocking may help to reach a diagnosis. All patients with myasthenia gravis should undergo a CT scan of the chest to look for thymoma or thymic hyperplasia.

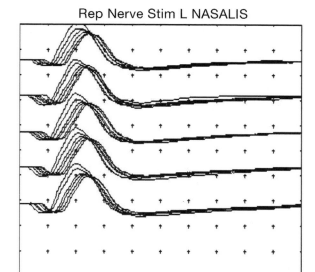

Rep Nerve Stim L NASALIS

Figure 10.2 Slow (3 Hz) repetitive nerve stimulation of the left facial nerve recording the nasalis. Six recordings are present in each of the five traces. Note the electrodecremental response suggestive of a disorder of neuromuscular transmission.

While symptomatic treatment with the acetylcholinesterase inhibitor pyridostigmine may improve symptoms of ocular myasthenia, it is not an effective treatment strategy for generalized myasthenia gravis. Almost all patients require immunosuppression with corticosteroids. Rapid steroid initiation, however, is often harmful to myasthenics, exacerbating their symptoms and sometimes leading to myasthenic crisis. A safer approach for patients with generalized myasthenia is to start prednisone at a dose of 10 mg/day and to titrate upwards to a goal of 60–80 mg/day over 4–6 weeks. The daily dose can be tapered by 5–10 mg each week after 6–8 weeks of high-dose treatment. Benefit from starting or increasing steroids in myasthenia is typically first seen at 2 weeks and becomes maximal at 1 or 2 months. In many cases, steroids by themselves are inadequate for the treatment of myasthenia gravis, and additional immunosuppressive agents such as mycophenolate mofetil (500 mg bid, titrated up to 1500 mg bid as needed) or azathioprine (50 mg qd, titrated up by 50 mg qd/week to a goal dose of 1–2 mg/kg qd) are needed. Mycophenolate mofetil and azathioprine may not produce any benefit until 3–6 months (or longer) after initiation.

Approximately 10% of patients with myasthenia gravis have thymoma, and those with thymoma should undergo thymectomy, usually within several weeks to months after detection, and sooner if there is evidence of malignant invasion. Patients with nonthymomatous myasthenia gravis may benefit from thymectomy, but the literature guiding this decision is murky at best.[12] I generally offer thymectomy to younger patients, as it may be curative and allow steroids to be discontinued. In order to optimize the perioperative course, thymectomy should be performed when symptoms are relatively stable and the daily dose of prednisone is 20 mg or less. I pretreat patients with severe myasthenia or history of myasthenic crisis with five plasma exchanges ending approximately 1 week before anticipated thymectomy.

Lambert–Eaton myasthenic syndrome

This disorder of neuromuscular transmission is produced by antibodies to presynaptic voltage-gated calcium channels. It usually occurs in middle-aged people with underlying neoplasms, most commonly small-cell lung cancer. Less frequently, LEMS is secondary to non-neoplastic autoimmune disorders such as rheumatoid arthritis, pernicious anemia, or hypothyroidism. The typical presentation of LEMS is subacute-to-chronic proximal weakness that is greater in the legs than in the arms. It may be associated with fatigability, but in many cases resembles a myopathy in that the symptoms do not fluctuate. Some patients have bulbar and extraocular muscle weakness, but if these are the most prominent or sole clinical features, consider an alternative diagnosis. Because voltage-gated calcium channels are also present on sensory and autonomic nerve terminals, patients with LEMS may also have mild sensory symptoms and autonomic dysfunction including dry mouth, constipation, and orthostatic hypotension. The cardinal examination finding in patients with LEMS is postexercise facilitation of strength and reflexes.

Confirm the diagnosis of LEMS by checking the blood for antibodies to voltage-gated calcium channels. For patients who require more rapid diagnosis (the antibodies usually require up to 2 weeks to return), the characteristic electrophysiological finding is a reduced compound muscle action potential amplitude that increases after 10 seconds of sustained exercise (Figure 10.3). Because small-cell lung cancer and LEMS coexist so commonly, order a CT scan of the chest for all patients with this disorder. Screen for other cancers as indicated by risk factors and physical examination. If you do not find a tumor or autoimmune disorder, repeat the surveillance scans every 3–6 months, as LEMS may predate cancer diagnosis by several years.

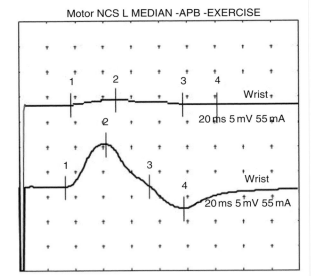

Figure 10.3 Motor nerve conduction study obtained by stimulating the left median nerve and recording the left abductor pollicis brevis (APB) in a patient with Lambert–Eaton myasthenic syndrome at rest (top trace). Ten seconds of sustained exercise followed by another stimulation produces an incremental response using the same recording parameters (bottom trace).

Treating LEMS is usually challenging. Obviously, addressing the underlying cancer or autoimmune disease is the first step. Most patients show an incomplete response to the acetylcholinesterase inhibitor pyridostigmine at a dose of 60 mg qid. The potassium channel blocker 3,4-diaminopyridine (which is available at a limited number of centers in the USA on a compassionate basis through Jacobus Pharmaceuticals) is also modestly effective. Patients with longer life expectancies require steroids, intravenous immunoglobulin, or other immunosuppressants.

Chronic inflammatory demyelinating polyradiculoneuropathy

As its name indicates, chronic inflammatory demyelinating polyradiculoneuropathy (CIDP) is an immune-mediated polyradiculoneuropathy that develops over several months. Although the association of neuropathy with distal weakness is widely known, most patients with CIDP present with simultaneous proximal and distal weakness. Weakness in CIDP is symmetric and, as a rule, accompanied by hyporeflexia or areflexia: increased reflexes should prompt investigation for alternative sources of weakness. Sensory deficits are usually present, but overshadowed by motor abnormalities. Nerve conduction studies demonstrate

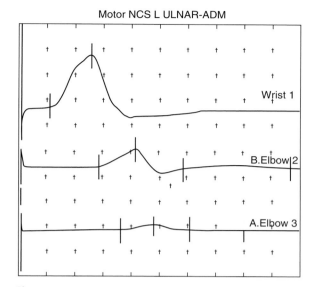

Motor NCS L ULNAR-ADM

Figure 10.4 Motor nerve conduction study (NCS) of the left ulnar nerve recording abductor digiti minimi (ADM). Note the drop in amplitude (measured from the baseline to the peak) with stimulation of the nerve above and below the elbow compared with the amplitude obtained by stimulating at the wrist. This is conduction block, a pathognomonic finding of inherited demyelinating neuropathies such as Guillain–Barré syndrome and chronic inflammatory demyelinating polyneuropathy.

changes consistent with demyelination including slow nerve conduction velocities, abnormal temporal dispersion, and conduction block (Figure 10.4). Similar to Guillain–Barré syndrome (Chapter 12), the CSF in CIDP shows albuminocytological dissociation in which the white blood cell count is low and the protein level is high. HIV, Lyme disease, sarcoidosis, and lymphoma or leukemia should be considered for patients with a CIDP-type presentation and >10 cells/mm³. While CIDP is usually idiopathic, it may be associated with systemic diseases, the most widely known of which are HIV infection and osteosclerotic myeloma. Patients with osteosclerotic myeloma develop the POEMS syndrome characterized by polyneuropathy, organomegaly, endocrinopathy, monoclonal gammopathy, and skin changes. This syndrome is often incomplete. The first steps in evaluating for the possibility of myeloma include serum protein electrophoresis, urine protein electrophoresis, immunofixation, calcium levels, and a skeletal survey to evaluate for a possible myeloma. Corticosteroids and intravenous immunoglobulin (IVIg) are the two agents that are most commonly employed for patients with CIDP. Because IVIg causes fewer side effects, it is usually the treatment of first choice. Initiate IVIg at 2 mg/kg over

5 days, and follow with monthly supplemental doses of 0.4–1 mg/kg. For patients who do not respond to IVIg, start prednisone at a dose of 60 mg and taper by 5–10 mg per dose per week. Although most patients will benefit from either of these treatments, CIDP is a relapsing disease that gets worse when treatment is withdrawn. Plasmapheresis and other immunosuppressants may be used for patients with refractory CIDP.

Central nervous system dysfunction

Peripheral nervous system disease accounts for most cases of proximal muscle weakness. The classic example of CNS dysfunction that breaks this rule is infarction in the border zone or watershed between the anterior and middle cerebral arteries (Chapter 21). Cervical spine disease (Chapter 17) may also lead to predominantly proximal weakness of both arms and legs, sometimes without much sensory dysfunction.

Amyotrophic lateral sclerosis

Amyotrophic lateral sclerosis (ALS) is a degenerative disease of motor neurons characterized by progressive muscle wasting and weakness. Although people of any age may develop ALS, the typical patient is in their 50s or 60s and presents initially with hand clumsiness, gait difficulty, or dysphagia. Patients may not complain specifically of weakness. In the earliest stages, symptoms are quite subtle, and may be overlooked or assigned to more common conditions such as radiculopathy, compression mononeuropathies, or musculoskeletal disorders. Because essentially any subacute-to-chronic-onset focal-or-generalized pattern of weakness described in this or the next chapter may be secondary to ALS, it is important always to consider the diagnosis in patients with painless muscle weakness.

The findings in ALS are best explained with reference to the motor neuron pool. The upper motor neurons begin in the cerebral cortex and descend through the corticospinal tract, while the lower motor neurons begin in the anterior horn cell in the spinal cord. Amyotrophic lateral sclerosis causes degeneration of both upper and lower motor neurons, although lower motor neuron symptoms including multifocal weakness, wasting, and fasciculations often predominate in the initial stages of the disease. While fasciculations are often present, they are not pathognomonic for the diagnosis, nor does their absence exclude ALS. Upper motor neuron findings include dysarthria, spasticity, and hyperreflexia. Sphincter function and extraocular movements are unimpaired. On the surface, cognition is preserved, but most patients eventually show signs of frontal dysfunction if they are tested carefully enough. Sensation should be preserved. Variations of ALS include progressive muscular atrophy in which exclusively lower motor neuron findings are present and primary lateral sclerosis in which exclusively upper motor neuron findings are present. These variants are associated with better long-term prognoses than ALS, although both still lead to disability.

Patients with suspected ALS should undergo EMG: fibrillations, positive sharp waves, and large motor units establish more widespread lower motor neuron involvement than may be evident from bedside examination. The use of EMG also helps to distinguish ALS from multifocal motor neuropathy with conduction block, the condition that most frequently mimics it (Chapter 11). MRI of the brain and spine should be performed to exclude structural processes that may lead to weakness and wasting.

Unfortunately, ALS is a relentlessly progressive condition that leaves patients paralyzed, unable to speak, eat, or breathe, and confined to bed requiring 24-hour care. Patients ultimately die of respiratory failure unless they choose long-term mechanical ventilation. The one medication that is approved for the treatment of ALS, the glutamate antagonist riluzole (50 mg bid), is only marginally effective at prolonging lifespan, and has an unclear benefit on delaying functional decline.[13] Care, therefore, is largely supportive and involves a multidisciplinary team of physical and occupational therapists, speech and swallowing specialists, social workers, and nutritionists.

References

1. *Aids to the Examination of the Peripheral Nervous System.* Edinburgh: WB Saunders; 2000.

2. Brewster LM, Mairuhu G, Sturk A, van Montfrans GA. Distribution of creatine kinase in the general population: implications for statin therapy. *Am Heart J* 2007;**154**:655–661.

3. Prelle A, Tancredi L, Sciacco M, et al. Retrospective study of a large population of patients with asymptomatic or minimally symptomatic raised serum creatine kinase levels. *J Neurol* 2002;**249**:305–311.

4. Nardin RA, Rutkove SB, Raynor EM. Diagnostic accuracy of electrodiagnostic testing in the evaluation of weakness. *Muscle Nerve* 2002;**26**:201–205.

5. Preston DC, Shapiro BE. *Electromyography and Neuromuscular Disorders: Clinical–Electrophysiologic Correlations.* Boston: Butterworth-Heineman; 1998.

6. Callen JP. Dermatomyositis. *Lancet* 2000;**355**:53–57.

7. Wada Y, Itoh Y, Furukawa T, Tsukagoshi H, Arahata K. Quadriceps myopathy: a clinical variant form of Becker muscular dystrophy. *J Neurol* 1990;**237**: 310–312.

8. Hoffman EP, Arahata K, Minetti C, Bonilla E, Rowland LP. Dystrophinopathy in isolated cases of myopathy in females. *Neurology* 1992;**42**:967–975.

9. Thompson PD, Clarkson P, Karas RH. Statin-associated myopathy. *JAMA* 2003;**289**:1681–1690.

10. Evans M, Rees A. Effects of HMG-CoA reductase inhibitors on skeletal muscle: are all statins the same? *Drug Saf* 2002;**25**:649–663.

11. Winkel LPF, Van den Hout JMP, Kamphoven JHJ, et al. Enzyme replacement therapy in late-onset Pompe's disease: a three-year follow-up. *Ann Neurol* 2004;**55**:495–502.

12. Gronseth GS, Barohn RJ. Practice parameter: thymectomy for autoimmune myasthenia gravis (an evidence-based review). *Neurology* 2000;**55**:7–15.

13. Bensimon G, Lacomblez L, Meininger V. A controlled trial of riluzole in amyotrophic lateral sclerosis. *N Engl J Med* 1994;**330**:585–591.

Chapter

11

Focal limb weakness

Anatomy

Asymmetric limb weakness generally conforms to one of several common patterns (Table 11.1). The ability to recognize these patterns and the three to five most common causes of each pattern is a powerful clinical tool that will help in localizing and diagnosing most patients with focal limb weakness. However, any pattern-matching algorithm has limitations, and a firm grounding in the anatomy of the motor system (see also Chapter 10) becomes necessary when evaluating patients with asymmetric weakness, especially for those patients with atypical or multifocal deficits.

The motor pathways that control the extremities begin in the precentral gyrus of the contralateral motor cortex (Figure 11.1). Fibers controlling the leg are located medially within the cortex, while those controlling the arm are found superiorly and laterally. From the cortex, motor fibers descend through the subcortical white matter and the posterior limb of the internal capsule. The motor pathways continue in the cerebral peduncle and then in the ventral pons, crossing within the pyramids of the medulla. Motor fibers descend predominantly through the lateral corticospinal tract to reach the anterior horn cells. The nerve roots are derived from the anterior horn cells, and form the brachial or lumbosacral plexi, which give rise to the named nerves. These nerves innervate the muscles via the neuromuscular junctions. Although focal weakness may be derived from any of these structures, problems at the level of the neuromuscular junction and the muscles usually lead to proximal or generalized rather than focal weakness of the extremities.

Shoulder weakness

C5–6 radiculopathy

Pain and paresthesias are usually the most prominent symptoms of cervical radiculopathy. Because there is a substantial degree of overlap among adjacent myotomes, weakness secondary to radiculopathy is often subtle and involves arm abduction, arm flexion, and external rotation. Biceps and brachioradialis reflexes may be diminished or lost. Sensation is decreased over the lateral shoulder and arm. Patients with C5–6 radiculopathy substantial enough to produce weakness should undergo evaluation and treatment as discussed in Chapter 17.

Brachial plexopathy

It is important to maintain a healthy skepticism when considering the possibility of a brachial plexopathy, as lesions of the plexus are rare in comparison with radiculopathy and musculoskeletal conditions such as rotator cuff tendonitis. Brachial plexus lesions occur most commonly in the setting of trauma, cancer, and idiopathic brachial neuritis. They are usually quite painful, and for this reason, they are discussed in more detail in Chapter 16. Although memorizing the structure of the brachial plexus is among the most time-consuming tasks in learning neuroanatomy, detailed anatomic knowledge is often not necessary because most plexus lesions conform to one of three common patterns:

1. Upper trunk brachial plexopathy produces proximal arm weakness involving the suprascapular (infraspinatus/external rotation), axillary (deltoid/shoulder abduction), and musculocutaneous (biceps/elbow flexion) nerves. Sensory signs and symptoms involve the lateral shoulder, arm, forearm, and hand. It is often difficult to distinguish weakness due to an upper trunk lesion from a C5–6 radiculopathy: both imaging and electrophysiological studies are often necessary.

2. Lower trunk brachial plexopathy produces weakness of the hand muscles and sensory symptoms involving the medial hand, forearm, and arm. Patients with lower trunk plexopathies often have accompanying Horner's syndrome.

Table 11.1 Patterns of focal limb weakness

Location of weakness	Most common sites of pathology
Shoulder	C5–6 nerve roots, upper trunk of brachial plexus
Periscapular region	Long thoracic nerve, accessory nerve
Intrinsic hand muscles	Anterior horn cells, ulnar nerve, cerebral cortex, internal capsule
Wrist drop	Radial nerve, cerebral cortex
Hip and proximal leg	Lumbosacral plexus, femoral nerve, obturator nerve
Foot drop	Peroneal nerve, sciatic nerve, L5 nerve root, cerebral cortex, anterior horn cells
Hemiparesis	Cerebral cortex, subcortical white matter, internal capsule
Multifocal	White matter of the brain and spine, multiple nerve roots, multiple nerves

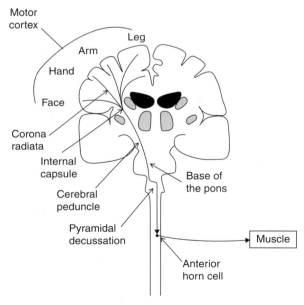

Figure 11.1 Schematic of the motor system.

3. Pan-plexopathy produces widespread weakness and sensory disturbances in the upper extremity. It is among the most common patterns of plexus lesions, especially in the context of trauma or neoplastic infiltration.

Periscapular weakness (scapular winging)

Long thoracic neuropathy

The long thoracic nerve innervates the serratus anterior, which stabilizes the scapula. A lesion of this nerve leads to medial scapular winging. This can be elicited on physical examination by examining the patient from behind while they attempt to do a pushup against a wall with their arms adducted to their trunk. The medial border of the scapula will elevate away from the posterior thoracic wall. Although isolated long thoracic neuropathy is a mononeuropathy, it is commonly produced by conditions that lead to brachial plexopathy such as idiopathic brachial neuritis.

Spinal accessory neuropathy

The other common cause of asymmetric scapular winging is spinal accessory neuropathy. This scapular winging is characterized by lifting of the superolateral border of the scapula away from the posterior thoracic wall upon attempted abduction and external rotation of the arm. In addition to scapular winging, spinal accessory neuropathy produces weakness of ipsilateral shoulder shrug (trapezius) and contralateral head turning (sternocleidomastoid). Common sites of spinal accessory nerve entrapment include the jugular foramen (in which case the glossopharyngeal and vagus nerves will also be involved; see Chapter 8) and the posterior cervical triangle.

Hand and finger weakness

Ulnar neuropathy

The ulnar nerve innervates most of the intrinsic hand muscles, and is therefore the mononeuropathy most likely to lead to hand muscle weakness. The usual cause of ulnar neuropathy is compression of the nerve at the elbow, a site at which it is relatively exposed to wear-and-tear trauma. Less common sites of ulnar nerve damage are in the forearm (especially in patients with diabetes[1]), and at the wrist in cyclists or in heavy older men who rest their weight on their wrists while using walkers. Numbness and paresthesias are usually present in the fourth and fifth digits, but in some cases, sensory complaints are completely absent. On examination, the hypothenar eminence and first dorsal interosseous (the fleshy muscle between the thumb and index finger) may be atrophic. Weakness of abduction of digits two and five is tested appropriately by applying finger pressure from the side and not by forcefully squeezing the fingers together. Flexion of the distal interphalangeal joints of digits four and five may be weak. Sensory loss is classically noted in the fifth digit and in the ulnar half of the fourth digit on both the palmar and dorsal aspects of the hand. Confirm the localization of a suspected ulnar neuropathy with nerve conduction studies. Mild ulnar neuropathies may respond to conservative measures such as wearing an elbow pad. More severe ones, particularly those that produce prominent weakness, are likely to require surgical release and transposition of the ulnar nerve.

Motor neuron disease

Focal hand weakness and wasting are often the first symptoms of amyotrophic lateral sclerosis, a disorder discussed in more detail in Chapter 10.

C8–T1 radiculopathy

A C8 or T1 radiculopathy may produce focal hand weakness, usually in association with neck pain and paresthesias radiating into the arm and hand. In general, the C8 and T1 nerve roots are relatively protected from degenerative spine disease, making this cause of hand weakness uncommon.

Central causes of hand weakness

Two common stroke syndromes lead to prominent hand weakness. The first is infarction of the contralateral cortical hand area, which produces weakness resembling an ulnar or radial neuropathy.[2] The second is the dysarthria–clumsy hand syndrome, which results from lacunar infarction in the subcortical white matter, internal capsule, or pons.[3] Contralateral cerebral cortical or subcortical lesions such as neoplasms, abscesses, or demyelinating lesions may also produce hand weakness. Many patients with parkinsonism come to neurological attention advertised as having hand weakness. Careful examination, however, reveals that the actual problems are bradykinesia and rigidity rather than weakness (Chapter 13).

Wrist and finger drop

Wrist and finger drop are special kinds of hand weakness that develop acutely and are characterized by weakness of extension at the wrist and fingers. The most common causes of wrist and finger drop are stroke and radial neuropathy.

Stroke

Middle cerebral artery infarction is the most common cause of hand and arm weakness secondary to stroke. Because the cortical representations of the hand and face are adjacent to each other in the motor homunculus, hand weakness is often (but not always) accompanied by facial weakness.

Radial neuropathy

"Saturday night palsy" is the classic radial neuropathy: an intoxicated patient, after a night of heavy sleep with their arm draped over a chair, awakens and finds that they cannot extend their wrist or fingers. Intoxication is not a prerequisite for acquiring a pressure palsy of the radial nerve, and it may develop in any state of prolonged immobilization such as surgery or even normal deep sleep. Other than compression of the radial nerve, the other common etiologies for radial neuropathy include vasculitis related to mononeuropathy multiplex and multifocal motor neuropathy with conduction block (see below).

Differentiating between stroke and radial neuropathy

The following examination techniques may help to distinguish between stroke and radial neuropathy:

1. Most compressive radial neuropathies occur at the level of the spiral groove, distal to the branches that innervate the triceps. Thus, a patient with a compressive radial neuropathy usually has profound weakness of wrist and finger extension with preserved arm extension. A patient with stroke may have triceps weakness in addition to wrist drop.

2. Testing extension of the interphalangeal joints may also help to differentiate between the two localizations. The prime extensors at these joints are the lumbricals, which are innervated by the median (digits two and three) and ulnar (digits four and five) nerves. Thus, extension of the distal interphalangeal joints should be preserved in a patient with radial neuropathy, but may be weak in a patient with stroke.

3. The pattern of sensory loss is also helpful in differentiating radial neuropathy from stroke. In a patient with radial neuropathy, sensory loss affects

---

Box 11.1 Postpartum leg weakness

Leg weakness following delivery occurs in approximately 1% of women.[4] The etiologies are usually benign, and self-resolving, but some may be more serious:

- Femoral neuropathy is produced by excessive thigh abduction and external rotation during delivery. It produces weakness of hip flexion and knee extension with sensory loss in the anteromedial thigh and leg. Despite common belief, the femoral nerve is not actually compressed by the baby's head, as the nerve does not enter the true pelvis.

- Obturator neuropathy is usually the result of compression of the nerve by the baby as it descends through the pelvis. It leads to weakness of thigh adduction and sensory loss in the medial thigh. Risk factors for compression include prolonged labor and cephalopelvic disproportion.

- Lumbosacral plexopathy is also caused by the descent of the baby through the pelvis. Due to the positioning of the component nerves within the pelvis, the peroneal nerve is often affected out of proportion to the other nerves of the lumbosacral plexus.

- Peroneal neuropathy may also result from compression of the fibular neck against stirrups during delivery. Deficits include weakness of foot dorsiflexion and eversion with sensory changes on the dorsum of the foot and lateral leg.

- Conus medullaris and cauda equina syndromes (Chapter 17) are exceedingly rare complications of epidural anesthesia. Because many women have back pain after delivery, new neurological deficits are often ascribed to the injection. Careful neurological examination, and in some cases imaging of the lumbosacral spine, however, discloses that procedure-related lesions of the conus medullaris or cauda equina are almost never responsible.

- Central nervous system processes, particularly superior sagittal sinus thrombosis, are important causes of postpartum leg weakness, especially when associated with headache, encephalopathy, or seizures. Women with suspected venous sinus thrombosis should undergo MRI and magnetic resonance venography (MRV) of the brain. Venous sinus thrombosis is discussed further in Chapter 19.

Peripheral nerve and plexus lesions acquired during delivery are usually self-resolving and should be managed with the expectation that they will improve. Patients with atypical examination findings may require imaging studies of the pelvis, lumbosacral spine, or brain. If symptoms do not improve by 3 weeks postpartum, nerve conduction studies and EMG help to localize the lesion and guide prognosis.

---

the dorsal hand, while in stroke sensory loss is typically greater in the palm.

Should any difficulty remain in distinguishing between radial neuropathy and ischemic stroke, head MRI with diffusion-weighted imaging or electromyography (EMG) should be performed.

Hip and proximal leg weakness

L2–3 radiculopathy

Spinal stenosis commonly involves the L2 or L3 nerve roots in older adults. Pain and paresthesias radiating from the back into the hip and thigh are usually more prominent in patients with upper lumbar radiculopathies, but in some cases, proximal leg weakness is the chief complaint. Because spinal stenosis is such a common radiological finding in older patients, it is often difficult to determine whether it is the true cause of weakness or if it is only an incidental finding. Upper lumbar radiculopathy is discussed in greater detail in Chapters 16 and 17.

Lumbosacral plexopathy

Like brachial plexopathy, lumbosacral plexopathy is usually associated with exquisite pain, and is therefore discussed in greater detail in Chapter 16. Common causes of lumbosacral plexopathy include trauma (including childbirth, see Box 11.1), neoplastic infiltration, diabetic amyotrophy, and retroperitoneal hematoma.

Foot drop

Weakness of the tibialis anterior, the principal dorsiflexor of the foot, results in foot drop. From distal to proximal, possible responsible lesion sites include the peroneal nerve, sciatic nerve, lumbosacral plexus, L4–5 nerve roots, and the CNS. In most cases, the cause is in the peripheral nervous system, and the localization of foot drop is determined by the presence or absence of weakness of other lower extremity muscles (Table 11.2).

Table 11.2 Distinguishing among peripheral nervous system sources of foot drop

	Dorsiflexion: tibialis anterior	Eversion: peroneus longus	Inversion: tibialis posterior	Plantarflexion: gastrocnemius	Hip abduction: gluteus medius
Peroneal nerve	+	+	−	−	−
Sciatic nerve	+	+	+	+	−
L5 radiculopathy	+	+	+	−	+

Peroneal neuropathy

Peroneal nerve damage results in weakness of dorsiflexion and eversion. Although foot inversion (mediated by the tibial nerve and tibialis posterior) is spared, it often appears to be involved in patients with severe dorsiflexion weakness. To properly test for inversion weakness in patients with severe dorsiflexion weakness, the foot must be passively dorsiflexed: in patients with peroneal neuropathy, it will become immediately obvious that inversion is much stronger than eversion. Damage to the peroneal nerve usually occurs as a result of trauma or prolonged immobilization. Sometimes, there is no clear precipitant. In patients without a relevant history of trauma, consider the possibilities of mononeuropathy multiplex, and multifocal motor neuropathy with conduction block.

Sciatic neuropathy

The sciatic nerve divides into the common peroneal and tibial nerves at the knee. Weakness should therefore involve dorsiflexion, plantarflexion, foot inversion, and foot eversion. Many cases of sciatic neuropathy, however, preferentially involve the peroneal fascicles while sparing the tibial fascicles. Sciatic neuropathy is distinguished from L5 radiculopathy by sparing of hip abduction. In such cases, a sciatic neuropathy may only be distinguishable from a peroneal neuropathy by EMG. The etiologies of sciatic neuropathy, like peroneal neuropathy, include trauma, immobilization, mononeuropathy multiplex, and multifocal motor neuropathy with conduction block.

L5 radiculopathy

Most L5 radiculopathies are associated with lower back pain. The pattern of motor abnormalities helps to distinguish L5 radiculopathy from peroneal or sciatic neuropathy when pain is absent: an L5 radiculopathy would be expected to produce weakness of dorsiflexion, inversion, eversion, and hip abduction, while sparing plantarflexion. L5 radiculopathy should be confirmed with MRI of the lumbosacral spine. Strongly consider surgery for patients with structural disc disease sufficient to produce a foot drop.

Motor neuron disease

Isolated foot drop may be the first abnormality in amyotrophic lateral sclerosis (ALS). Careful examination may disclose weakness of other muscles, fasciculations, and hyperreflexia, which support the diagnosis. Confirmation of the diagnosis by EMG is usually required for patients with ALS.

Central nervous system localizations

While more widespread lower extremity weakness might be expected with CNS disease, medial frontal lesions may also produce isolated or predominant foot drop. Clues to a CNS source include the presence of headache and, in some cases, transcortical motor aphasia (Chapter 3). Anterior cerebral artery stroke, dural sinus thrombosis, tumor, and hemorrhage are among the most common CNS etiologies of foot drop.

Treating foot drop

Treatment of foot drop begins by addressing the underlying cause. In many cases, however, supportive care including physical therapy and wearing an ankle foot orthosis to keep the foot passively dorsiflexed while the patient recovers is the only available treatment option. It is important to counsel patients on the prolonged (up to 2 years) and sometimes incomplete recovery from foot drop due to peripheral nerve lesions. Electromyography is often helpful for prognostication.

Hemiparesis and hemiplegia

Hemiparesis essentially always reflects dysfunction of the CNS. Common causes include ischemic stroke, hemorrhage, tumor, demyelination, or abscess. In exceptional cases, multiple simultaneous peripheral nervous system lesions may produce multifocal problems that masquerade as hemiparesis. The following five rules help to pinpoint the site of pathology:

1. Cerebral cortical lesions producing simultaneous weakness of the face, arm, and leg should always be accompanied by some behavioral manifestation. It would be unusual for a right-handed patient with a left cortical lesion, for example, to have severe hemiparesis without aphasia.

2. Large subcortical lesions, particularly within the internal capsule, produce severe hemiparesis that is usually unassociated with behavioral deficits. The most common etiology of hemiplegia secondary to an internal capsule lesion is infarction in the territory of the medial lenticulostriate arteries (Chapter 21).

3. A brainstem lesion often produces a "crossed hemiparesis" in which an ipsilateral cranial nerve deficit is accompanied by contralateral hemiparesis:

    a. A midbrain lesion produces ipsilateral third-nerve palsy and contralateral hemiparesis (Chapter 6).

    b. A pontine lesion produces ipsilateral sixth- and/or seventh-nerve palsy and contralateral hemiparesis (Chapters 6 and 8).

    c. A medullary lesion produces ipsilateral twelfth-nerve palsy and contralateral hemiparesis (Chapter 8).

4. Small lacunar infarcts of the contralateral corona radiata, internal capsule, or pons may lead to the syndrome of ataxic hemiparesis (Chapter 21). As its name suggests, the limbs are both clumsy and weak.

5. Hemiparesis that spares the face is generally the result of an ipsilateral cervical spinal cord lesion (Chapter 17).

Multifocal weakness

Multifocal weakness is always due to multifocal nervous system disease. The common localizations of multifocal weakness are the CNS white matter, anterior horn cells, nerve roots, and peripheral nerves. Common conditions that produce multifocal weakness include multiple sclerosis (Chapter 22), motor neuron disease (Chapter 10), and cervical and lumbosacral polyradiculopathy (Chapter 17). In some cases, multiple simultaneous embolic strokes may lead to multifocal weakness. The following are three disorders of the peripheral nervous system that produce multifocal weakness.

Vasculitic mononeuropathy multiplex

Mononeuropathy multiplex is an uncommon diagnosis, usually associated with vasculitis. Although rheumatologists often refer patients with vague pain syndromes for mononeuropathy multiplex evaluation, true mononeuropathy multiplex is not subtle, and patients often have profound multifocal weakness. In many cases, the first mononeuropathy of mononeuropathy multiplex clinically resembles an ischemic stroke rather than a peripheral nerve disorder. The nerves that are most commonly affected include the sciatic, peroneal, radial, and ulnar. The site of nerve involvement is usually at the vascular watershed territories in the middle of the femur or humerus. Attacks of mononeuropathy multiplex are usually painful and result in flaccid weakness. A generalized polyneuropathy often accompanies the motor symptoms (Chapter 15). The diagnosis of vasculitic mononeuropathy multiplex is established by finding lymphocytic infiltration of blood vessels with fibrinoid necrosis on nerve biopsy. Laboratory studies should include erythrocyte sedimentation rate, rheumatoid factor, double-stranded DNA antibodies, anti-Smith antibodies, Sjögren's antibodies, and cryoglobulins. Mononeuropathy multiplex should be treated with a combination of steroids and cyclophosphamide. Recovery is often very slow and incomplete.

Multifocal motor neuropathy with conduction block

Patients with multifocal motor neuropathy with conduction block (MMNCB) are typically younger to middle-aged men who develop focal arm weakness in the distribution of a named nerve.[5] Because the weakness begins so suddenly and is usually not associated with pain, patients are often evaluated for stroke. As the disease progresses, additional motor nerves become involved, and, at this stage, MMNCB may resemble motor neuron disease. Nerve conduction studies confirm the presence of conduction block. Approximately 50% of patients with MMNCB will have antibodies to the ganglioside GM_1. Intravenous immunoglobulin is the standard first-line treatment for MMNCB.

Hereditary neuropathy with liability to pressure palsies

Hereditary neuropathy with liability to pressure palsies (HNPP) is an autosomal dominantly inherited neuropathy characterized, as its name suggests, by the development of multiple pressure palsies. Recurrent carpal tunnel syndrome, ulnar neuropathy, and peroneal neuropathy are separated in space and time over many years. The diagnosis is established by testing for the responsible mutation in the *PMP22* gene. The mainstay of treating HNPP is counseling the patient to avoid activities that precipitate pressure palsies.

References

1. Acosta JA, Hoffman SN, Raynor EM, Nardin RA, Rutkove SB. Ulnar neuropathy in the forearm: a possible complication of diabetes mellitus. *Muscle Nerve* 2003;**28**:40–45.

2. Gass A, Szabo K, Behrens S, Rossmanith C, Hennerici M. A diffusion-weighted MRI study of acute ischemic distal arm paresis. *Neurology* 2001;**57**:1589–1594.

3. Fisher CM. Lacunar strokes and infarcts: a review. *Neurology* 1982;**32**:871–876.

4. Wong CA. Neurologic deficits and labor analgesia. *Regional Anesth Pain Med* 2004;**29**:341–351.

5. Nobile-Orazio E, Cappelari A, Priori A. Multifocal motor neuropathy: current concepts and controversies. *Muscle Nerve* 2005;**31**:663–680.

Chapter 12 · Rapidly progressive weakness

Neuromuscular respiratory failure

The first priority in evaluating the patient with rapidly progressive weakness is to determine whether they will require immediate intubation. Warning signs of impending respiratory disaster include tachypnea, punctuated speech, and accessory respiratory muscle use. Check inspiratory muscle strength at the bedside by asking the patient to count to 30 as quickly as possible. The ability to do so in a single breath suggests sufficient diaphragmatic strength to maintain adequate gas exchange. While performing the initial bedside assessment, check for a strong, forceful cough, which indicates the ability to "clear the airway."

Unlike most cardiopulmonary sources of respiratory distress, early neuromuscular respiratory failure is usually not accompanied by a decline in oxygen saturation. Similarly, typical arterial blood gas abnormalities that reflect hypoventilation (low P_{O2} and high P_{CO2}) do not appear early enough to predict the need for intubation. Rather, bedside spirometry is the most important quantitative measurement of neuromuscular respiratory failure. The two most important spirometry values are the negative inspiratory force (NIF) and forced vital capacity (FVC). Values that should prompt you to consider intubation or at least monitoring in an intensive care unit setting are a NIF <40 cmH$_2$O and a FVC <1 liter. Use clinical judgment in interpreting these numbers, as poor patient effort and bulbar weakness (resulting in inability to form an adequate seal around the spirometer) lead to false-positive results.

Initial pattern of weakness

All severe generalized weakness ultimately produces a flaccid, intubated patient. It is the initial pattern of weakness, therefore, that helps to determine the etiology. Severe weakness beginning in the extraocular muscles and descending over a period of hours suggests botulism. Fluctuating extraocular weakness with ptosis for several weeks or more prior to the onset of generalized weakness is most consistent with myasthenia gravis. Weakness that begins in the bulbar muscles, descends rapidly, and is accompanied by a pharyngeal exudate is classic for diphtheria. Limb weakness sparing the face is most consistent with pathology at the level of the cervical spine. Weakness that begins in the legs and ascends rapidly over several days to a few weeks is the classic (but not exclusive) presentation of Guillain–Barré syndrome (GBS; acute inflammatory demyelinating polyradiculoneuropathy). Generalized weakness that develops over seconds is most consistent with infarction or hemorrhage of the ventral pons.

Neurological examination

Although many patients with rapidly progressive weakness are intubated and incapable of cooperating with the neurological examination, it is essential to perform as careful an assessment as the circumstances will allow. Mental status should be tested in as much detail as possible in order to exclude coma and severe encephalopathy masquerading as weakness (see Chapters 1 and 2). Important components of cranial nerve examination include pupillary reactions and eye movements. Absent pupillary reactions are characteristic of but not universal in botulism: more than half of patients with botulism actually have normal, reactive pupils.[1] While diplopia and ptosis are common to many causes of rapidly progressive weakness, fluctuating rather than fixed extraocular muscle weakness strongly suggests myasthenia gravis. Preserved vertical eye movements in a tetraplegic, seemingly unresponsive patient point to a locked-in state caused by pontine hemorrhage or infarction. Deep tendon reflex testing assumes utmost importance in patients with rapidly progressive weakness. Hyporeflexia or areflexia are prerequisites for the diagnosis of GBS. While spasticity and hyperreflexia might be expected in CNS disorders, patients with spinal cord lesions sufficient to produce spinal shock are flaccid and areflexic. Sensory examination is often unhelpful in patients with rapidly progressive weakness, as cooperation is usually limited. In a patient who is sufficiently awake, decreased sensation points to a peripheral nerve or spinal cord lesion, whereas preserved sensation makes the muscle or neuromuscular junction more likely localizations.

Diagnostic studies

If there are signs of a specific etiology of rapidly progressive weakness, investigations should be tailored to confirm that diagnosis. In many cases, however, a broad spectrum of studies is required, as the diagnosis is not apparent from the clinical history and examination. Although this "shotgun" approach may appear inelegant, the gravity of rapidly progressive weakness and limitations in the examination necessitate a thorough battery of tests in many cases. The most important diagnostic tools are neuroimaging studies of the brain and spine, nerve conduction studies (NCS) and electromyography (EMG), and lumbar puncture.

Neuroimaging studies

In most cases, rapidly progressive weakness results from injury to the peripheral nervous system rather than the CNS. In some cases, however, ischemic, inflammatory, or space-occupying lesions of the CNS may produce acute-onset weakness. MRI of the brain and entire spine with and without contrast should be performed if CNS injury is suspected or if evaluation of the peripheral nervous system is unrevealing.

Electromyography and nerve conduction studies

These are the most useful diagnostic studies for localizing the source of rapidly progressive weakness. Nerve conduction studies involve stimulating and recording from a select group of sensory and motor nerves, thereby allowing measurement of the amplitude and velocity of peripheral nerve responses. Needle EMG allows recording of spontaneous activity from muscles and motor unit analysis, and is helpful in patients with muscle, nerve, and nerve root disease. Repetitive nerve stimulation and single-fiber EMG are special studies that assess the neuromuscular junction.

Neurophysiological testing has several important limitations when used for evaluation of patients with severe generalized weakness. First, a fair amount of cooperation is required for needle EMG, and single-fiber EMG is essentially impossible in severely weak patients. Secondly, many patients with severe weakness are intubated and have a variety of intravenous lines and other catheters that prevent adequate exposure for electrode placement. Finally, electrical interference from intensive care unit equipment creates excessive electrical noise.

The following is a brief summary of the most important patterns of EMG and NCS abnormalities in patients with rapidly progressive weakness.

Demyelinating neuropathy

The neurophysiological hallmark of GBS is acquired demyelination: NCS show prolonged distal latencies, markedly slowed conduction velocities (<75% of normal values), abnormal temporal dispersion, conduction block, and prolonged late responses (see Chapter 10, Figure 10.4). As discussed below, many of the findings of primary demyelination are not present in early GBS. Needle EMG showing decreased motor unit recruitment may be the only electrophysiological abnormality in the first week of the disease.

Axonal neuropathy

Axonal neuropathies are less likely to lead to rapidly progressive weakness than are demyelinating ones. Neurophysiological characteristics of axonal neuropathy include low response amplitudes and mildly reduced (never below 75% of normal) conduction velocities. Electromyography shows decreased motor unit recruitment and fibrillation potentials. Rapidly progressive weakness produced by an axonal polyneuropathy should prompt investigation for heavy metal intoxication, porphyria, and vasculitis. Axonal variants of GBS are less common outside China.

Presynaptic neuromuscular junction dysfunction

Botulism is the most important presynaptic neuromuscular junction disorder leading to rapidly progressive weakness. The hallmark of presynaptic neuromuscular junction dysfunction is that exercise or fast repetitive nerve stimulation results in an increase in motor amplitudes (see Chapter 10, Figure 10.3).

Postsynaptic neuromuscular junction dysfunction

Myasthenia gravis and other postsynaptic neuromuscular junction transmission disorders are accompanied by abnormal decremental responses with repetitive nerve stimulation (Chapter 10, Figure 10.2). If it is technically possible in the intensive care unit, perform single-fiber EMG to investigate for increased jitter and blocking.

Myopathy

Muscle diseases uncommonly cause rapidly progressive weakness, but may cause failure to wean from the ventilator (see below). The EMG characteristics of myopathy are short-duration, small-amplitude, polyphasic motor units with early recruitment. Motor NCS may show decreased response amplitudes, while sensory NCS are normal.

CSF analysis

The characteristic CSF finding in GBS is albuminocytological dissociation in which elevated protein is accompanied by a normal cell count. This abnormality, however, is present in only 70% of patients within 1 week of symptom onset.[2] The spinal fluid in acute disseminated encephalomyelitis and other inflammatory myelopathies shows increased white blood cell counts and protein. Viral antibodies are present in patients with poliomyelitis caused by West Nile virus. CSF protein may be slightly elevated in patients with botulism.

Blood, urine, and stool examination

Abnormalities in blood, urine, and stool may help to reach a diagnosis in some patients with rapidly progressive weakness. Patients with lead, arsenic, or thallium poisoning will have elevated levels of the relevant heavy metal. Antibodies to West Nile virus are seen in some patients with poliomyelitis. Antibodies to the acetylcholine receptor are present in the majority of patients with myasthenic crisis. If tested early enough, botulinum toxin is detectable in the stool or serum of patients with botulism.[1] Elevated levels of 24-hour urine porphobilinogen excretion are diagnostic of porphyria.

Causes of acute paralysis

Guillain–Barré syndrome

Guillain–Barré syndrome (GBS), or acute inflammatory demyelinating polyradiculoneuropathy (AIDP), is the most common source of acute-onset generalized paralysis in the industrialized world. As its name suggests, it is an autoimmune demyelinating disorder of the peripheral nerves and roots. The classical clinical history begins with a prodrome of gastrointestinal or respiratory illness or vaccination, which is followed several weeks later by numbness and tingling in the extremities and weakness that begins in the feet and spreads upwards to the legs, arms, face, and respiratory muscles. Many cases of GBS, however, do not conform

to this pattern, and weakness may also begin in the proximal muscles or even occasionally in the bulbar muscles. Back pain is often exquisite and may lead to exhaustive but fruitless investigation for structural spinal disease. The symptoms of GBS become maximal within 2–4 weeks of onset. Untreated, most patients develop rapidly progressive flaccid weakness, which often requires intubation. Occasional patients may develop only mild distal weakness and paresthesias.

The two most important physical examination findings are symmetric weakness and decreased reflexes. While there may be some side-to-side asymmetry in patients in the early stages of GBS, the left and right sides should be symmetrically weak as the disorder progresses. Consider a diagnosis other than GBS in the absence of hyporeflexia or areflexia. Bulbar weakness may be present in patients with more advanced weakness. Sensory loss is less severe than motor dysfunction, with large-fiber modalities such as vibration and proprioception typically more affected than small-fiber modalities such as pinprick and temperature.

In many cases, the diagnosis of GBS is obvious from the clinical history and examination. Lumbar puncture and EMG play a confirmatory role, but may be especially important in patients with very early disease in whom the syndrome is incomplete. Albuminocytological dissociation of the cerebrospinal fluid in which the protein is high and the white blood cell count is low (<10 cells/mm^3) is present in approximately 70% of patients with symptom duration of 1 week or less.[2] If >10 cells/mm^3 are present, consider HIV seroconversion as an alternative explanation.[3] Electromyography findings diagnostic of GBS (discussed above) are present in only 50% of patients within the first 5 days of symptoms.[2]

Plasmapheresis and intravenous immunoglobulin (IVIg) are the mainstays of the immunomodulatory treatment of GBS. Plasmapheresis is performed as a series of five exchanges every other day. Complications of plasmapheresis include those related to central line insertion and fluctuations in blood pressure due to large-volume fluid shifts. The IVIg is administered at a dose of 2 g/kg, usually divided over 2 days. Important side effects of IVIg include headache, aseptic meningitis, kidney failure, and hypercoaguability. Both plasmapheresis and IVIg reduce the time required to regain the ability the walk, and should be started as quickly as possible.[4,5] Although neither treatment is superior to the other, I choose IVIg more often, as it can be started more quickly, has fewer serious associated side effects, and, in at least one relatively large study, showed a trend towards producing faster improvement than plasmapheresis.[6]

Supportive care is also important in patients with GBS. Patients with airway compromise, cardiac arrhythmias, and blood pressure fluctuations should be treated in the intensive care unit. Patients with GBS often require narcotics (including patient-controlled anesthesia in some cases) and agents for neuropathic pain in order to obtain adequate pain control.

As might be guessed, the ultimate prognosis of GBS is correlated with the maximal severity of clinical deficits. Electrophysiologically, finding reduced compound muscle action potential (CMAP) amplitudes on NCS predicts slower and incomplete recovery. Some patients who are diagnosed and treated at an early enough stage may be able to walk out of the hospital unassisted. Recovery for patients with severe disease, however, usually takes 3–6 months or longer. Because improvement may be slow, there is often a temptation to treat patients with another course of IVIg or plasmapheresis, or to switch between treatments. There is no evidence, however, to support either of these approaches.

Myasthenic crisis

A myasthenic crisis characterized by respiratory muscle paralysis may occur at any stage of the disorder, even as its initial presentation. It may be differentiated from the other causes of rapid-onset weakness by the preceding weakness of extraocular and bulbar muscles. Precipitants of myasthenic crisis include infection and medications that are known to exacerbate myasthenia, especially aminoglycosides. High-dose corticosteroids prescribed for myasthenia gravis may paradoxically worsen symptoms within 1 or 2 weeks of initiation, often leading to crisis. The mechanism for this worsening is unclear, but corticosteroids are usually titrated slowly upwards to prevent this from happening.

Myasthenic crisis should be differentiated from the much less common cholinergic crisis caused by acetylcholinesterase inhibitors. Telltale signs of cholinergic crisis include excessive oral and nasal secretions, fasciculations, and gastrointestinal cramps. Unlike myasthenic crisis, cholinergic crisis resolves within several hours of stopping acetycholinesterase inhibitors. It is best, however, to anticipate the need to intubate all myasthenics with respiratory muscle weakness, rather than to assume that they will improve spontaneously.

Treating myasthenic crisis must obviously begin with pulmonary function testing and intubation as necessary. Superimposed respiratory, gastrointestinal, and urinary tract infections must be addressed. In rare cases, treating such an infection may resolve the crisis. Almost all patients, however, will require a series of five plasma exchanges or IVIg given at a dose of 2 mg/kg divided over 5 days. A response is typically noted within 1–3 weeks, if it does occur. I prefer to treat myasthenics in crisis with plasmapheresis based on personal experience and verified by the findings of Gajdos and colleagues, which suggested that patients who underwent plasmapheresis improved more quickly than those who received IVIg.[7] Larger doses of acetylcholinesterase inhibitors are not helpful in treating myasthenic crisis.

Because the benefits of IVIg and plasmapheresis are transient, disease-modifying regimens need to be augmented in patients with myasthenic crisis. Increase steroids to their goal doses while patients receive IVIg or plasmapheresis. In patients who are already taking steroids, start a steroid-sparing agent such as mycophenolate mofetil (500 mg bid to start, increase to 1000 mg bid in 1 week) or azathioprine (50 mg qd to start, increase by 50 mg per dose each week to a goal of 1–2 mg/kg). Be aware, however, that these agents will not provide any symptomatic benefit for several months.

Brainstem catastrophe

Large brainstem lesions, typically in the ventral pons, may produce severe, instantaneous weakness. The classic example is the locked-in state caused by basilar artery thrombosis or pontine hemorrhage. This state is characterized by complete paralysis of the face and limbs with sparing of vertical eye movements and blinking. Other causes of brainstem catastrophe include inflammatory, neoplastic, infectious mass lesions, and central pontine myelinolysis caused by overly rapid correction of hyponatremia. Patients with suspected brainstem catastrophe should undergo MRI with diffusion-weighted imaging and contrast, and treatment should be directed at the underlying cause.

Less common causes of acute paralysis

Botulism

Food-borne botulism is an uncommon form of acute-onset paralysis caused by ingestion of botulinum toxin, an inhibitor of presynaptic acetylcholine release.[1] Gastrointestinal distress usually begins 12–36 hours after toxin ingestion. Diplopia, ptosis, dysarthria, and

Table 12.1 Uncommon neuropathies causing rapidly progressive weakness

Condition	Diagnostic test	Treatment
Arsenic	Elevated serum arsenic levels	Dimercaprol
Lead	Elevated serum lead levels	Dimercaptosuccinic acid
Thallium	Elevated serum thallium levels	Prussian blue
Porphyria	Elevated 24-hour urine porphobilinogen	Hematin and glucose
Peripheral nerve vasculitis (polyarteritis nodosa, Churg–Strauss, rheumatoid arthritis)	Elevated erythrocyte sedimentation rate, rheumatoid factor Consider rheumatology consultation	Prednisone 60–80 mg qd plus cyclophosphamide 1–2 mg/kg qd
Diphtheria	Culture of pharyngeal membrane	Antitoxin plus penicillin
Beriberi	Decreased thiamine levels, often in alcoholics, undernourished people, or those who have undergone gastric bypass	Thiamine supplementation

dysphagia are the first neurological symptoms. Large unreactive pupils are present in approximately 50% of patients with botulism, distinguishing the disorder from other causes of acute paralysis. Weakness of the arms, respiratory apparatus, and legs follows within several hours to a few days. The toxin may be identified from the serum or stool if checked within 48–72 hours of symptom onset. Nerve conduction study findings of botulism include small motor amplitudes that increase in size with sustained exercise or rapid (50 Hz) repetitive nerve stimulation. If botulism is strongly suspected, then initiate treatment with antitoxin. Although this intervention will not reverse active symptoms, it may prevent new ones from developing. Recovery from botulism takes many months, but is usually complete if the comorbidities of chronic ventilation can be avoided.

Uncommon polyneuropathies

Several uncommon polyneuropathies may produce an acute paralysis that mimics GBS. Because these neuropathies are all rare, they will only be mentioned briefly (Table 12.1).

Poliomyelitis

While it is uncommon in the industrialized world, poliomyelitis due to poliovirus still affects patients in the developing world. After a viral prodrome, patients with poliomyelitis develop painful monoparesis followed by the rapid onset of flaccid paralysis. During the acute phase, the spinal fluid of patients with poliomyelitis shows an increased neutrophil count, which distinguishes it from GBS. West Nile virus is an important cause of poliomyelitis, and may be diagnosed by finding antibodies in the serum or spinal fluid.[8]

Spinal cord insults

Lesions of the high cervical spinal cord may produce acute paralysis of all four limbs while sparing the face. Trauma is the most important cause of severe cervical myelopathy. Other important spinal processes that cause rapidly progressive weakness include herniated intervertebral discs, transverse myelitis, and spinal cord stroke (Chapters 17 and 22).

Difficulty weaning from the ventilator

Difficulty weaning from the ventilator is usually due to cardiopulmonary disease.[9] In some cases, intensivists are not able to find a cardiopulmonary explanation for failure to wean, and neurologists are consulted. Begin the diagnostic process by addressing possible CNS processes such as coma and encephalopathy. Next, exclude disorders acquired prior to intubation such as GBS and myasthenia gravis. Finally, investigate for neuromuscular disorders acquired in the intensive care unit including critical illness polyneuropathy, critical illness myopathy, and prolonged neuromuscular junction blockade.

Critical illness polyneuropathy

Critical illness polyneuropathy (CIP) occurs in the setting of severe sepsis and multiorgan failure, usually in patients with intensive care unit stays of at least a week in duration.[10] Clinically, CIP is characterized by flaccid areflexic weakness and sensory loss. Nerve conduction studies show evidence for axonal polyneuropathy in the form of low sensory and motor response amplitudes. Electromyography shows fibrillations and positive sharp waves, which reflect denervation. Unfortunately, there is no specific treatment for CIP, and patients who have the condition usually need several months (or longer) to allow axonal regrowth and clinical recovery.

Critical illness myopathy

Critical illness myopathy (CIM) also occurs in the setting of severe sepsis. Use of corticosteroids and neuromuscular junction blocking agents are additional risk factors for CIM.[11] Patients with CIM are usually weak and areflexic, much like those with CIP. Unlike patients with CIP, the sensory examination (if assessable) should be normal in patients with CIM. Creatine kinase levels may be normal, modestly elevated, or markedly elevated. Nerve conduction studies show decreased motor response amplitudes with normal sensory response amplitudes. Like CIP, needle EMG shows signs of denervation including fibrillation potentials and positive sharp waves. If motor units can be activated, they are small, polyphasic, and show early recruitment. It is often difficult to distinguish between CIM and CIP by clinical examination and with standard neurophysiological assessment, and many patients have both conditions simultaneously. The best way to distinguish between the two is by finding electrical inexcitability upon direct muscle stimulation in CIM.[12] The distinction between CIP and CIM is not necessarily important, as neither has a specific treatment, and both require weeks to months of supportive care before a substantial improvement occurs.

Prolonged neuromuscular junction blockade

Neuromuscular junction blocking agents are used to paralyze patients for surgery or to maintain an airway in patients with cardiopulmonary disease who are resisting the ventilator. Unfortunately, weakness may persist for several days after these are withdrawn, especially in patients with hepatic or renal dysfunction.[13] Although this process is localized to the neuromuscular junction, creatine kinase levels are often elevated. Although abnormal repetitive nerve stimulation may help to diagnose prolonged neuromuscular junction blockade, interference from electrical equipment in the intensive care unit generally makes this technique unfeasible. Other than discontinuing the responsible agents and waiting for recovery, there is no specific treatment for prolonged neuromuscular junction

blockade. While most patients recover in a few days, some have prolonged deficits that may overlap clinically with CIM.

References

1. Hughes JM, Blumenthal JR, Merson MH, et al. Botulinum stool and serum testing – clinical features of types A and B food-borne botulism. *Ann Intern Med* 1981;**95**:442–445.
2. Gordon PH, Wilbourn AJ. Early electrodiagnostic findings in Guillain–Barré syndrome. *Arch Neurol* 2001;**58**:913–917.
3. Cornblath DR, McArthur JC, Kennedy PGE, Witte AS, Griffin JW. Inflammatory demyelinating peripheral neuropathies associated with human T-cell lymphotropic virus type III infection. *Ann Neurol* 1987;**21**:32–40.
4. Hughes RAC, Swan AV, van Doorn PA. Intravenous immunoglobulin for Guillain–Barré syndrome. *Cochrane Database Syst Rev* 2006;(1):CD002063.
5. Raphael JC, Chevret S, Hughes RAC, Annane D. Plasma exchange for Guillain–Barré syndrome. *Cochrane Database Syst Rev* 2002;(2):CD001798.
6. van der Meche FG, Schmitz PI. A randomized trial comparing intravenous immune globulin and plasma exchange in Guillain–Barré syndrome. Dutch Guillain–Barré Study Group. *N Engl J Med* 1992;**326**:1123–1129.
7. Gajdos P, Chevret S, Clair B, Tranchant C, Chastang C. Clinical trial of plasma exchange and high dose intravenous immunoglobulin in myasthenia gravis. *Ann Neurol* 1997;**41**:789–796.
8. Petersen LR, Marfin AA. West Nile virus: a primer for the clinician. *Ann Intern Med* 2002;**137**:173–179.
9. De Jonghe B, Sharshar T, Lefaucheur JP, et al. Paresis acquired in the intensive care unit. A prospective multicenter study. *JAMA* 2002;**288**:2859–2867.
10. Bolton CF, Gilbert JJ, Hahn AF, Sibbald WJ. Polyneuropathy in critically ill patients. *J Neurol Neurosurg Psychiatry* 1984;**47**:1223–1231.
11. Lacomis D, Giuliani MJ, Van Cott A, Kramer DJ. Acute myopathy of intensive care: clinical, electromyographic, and pathological aspects. *Ann Neurol* 1996;**40**:645–654.
12. Rich MM, Bird SJ, Raps EC, McCluskey LF, Teener JW. Direct muscle stimulation in acute quadriplegic myopathy. *Muscle Nerve* 1997;**20**:665–673.
13. Gooch JL. AAEM Case Report #29: prolonged paralysis after neuromuscular blockade. *Muscle Nerve* 1995;**18**:937–942.

Parkinsonism

History

Parkinsonism refers to the combination of bradykinesia (slowness of movement) and rigidity. It is the defining feature of Parkinson's disease (PD) and other disorders of the extrapyramidal system such as progressive supranuclear palsy (PSP), multisystem atrophy (MSA), and corticobasal degeneration (CBD). A patient with parkinsonism may describe their problem as slowness or stiffness, but may also say that they have no energy or that they are weak. Parkinsonism is often attributed to fatigue, normal aging, or depression for months or years, and a patient with parkinsonism may only come to neurological attention after developing a tremor or gait impairment. The following are the important elements of the history in patients with parkinsonism.

Age of onset

Parkinsonism is generally a problem of older patients. Symptoms beginning before the age of 40 suggest an early-onset or familial variant of PD, a toxin- or medication-related process, or Wilson's disease.

Pace of onset

Most forms of parkinsonism become clinically apparent over a course of months to years. Examples include PD, MSA, and PSP. Apoplectic symptom onset is exceptionally rare, and is usually due to bilateral caudate, putaminal, or thalamic infarcts.[1] Symptoms that develop over days to weeks may be due to drug-induced parkinsonism (a condition that may also develop over several years). Rapid progression over several weeks to months is most typical of Creutzfeldt–Jakob disease.

Presence of tremor

Asymmetric resting hand (or less likely, foot) tremor strongly suggests a diagnosis of PD. Other tremors that are characteristic of PD include resting jaw or lip tremors. Tremor is usually absent in atypical forms of parkinsonism – when present, it is often mild,

symmetric, and occurs with action rather than with rest. Large-amplitude action or intention tremors are more typical of Wilson's disease. Chapter 14 provides a more detailed discussion of the evaluation and treatment of tremor.

Gait dysfunction and falls

Almost all patients with parkinsonism eventually develop gait abnormalities, usually as a later feature of the disease. Gait difficulty at or shortly after symptom onset suggests PSP. Common descriptions of gait abnormalities in parkinsonism include stiff-leggedness, shuffling, slowness, and walking with a lack of arm movement.

Left–right symmetry

Parkinson's disease is usually asymmetric in its early stages. As the disease advances, however, both sides become involved, and most patients eventually develop more symmetric deficits. With the additional exception of CBD, most other forms of parkinsonism are relatively symmetric.

Autonomic symptoms

Autonomic dysfunction including dry mouth, decreased perspiration during exercise, lightheadedness, fainting, constipation, and urinary retention is prominent in MSA, and may be more impressive than either rigidity or bradykinesia. Autonomic symptoms are also common in PD, but do not usually bring the patient to clinical attention.

Ataxia

Ataxic symptoms including clumsiness, frequent spilling of food or liquids, and dropping things are common in MSA. These symptoms are often much more prominent than extrapyramidal ones, and patients are often referred for cerebellar strokes and tumors or hereditary ataxic disorders.

Medications and toxins

Dopamine antagonists used as antipsychotics and the promotility agent metoclopramide are the most commonly identified precipitants of drug-induced parkinsonism. Drugs of abuse are sometimes "cut" with substances that precipitate parkinsonism. Other uncommon toxins that may produce parkinsonism include manganese and carbon monoxide.

Family history

There are a number of genetic mutations, inherited in both autosomal dominant and recessive fashions that may produce familial forms of PD.[2] Huntington's disease (autosomal dominant) and Wilson's disease (autosomal recessive) are among the more common inherited forms of parkinsonism. In most patients, however, the family history is noncontributory.

Dementia

Memory loss and behavioral changes affect approximately 25–30% of patients with PD, but are not usually prominent at disease onset.[3] Dementia with Lewy bodies, Huntington's disease, PSP, and CBD are causes of parkinsonism that may initially present as dementia.

Activities of daily living

It is often helpful to ask the patient if it takes them more time to get ready in the morning, whether it is more difficult to turn over or get out of bed, and whether they have difficulty eating. Asking about activities of daily living, while not necessarily helpful in differentiating among the various forms of parkinsonism, helps to determine disease severity and guides treatment initiation.

Examination

Rigidity

Rigidity (often called "lead-pipe" rigidity) is an increase in tone that is independent of the velocity, displacement, and direction of movement. It is the form of hypertonicity produced by extrapyramidal disease. Rigidity may affect the appendicular or axial musculature. Evaluate for appendicular rigidity at the elbow, wrist, knee, and ankle. When testing for rigidity, look for an increase in tone in response to distraction: ask the patient to rapidly tap the opposite hand or foot, trace broad circles in the air, or recite the months of the year backwards. These maneuvers may uncover rigidity

that was not apparent at rest. Test for axial rigidity by examining tone in the neck and torso. With the patient sitting up straight but relaxed in a chair, grasp their head firmly by the sides and attempt to move it briskly in the anterior–posterior plane. Normally, the neck is quite loose and there will be little resistance to this movement. In a patient with axial rigidity, however, the whole trunk will move in unison with the head. One form of rigidity that is somewhat specific to PD is cogwheeling rigidity, in which a tremor is superimposed on a background of rigidity. This is most easily elicited by rotating the hand at the wrist and feeling for a ratchety resistance.

Bradykinesia

Bradykinesia, or slowness of movement, is often overlooked by primary care physicians or dismissed as a manifestation of normal aging. Masking of facial expression, reduced blinking frequency, and slowness of speech and gait are all signs of bradykinesia that may be observed without formal testing. Tests of bradykinesia should include asking the patient to rapidly tap their fingers together, alternately slap the palmar and dorsal surfaces of the hand against their thigh, and elevate the foot slightly and tap the ground with the tips of their toes. Observe for slowness, decomposition, or inability to perform these movements.

Tremor

Asymmetric resting tremor is one of the findings that most reliably distinguishes between PD and other forms of parkinsonism. Chapter 14 contains a detailed discussion of the tremor of PD and other movement disorders.

Gait

The typical features of an extrapyramidal gait are a relatively narrow base, slow initiation, shortened stride length, and slow turns. A patient with PD is characteristically hunched over at the shoulders, whereas a patient with PSP tends to be hyperextended throughout the trunk. The cerebellar form of MSA may be associated with an ataxic gait. Chapter 18 contains a more detailed discussion of the gait abnormalities in patients with extrapyramidal disease.

Speech

Dysarthria is discussed in further detail in Chapter 8. It may be a useful sign in differentiating among the various forms of parkinsonism. Hypophonia and slowness of speech are the most common speech abnormalities in PD. Early spastic dysarthria suggests atypical parkinsonism, especially PSP. A high-pitched quivering dysarthria may accompany MSA.

Mental status examination

Perform a complete mental status examination (Chapter 4) in all patients with parkinsonism, as cognitive abnormalities are common in patients with extrapyramidal disease, and specific abnormalities may help to differentiate among the various disorders. Dementia in parkinsonism is usually dominated by cognitive slowing rather than by the frank memory deficits that characterize Alzheimer's disease. Problems with processing speed and visuospatial abnormalities are the most common findings on mental status examination. Asymmetric limb apraxia is particularly suggestive of corticobasal ganglionic degeneration, and may be the presenting feature in some patients. Dementia with Lewy bodies is discussed further in Chapter 4.

Eye movements

Examining eye movements is essential in patients with suspected PSP, as it is often difficult to establish the diagnosis without abnormalities of saccadic movements. To test saccades, instruct the patient first to look at your nose. Next, ask them to quickly shift their gaze up, down, to the left, and to the right. Poor initiation, decreased velocity, and decreased amplitude of downward saccades are classical but not universal features of PSP. If downward saccades are absent, attempt to prove that the saccadic disorder results from supranuclear dysfunction by looking for a preserved oculocephalic reflex: quickly thrust the head in each of the four cardinal directions and observe for an intact vestibulo-ocular response in the opposite direction.

Orthostasis

Autonomic dysfunction is the main problem in many patients with MSA, and may also be a disabling component of PD. Testing for orthostatic hypotension is described in further detail in Chapter 9.

Laboratory and neuroimaging studies

Brain MRI

In most cases, neuroimaging is of limited utility in evaluating parkinsonism. Brain MRI is mainly employed to exclude the possibilities of vascular parkinsonism, tumors, and hydrocephalus. Patients with rapid-onset disease should undergo diffusion-weighted imaging to look for ischemic lesions or evidence of Creutzfeldt–Jakob disease. In some cases, MRI may help to distinguish among the different forms of parkinsonism. Brain MRI of a patient with MSA may show atrophy of the pons and cerebellum and the "hot cross bun" sign (crossed T2 hyperintensities) in the pons (Figure 13.1). Huntington's disease leads to prominent atrophy of the caudate nuclei (Chapter 14, Figure 14.1). Other neuroimaging studies including single photon emission computed tomography (SPECT) and positron emission tomography (PET) scanning are used for research purposes but are not employed routinely in the clinical setting.

Other studies

In younger patients, check for reduced serum ceruloplasmin levels or increased 24-hour urinary copper

(a)

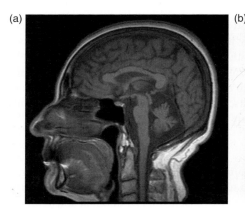

(b)

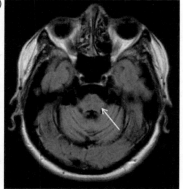

Figure 13.1 In general, neuroimaging studies are not particularly helpful in the diagnosis of parkinsonism. In this patient with multisystem atrophy, however, atrophy of the pons and cerebellum is shown in (A), while (B) shows the pathognomonic "hot cross bun" sign in the pons (arrow).

excretion diagnostic of Wilson's disease (Chapter 14). A variety of commercial genetic studies is available to evaluate patients with familial forms of PD. Autonomic testing to document orthostatic hypotension and other autonomic abnormalities is essential to the diagnosis of MSA. Anal sphincter electromyography is often performed in an attempt to distinguish MSA from PD, but it is generally less helpful than history and autonomic testing.

Parkinson's disease

Idiopathic PD is the most common form of parkinsonism. Patients usually develop the disorder between their 50s and 70s, although symptoms will begin before the age of 40 in 5–10% of patients.[4] The cardinal features of PD are tremor, rigidity, and bradykinesia. Unfortunately, there is no laboratory test or neuroimaging study that definitively confirms PD, and the diagnosis must be made clinically. The features that most reliably distinguish PD from other forms of parkinsonism are asymmetric resting tremor and symptomatic improvement with levodopa.[5] Because up to 30% of patients lack a tremor, a trial of levodopa is often necessary in unclear cases.[5] Parkinson's disease may be divided into three stages: an early, levodopa-responsive stage in which disability is minimal, a middle stage in which responsiveness to levodopa decreases and disability becomes more prominent, and an end stage in which the benefits from levodopa are minimal and disability becomes severe, leading to death in some cases.

Treatment of early Parkinson's disease

Tremor is often the most prominent symptom in the early stages of PD, and some patients may have a milder, tremor-predominant form of the disease for many years. The anticholinergic agent trihexyphenidyl (started at 1 mg qd and titrated up to 2–3 mg tid as needed) is the preferred treatment for a patient with isolated or predominant tremor. Side effects of this medication include sedation and dry mouth. Other options for tremor-predominant PD include benzodiazepines such as clonazepam (0.5–1.0 mg bid) and the anticonvulsant zonisamide (50–100 mg qd).

The treatment options for a patient with symptomatic bradykinesia or rigidity include dopamine agonists, levodopa, and monoamine oxidase B (MAO-B) inhibitors. Because early exposure to levodopa theoretically

increases the long-term risk for developing dyskinesias, I usually treat younger patients or those with mild disability with a dopamine agonist. The two most commonly used agents are ropinirole (starting dose 0.25 mg tid, usual effective dose 1–3 mg tid) and pramipexole (starting dose 0.125 mg tid, usual effective dose 0.5 mg tid). Side effects of these agents include nausea, vomiting, and hypotension. Excessive daytime sleepiness, sleep attacks, and compulsive behaviors such as gambling and shopping are important, but less common side effects of dopamine agonists.

Use levodopa for patients who do not tolerate dopamine agonists, do not respond to therapeutic doses after 3 months of treatment, or have at least moderate disability at presentation. Peripheral side effects from levodopa include nausea, vomiting, and orthostasis, and may be avoided by using levodopa in combination with the dopamine decarboxylase inhibitor carbidopa. Carbidopa/levodopa combinations come in 10 mg/100 mg, 25 mg/100 mg, and 25 mg/250 mg doses. I usually initiate treatment with one half of a 25 mg/100 mg pill three times a day and titrate it to a full pill three times a day over 2–3 weeks in order to avoid side effects such as confusion, hallucinations, and orthostatic hypotension. Most patients respond by the time the daily levodopa dose reaches 300–600 mg.

The MAO-B inhibitors rasagiline (1–2 mg qd) and selegiline (5 mg bid) are the third main option for treating early parkinsonism. There are two important interactions to keep in mind when prescribing MAO-B inhibitors: when combined with a selective serotonin reuptake inhibitor, they may lead to the serotonin syndrome characterized by confusion, autonomic instability, and myoclonus, and when combined with tyramine-rich foods such as red wine, aged cheese, or aged meat, they may precipitate a hypertensive crisis. Inhibitors of MAO-B may provide mild symptomatic relief. Their capacity to provide neuroprotection is of great interest but is not necessarily supported by available evidence.

Treatment of intermediate Parkinson's disease

Patients with PD almost inevitably progress over a period of months to years. During the intermediate stage of PD, bradykinesia and rigidity worsen. Responsiveness to levodopa decreases, while side effects secondary to the medication increase. Motor fluctuations and the "wearing-off" phenomenon begin in the intermediate stages of PD: after several hours of symptomatic response to levodopa, the benefit disappears before the next scheduled dose is administered and the patient enters the "off" state. Address the wearing-off phenomenon by decreasing the interval between levodopa doses or by adding the catechol-O-methyltransferase (COMT) inhibitor entacapone (200 mg with each dose of levodopa) to extend the half-life of levodopa. The main side effect of entacapone is diarrhea. Liver dysfunction, a concern with the older COMT inhibitor tolcapone, is not a side effect of entacapone. Other options to treat wearing off include adding dopamine agonists or MAO-B inhibitors. Controlled-release formulations of carbidopa/levodopa are not terribly effective at extending "on" time and reducing wearing-off symptoms.[6]

In addition to experiencing motor fluctuations and wearing off, patients in the intermediate stage of PD also derive less benefit from each individual levodopa dose. Higher doses of levodopa, even up to a total daily dose of 1000–1200 mg, may be ineffective. It is important to determine at what times of day the patient is most symptomatic, and to make sure that the levodopa is dosed adequately in anticipation of these dips. Most patients require additional medication early in the day to get through their morning routines. Others might require more levodopa at night in order to avoid nocturnal akinesia that prevents them from getting to the bathroom. For some patients, the problem might be eating high-protein meals that interfere with the intestinal absorption of levodopa. Address this problem by instructing the patient to take their levodopa an hour before or after meals, or to eat low-protein meals in the morning. Dopamine agonists and MAO-B inhibitors may be effective as adjuncts to levodopa.

Dyskinesias secondary to long-term levodopa use also develop in the intermediate stage of PD. Dyskinesias may affect any part of the body and are usually choreiform in nature, but may take the form of any of the hyperkinetic movements (Chapter 14). Dyskinesias are generally more prominent at the time of peak levodopa effect, but may also be more pronounced in the "off" state. In some patients, decreasing the levodopa dose reduces peak-dose dyskinesias. Obviously, though, this reduces any symptomatic benefit from levodopa and increases time spent in the "off" state. Amantadine (100 mg bid–tid) may provide modest benefit in reducing dyskinesias, but should be used cautiously in older patients, as it may precipitate confusion.

Deep brain stimulation (DBS) of the subthalamic nucleus is a surgical option for patients with intermediate PD, and may improve any of the symptoms of PD, decrease the time spent in the "off" state, and reduce dyskinesias. Candidates for DBS must be selected carefully and evaluated by a multidisciplinary team. The response to DBS is generally equivalent to the maximum improvement that the patient derives from medical treatment: patients with no response to levodopa are therefore not eligible for treatment. Patients with severe cognitive impairment are also poor candidates and are usually excluded. Possible side effects of DBS include infection, hemorrhage, seizure, and misplacement of the stimulator leads, requiring reoperation. Deep brain stimulation requires frequent follow-up visits for stimulator testing and programming. Other less commonly employed surgical options include thalamotomy or thalamic DBS (for patients with disabling tremor) and pallidotomy.

Treatment of advanced Parkinson's disease

In the advanced stage of PD, bradykinesia and rigidity worsen. Further increases in levodopa doses or addition of other symptomatic treatments for PD are generally unhelpful. Gait freezing and other forms of akinesia also become problematic in advanced PD. Falls become more frequent as postural reflexes become impaired. As a result, patients often need to use walkers or wheelchairs or become bed bound. Medical and surgical treatment of freezing gait and falls are generally ineffective. Supportive care, including management of nonmotor symptoms, becomes the mainstay of treatment at this stage. Unfortunately, many patients with later-stage PD die from pneumonia or as a result of a traumatic injury from a fall.

Treatment of nonmotor symptoms

As PD progresses, treating nonmotor symptoms becomes increasingly important. Cognitive and autonomic functions generally worsen as motor symptoms become more severe. The following are among the most important of the nonmotor symptoms of PD.

Depression

Disentangling psychomotor slowing produced by depression and bradykinesia secondary to PD is often challenging and in some cases requires formal neuropsychological or psychiatric evaluation. Depressive symptoms may affect as many as 50% of patients with

PD, and generally parallel the severity of intellectual impairment.[7] Selective serotonin reuptake inhibitors (SSRIs) are usually the first line of treatment, but must be avoided in patients who are taking MAO-B inhibitors. Tricyclic antidepressants are also helpful, but their anticholinergic properties may worsen cognitive dysfunction. Electroconvulsive therapy is often effective for treating severe depression in PD, and offers the additional benefit of temporary PD symptom relief.[8]

Dementia

Approximately 25–30% of patients with PD develop dementia. Executive function, processing speed, and visuospatial abilities are the cognitive domains that tend to be most severely affected. Memory and language deficits may be later occurrences. Because medications used to treat PD may contribute to cognitive deficits, a trial of decreasing or discontinuing medications may help to improve symptoms. The medications used for PD in descending order of cognitive side effect likelihood (and thus the recommended sequence of discontinuation) are:

- anticholinergic agents
- amantadine
- MAO-B inhibitors
- COMT inhibitors
- dopamine agonists
- levodopa

Acetylcholinesterase inhibitors such as donepezil or rivastigmine are somewhat effective for patients with dementia associated with PD.[9]

Hallucinations and psychosis

Hallucinations and psychosis are features of intermediate and advanced PD. They often occur as side effects of one of the medications used to treat motor symptoms, and may lead to hospitalization or, in severe cases, institutionalization. The first step in evaluating and treating psychotic symptoms is to screen for metabolic disturbances that may cause confusion, as described in Chapter 1. Try to decrease psychoactive antiparkinsonian medications as described above. If excluding metabolic derangements and tapering medications still does not improve symptoms, consider antipsychotics with minimal extrapyramidal side effects such as clozapine (25–75 mg qd) or quetiapine (25 mg qd–qid). Although clozapine improves psychosis, it may cause agranulocytosis and, for this reason, requires frequent white blood count monitoring and registration with a clozapine provider program.

Constipation

Constipation occurs in approximately half of patients with PD, and may be a disabling symptom.[10] The first step in evaluating and treating constipation is to exclude treatable medical causes. Although constipation may be related to agents used for PD including anticholinergics and levodopa, discontinuing these medications usually does not help to reverse symptoms. Laxatives such as lactulose (30–45 ml tid–qid) and polyethylene glycol (17 g qd) are usually the agents of first choice. Consider referring patients with refractory symptoms to a gastroenterologist.

Dysphagia

Oropharyngeal bradykinesia leads to difficulty with eating and swallowing pills, and puts patients at risk of aspiration. Formal swallowing studies may help to clarify the problem if there is any doubt about the presence or severity of dysphagia. Dysphagia often responds to levodopa, provided that the patient has enough residual swallowing function to take their pills. Parcopa is an orally disintegrating carbidopa/levodopa formulation that dissolves on the tongue, allowing patients with severe dysphagia access to adequate levodopa. Percutaneous enteric gastrostomy tubes may be necessary for patients with severe dysphagia.

Dysarthria

Dysarthria affects up to 70% of patients with PD and is characterized by a slow, monotonous, hypophonic voice.[11] Although dysarthria may improve initially with levodopa, as the disease progresses the response of this symptom to levodopa also decreases. Deep brain stimulation of the subthalamic nucleus is similarly disappointing. While speech therapy may help marginally, the treatment of dysarthria related to PD is often unsatisfactory and may ultimately require assistive communication devices.

Atypical parkinsonism

Progressive supranuclear palsy

Although there is considerable clinical heterogeneity, PSP most commonly presents with bradykinesia and rigidity without tremor.[12] Other common presentations include dementia, gait dysfunction, and bulbar dysfunction. It may be difficult to differentiate PSP from other forms of parkinsonism, but the following features are the most valuable in making the diagnosis:

- Prominent gait instability at disease onset. Falls and other gait disturbances that occur within the first year of disease presentation are more consistent with PSP than with any of the other extrapyramidal syndromes. Patients with PSP tend to be hyperextended at the trunk, unlike those with PD who tend to be hunched over at the shoulders.
- Spastic dysarthria. Patients with PSP may have a harsh, strangled quality to their speech or may sound robotic. Amyotrophic lateral sclerosis and the pseudobulbar state affect speech in similar ways (Chapter 8).
- Supranuclear gaze palsy or slowing of vertical saccades. This is the most specific feature for PSP, but its frequent absence at disease onset often prevents definitive diagnosis. Patients with PSP have most difficulty with looking downwards, often leading to problems with reading or with spilling food. Examination of saccadic eye movements is discussed above.
- Eyelid-opening apraxia. This disorder is often confused with blepharospasm, and is discussed in further detail in Chapter 7. Briefly, patients have difficulty opening their eyelids, in some cases leading to functional blindness.
- Axial rigidity. Unlike PD, rigidity is greater in the axial relative to the appendicular musculature. This results in slow head turning and difficulty with truncal stability.

There is no single neuroimaging or laboratory test that confirms the diagnosis of PSP. Rather, the diagnosis is established by suggestive clinical features and by exclusion of other extrapyramidal disorders. Patients in the early stages of PSP may derive mild benefit from levodopa, and a trial up to a total daily dose of 1000 mg is justifiable. As the disease progresses, supportive care becomes the mainstay of treatment. Physical therapy and occupational therapy are important for patients with PSP. Unfortunately, patients with PSP have a poor prognosis, surviving for 5–6 years, on average.[12]

Multisystem atrophy

Multisystem atrophy is characterized by extrapyramidal dysfunction in combination with autonomic, cerebellar, or pyramidal dysfunction. Extrapyramidal features may be the initial and often sole manifestations of MSA for many years (MSA-P subtype), in which case it may

be difficult to separate MSA from PD. Other patients present with primary autonomic dysfunction including orthostatic hypotension, hypohydrosis, and sphincter dysfunction (MSA-A subtype). Finally, the initial symptoms may be cerebellar ataxia, in which case the disorder may be difficult to distinguish from an inherited spinocerebellar ataxia (MSA-C subtype). The diagnosis of MSA is usually established by clinical history and examination. Autonomic testing may help to confirm the diagnosis in patients with MSA-A. Brain MRI demonstrating atrophy of the pons and cerebellum or the "hot cross bun" sign (Figure 13.1) is often useful in patients with the MSA-P and MSA-C variants. Patients may respond to levodopa in the early stages of MSA, but this response declines as the disease progresses. The mainstays of treatment are symptomatic therapy for orthostatic hypotension (Chapter 9) and other autonomic nervous system problems, and physical therapy and occupational therapy for the cerebellar components. Unfortunately, MSA is a progressive disabling disease, with a median survival of 6–9 years.[13]

Corticobasal ganglionic degeneration

Corticobasal ganglionic degeneration (CBD) is an uncommon condition that is often confused with another extrapyramidal disorder such as PD or PSP, or with a primary dementing disorder.[14] Similar to PD, CBD is usually characterized by asymmetric rigidity and bradykinesia. Tremor, however, is usually absent. Two important findings in CBD that are unusual at presentation in the other movement disorders are asymmetric limb apraxia (Chapter 4) and cortical sensory loss (Chapter 15). Limb apraxia may be accompanied by an unusual finding known as the "alien hand" phenomenon in which the affected limb seems to act of its own volition without the input of the patient. Many patients with CBD are demented at presentation. Unlike dementia in other extrapyramidal disorders, the dementia in CBD affects cortical function such as memory and language. Dysarthria and vertical gaze impairments may lead to confusion of CBD with PSP. Patients with CBD respond minimally to levodopa, and supportive therapy is the mainstay of treatment.

Other causes of parkinsonism

Drug-induced parkinsonism

Dopamine antagonists including antipsychotics and the antiemetic metoclopramide may precipitate parkinsonism. Although symptoms tend to be relatively symmetric in drug-induced parkinsonism, almost half of patients with drug-induced PD will have a degree of asymmetry suggestive of idiopathic PD.[15] Only a minority, however, will have resting tremor. Removing the offending agent may lead to mild symptomatic improvement. Treating symptoms with levodopa or with a dopamine agonist is usually not effective and should be avoided.

Vascular parkinsonism

Parkinsonism due to cerebrovascular disease is perhaps only 5% as common as idiopathic PD.[16] Although patients often have a history of prior acute ischemic stroke, this is not a requirement for diagnosis. The lower half of the body is more commonly affected in vascular parkinsonism than it is in PD, and gait disturbances are often the presenting symptoms. Tremor is usually absent, and symptoms tend to be relatively symmetric. Dementia, corticospinal tract findings such as spasticity and hyperreflexia, and urinary incontinence commonly accompany vascular parkinsonism. Unfortunately, vascular parkinsonism does not respond to levodopa, making supportive care the mainstay of treatment.

Other extrapyramidal disorders

Other common disorders leading to parkinsonism include those that have more prominent hyperkinetic features (Huntington's disease and Wilson's disease, Chapter 14) or dementia (dementia with Lewy bodies, Chapter 4) at onset.

References

1. Ghika J, Bogousslavsky J. Abnormal movements. In: Bogousslavsky J, Caplan L, eds. *Stroke Syndromes*. Cambridge: Cambridge University Press; 2001; 162–181.

2. Hardy J, Cai H, Cookson MR, Gwinn-Hardy K, Singleton A. Genetics of Parkinson's disease and parkinsonism. *Ann Neurol* 2006;**60**:389–398.

3. Aarsland D, Zaccai J, Brayne C. A systematic review of prevalence studies of dementia in Parkinson's disease. *Mov Disord* 2006;**20**:1255–1263.

4. Schrag A, Ben-Shlomo Y, Brown R, Marsden CD, Quinn N. Young-onset Parkinson's disease revisited – clinical features, natural history, and mortality. *Mov Disord* 1998;**13**:885–894.

5. Hughes AJ, Ben-Shlomo Y, Daniel SE, Lees AJ. What features improve the accuracy of clinical diagnosis in Parkinson's disease: a clinicopathologic study. *Neurology* 1992;**42**:1142–1146.

6. Jankovic J, Schwartz J, Vander Linden C. Comparison of sinemet CR4 and standard sinemet: double blind and long-term open trial in parkinsonian patients with motor fluctuations. *Mov Disord* 1989;**4**:303–309.

7. Mayeux R, Stern Y, Rosen J, Leventhal J. Depression, intellectual impairment, and Parkinson disease. *Neurology* 1981;**31**:645–650.

8. Faber R, Trimble MR. Electroconvulsive therapy in Parkinson's disease and other movement disorders. *Mov Disord* 1991;**6**:293–303.

9. Miyasaki JM, Shannon K, Voon V, et al. Practice parameter: evaluation and treatment of depression, psychosis, and dementia in Parkinson disease (an evidence-based review). *Neurology* 2006;**66**:996–1002.

10. Winge K, Rasmussen D, Werdelin LM. Constipation in neurological diseases. *J Neurol Neurosurg Psychiatry* 2003;**74**:13–19.

11. Pinto S, Ozsancak C, Tripoliti E, et al. Treatments for dysarthria in Parkinson's disease. *Lancet Neurol* 2004;**3**:547–556.

12. Nath U, Ben-Shlomo Y, Thomson RG, Lees AJ, Burn DJ. Clinical features and natural history of progressive supranuclear palsy. A clinical cohort study. *Neurology* 2003;**60**:910–916.

13. Wenning GK, Colosimo C, Geser F, Poewe W. Multiple system atrophy. *Lancet Neurol* 2004;**3**: 93–103.

14. Wenning GK, Litvan I, Jankovic J, et al. Natural history and survival of 14 patients with corticobasal degeneration confirmed at postmortem examination. *J Neurol Neurosurg Psychiatry* 1998;**64**:184–189.

15. Hardie RJ, Lees AJ. Neuroleptic-induced Parkinson's syndrome: clinical features and results of treatment with levodopa. *J Neurol Neurosurg Psychiatry* 1988;**51**:850–854.

16. Winikates J, Jankovic J. Clinical correlates of vascular parkinsonism. *Arch Neurol* 1999;**56**:98–102.

14

Chapter

Hyperkinetic movement disorders

Introduction

Hyperkinetic movement disorder may reflect pathology at several levels of the nervous system including the cerebral cortex, basal ganglia, cerebellum, and even the peripheral nerve. The first step in approaching a patient with a hyperkinetic movement is to classify the movement. Observation of the patient while sitting face to face and taking their history is often sufficient. If the movement is not present, then it is usually best to ask the patient to demonstrate it, as verbal descriptions are often vague or inaccurate. When examining a patient with a hyperkinetic movement disorder, it is important not only to describe and classify the movement, but also to perform a comprehensive neurological history and examination to determine whether the abnormality is a sign of a systemic metabolic process or neurodegenerative disease.

Tremor

Tremor is the rhythmic oscillation of a body part caused by alternating contraction of agonist and antagonist muscles. Patients describe tremor as shaking or trembling, or may specifically use the word tremor. Some may even diagnose themselves (usually incorrectly) with Parkinson's disease. When examining a tremor, note its location, presence with rest or activity, frequency, amplitude, and direction.

Most tremors involve the upper extremities. Important exceptions include essential tremor involving the head and voice, oculopalatal myoclonus, resting leg tremor in Parkinson's disease, and leg tremor upon standing in patients with orthostatic tremor. Beyond location, the most important step in diagnosing tremor is to classify it as a resting tremor, action (or postural) tremor, or intention tremor. Resting tremor is present with rest and improves or disappears with movement. Action or postural tremor develops when moving or holding a body part against gravity. Intention tremor worsens with precise, target-directed movements. In order to determine the tremor type, examine the affected body part in the following positions:

- completely still
- extended in front of the patient
- as the patient moves it rapidly back and forth between two targets
- as the patient attempts to bear weight (e.g. reaching out for a cup of water and then bringing it to their lips)

Action tremor

Essential tremor

Essential or benign familial tremor is the most common type of tremor, and indeed the most common movement disorder. It typically begins in early middle age and is transmitted from generation to generation with an autosomal-dominant pattern of inheritance. The tremor is principally an intermediate-frequency, small-to-medium amplitude, symmetric action tremor of the hands. Involvement of the head (including "yes–yes" or "no–no" forms) and voice is common. The feet and legs are usually spared. Patients may report an improvement in the tremor with alcohol ingestion and an exacerbation of the tremor with stress or anxiety.

Many patients with essential tremor have mild symptoms and do not require treatment. A number of options are available for patients with disabling or socially embarrassing symptoms. Primidone and propranolol are the first-line medications, and are effective in about two-thirds of patients with essential tremor. Other treatment options are listed in Table 14.1. Deep brain stimulation of the ventral intermediate nucleus of the thalamus is an option for patients with refractory tremor. Botulinum toxin injections may be useful for patients with vocal or head tremors.

Wilson's disease

Wilson's disease is an autosomal-recessive disorder of copper metabolism that produces a combination of neurological, psychiatric, and hepatic dysfunction.

Table 14.1 Medications used to treat essential tremor

Medication	Starting dose	Titration instructions	Side effects
Clonazepam	0.5 mg qhs	Increase to goal dose of 1–2 mg bid over 3–4 weeks	Sedation
Gabapentin	100 mg tid	Increase by 100 mg tid every 3 days to goal dose of 600–1200 mg tid	Sedation, ataxia, peripheral edema
Primidone[a]	25 mg qd	Increase by 25 mg qd each week to goal dose of 100 mg, then increase by 50 mg qd each week to goal dose of 750–1000 mg qd	Sedation, ataxia
Propranolol[a]	10 mg qd	Increase by 10 mg qd each week to goal dose of 120–640 mg qd	Orthostatic hypotension, bradycardia, fatigue, depression
Topiramate	25 mg qd	Increase by 25 mg qd each week to goal dose of 100–200 mg bid	Weight loss, anomia, nephrolithiasis, acral paresthesias
Zonisamide	50 mg qd	Increase by 50 mg qd each week to goal dose of 100–200 mg qd	Nephrolithiasis, weight loss

[a] First-line agent.

Although symptoms usually develop in children and young adults, rare patients may first come to clinical attention in middle age or later. The most prominent initial neurological symptom is usually an action tremor, which may resemble essential tremor, but in many cases is of much larger amplitude (wing-beating tremor). Some patients present with rigidity and bradykinesia or ataxia rather than tremor. Kayser–Fleischer (KF) rings, brownish-green copper deposits in Descemet's membrane of the cornea, are the tell-tale physical examination sign of Wilson's disease. If not visible by simple visual inspection, slit-lamp examination may be used to confirm the presence of KF rings. The characteristic laboratory findings of Wilson's disease are reduced serum ceruloplasmin (<20 mg/dl), and elevated urine 24-hour copper excretion (>40 μg/ml).[1] If clinical suspicion for Wilson's disease remains despite normal or equivocal test results, refer the patient for molecular testing or liver biopsy. Treatment with the copper-chelating agents trientine and penicillamine help both the neuropsychiatric and hepatic components of the disease.[1] Wilson's disease should be evaluated and treated in conjunction with a hepatologist.

Enhanced physiological tremor

Every person has a small-amplitude, high-frequency tremor that is usually imperceptible in day-to-day activities. Some patients, however, experience an enhanced physiological tremor, which has a very high frequency, usually involves the hands, and appears with stress

Table 14.2 Common medications that produce tremor

Amiodarone
Beta-agonists
Cyclosporine
Levothyroxine
Lithium
Neuroleptics
Theophylline
Valproic acid

such as performance anxiety. Patients with this type of tremor usually respond to a small dose of propranolol (10–40 mg prn) prior to stress exposure. Treat those who do not respond to propranolol with clonazepam (0.5–1 mg prn) or lorazepam (0.5–1 mg prn).

Secondary tremor

A variety of medications, toxins, and metabolic disturbances lead to a tremor that appears quite similar to essential tremor. Table 14.2 lists common medications that lead to tremor. Intoxication with caffeine, cocaine, and phencyclidine and withdrawal from ethanol and benzodiazepines are other important causes of secondary tremor. Hyperthyroidism, hypoglycemia, uremia, and hepatic dysfunction are the common medical precipitants. Correction of the responsible problem or withdrawal of the offending medication usually results in tremor resolution or improvement.

Resting tremor

Parkinsonian tremor

Up to 75% of patients with Parkinson's disease will develop a tremor, and it is the most prominent feature in approximately 15%.[2] Parkinsonian tremor is a low-frequency, small-to-medium amplitude, resting tremor that most commonly involves one hand or foot in an asymmetric fashion. It may change in appearance and distribution, even during the course of a single office visit. Classical parkinsonian tremors include:

- flexion–extension of the wrist
- pronation–supination of the wrist
- pill-rolling involving the thumbs and fingers
- foot tapping
- internal–external rotation at the hip
- up-and-down jaw movements
- "rabbit tremor" characterized by repetitive perioral and nasal muscle contractions

Anticholinergic medications such as trihexyphenidyl are the mainstays of treatment of parkinsonian tremor. Levodopa and dopamine agonists tend to be less effective in treating parkinsonian tremor than they are for bradykinesia and rigidity. Deep brain stimulation of the ventral intermediate nucleus of the thalamus or the subthalamic nucleus may help in refractory cases.[3] Treatment of Parkinson's disease is discussed in further detail in Chapter 13.

Intention tremor

Cerebellar outflow tremor

Lesions of the dentate nucleus of the cerebellum and its connections within the cerebellum and brainstem produce very striking low-frequency, large-amplitude intention tremor. This tremor may have a postural element, but becomes much worse when attempting to reach out for a target. Ataxia and other signs of cerebellar dysfunction usually accompany the tremor. Common pathologies that produce cerebellar outflow tremor include stroke, demyelination, neoplasm, and trauma. Unfortunately, this type of tremor responds poorly to treatment.

Other tremors

Palatal tremor

Palatal tremor (also called palatal myoclonus) is a low-frequency tremor of the palatal and pharyngeal muscles. It is usually secondary to a lesion of the Guillain–Mollaret triangle, which connects the red nucleus, inferior olivary nucleus, and dentate nucleus. In many cases, the palatal tremor is accompanied by tremor of the extraocular muscles (oculopalatal myoclonus), diaphragm, head, and neck.

Dystonic tremor

Focal or generalized dystonia is often accompanied by a mild, superimposed tremor that is usually worsened by movement. Dystonic tremor, like other aspects of dystonia, responds best to botulinum toxin injection.

Neuropathic tremor

Neuropathic tremor is usually a large-amplitude, low-frequency action tremor. It is most common in patients with demyelinating neuropathies, especially those caused by monoclonal gammopathies (Chapter 15).[4]

Psychogenic tremor

Psychogenic tremor should be included in the differential diagnosis of any tremor. This may be a resting or action tremor, and may have any amplitude or frequency. The tremor improves with distraction and worsens when the patient focuses on it. One feature of psychogenic tremor that may help to distinguish it from other tremors is entrainment: the patient will not be able to continue to feign a tremor in a hand (or other affected body part) when asked to tap out a complex rhythmic pattern with another body part.

Jerking movements

Myoclonus

Myoclonus is defined as a sudden-onset, brief-duration jerking movement of a muscle or group of muscles. It may be a manifestation of a systemic disease, associated with an epilepsy syndrome, or occur as a benign phenomenon. Essentially any part of the CNS may generate myoclonus. Unfortunately, because myoclonus often looks quite similar regardless of its cause, it may be difficult to start with the movement and work backwards toward the diagnosis. Rather, the best way to classify myoclonus at the bedside is by looking for neighborhood signs of medical or neurological disease.

Toxic and metabolic myoclonus

The metabolic disturbances that produce myoclonus include uremia, hepatic encephalopathy, and thyroid dysfunction. Commonly used medications that precipitate myoclonus include narcotics, anticonvulsants, antidepressants, calcium channel blockers, and lithium. Correction of the responsible toxic exposure or metabolic abnormality reverses the myoclonus.

Anoxic myoclonus

Acute postanoxic myoclonus

Many patients in coma following cardiac arrest develop myoclonus, often diffuse and continuous.[5] The myoclonus may be quite violent and disturbing to family members, and may persist despite all efforts short of neuromuscular junction blockade. Acute anoxic myoclonus portends a uniformly poor prognosis (Chapter 2), and should prompt serious discussions about the direction of care with family members and intensive care unit physicians.

Chronic postanoxic myoclonus (Lance–Adams myoclonus)

A patient who *recovers* from anoxic brain injury may develop myoclonus that is absent at rest and develops with movement. For this reason, it is often called intention myoclonus. Chronic postanoxic myoclonus is difficult to control, but may respond to clonazepam (0.5–2 mg bid) or valproate (500–1000 mg bid).

Myoclonus associated with dementia

Myoclonus is often an early feature of Creutzfeldt–Jakob disease (Chapter 4). It is important, however, to understand that myoclonus in a demented patient is not pathognomonic for Creutzfeldt–Jakob disease, and may develop in the later stages of any of the degenerative dementias.

Myoclonic epilepsy

Juvenile myoclonic epilepsy (Chapter 20) is the most common of the epilepsies associated with myoclonus. Rare myoclonic epilepsies include neuronal ceroid lipofuscinosis, Lafora body disease, and myoclonic epilepsy with ragged red fibers (MERRF), all of which tend to occur primarily in children.

Opsoclonus–myoclonus syndrome

This condition, characterized by fast, chaotic, multidirectional eye movements and myoclonus, is classically associated with neuroblastoma in children. In adults, opsoclonus–myoclonus syndrome may be a paraneoplastic process or may be associated with a variety of other inflammatory, autoimmune disorders.[6] Like other forms of myoclonus, opsoclonus–myoclonus syndrome often responds to clonazepam or valproate. Adrenocorticotropic hormone infusions are effective in children, but tend not to work in adults.

Segmental myoclonus

Segmental myoclonus involves muscle groups supplied by one or more contiguous segments of the brainstem or spinal cord.[7] It may be misdiagnosed as another abnormal movement, usually tics or hemiballismus. Common causes include multiple sclerosis, tumors, and encephalomyelitis. Clonazepam and valproic acid often provide good symptomatic control, but treating the responsible cause is the most important step in therapy.

Physiological myoclonus

The two most common examples of physiological myoclonus are hypnic jerks (sleep starts that occur just upon falling asleep) and hiccoughs (diaphragmatic myoclonus). With rare exception, physiological myoclonus does not require any further evaluation or treatment.

Essential myoclonus

Essential myoclonus is a benign condition, often inherited in an autosomal-dominant fashion, which begins in childhood or young adulthood.[8] Exhaustive evaluation discloses no underlying structural or metabolic abnormalities. Essential myoclonus improves considerably with ethanol ingestion, which obviously cannot be recommended as long-term therapy. Many patients are not bothered by their symptoms and some note an improvement over time. For patients with disabling myoclonus, clonazepam is often helpful.

Ballismus

Ballismus is a violent, involuntary flinging movement of a limb, which may be difficult to distinguish from myoclonus. It usually involves one side of the body, in which case it is called hemiballismus. Although hemiballismus is classically associated with strokes involving the subthalamic nucleus, this is the lesion site in only a minority of cases – other subcortical structures are often involved.[9] Hemiballismus is quite disruptive to the patient, and should be treated with haloperidol in divided doses up to 15 mg. Most patients need treatment for about 3 months, at which point a trial of discontinuing the haloperidol may be attempted.

Twitching

Fasciculations

Fasciculations are visible muscle twitches that are generated at the level of the motor neuron, nerve root, or peripheral nerve. They may affect the face, eyes, tongue, and limbs. Most patients with fasciculations have otherwise normal neurological examinations and a diagnosis of benign fasciculations or cramp-fasciculation syndrome, both of which reflect disorders of peripheral nerve hyperexcitability.[10] The association of fasciculations with amyotrophic lateral sclerosis (ALS) (Chapter 10) is widely known, and many patients with benign fasciculations are worried that they have ALS. Reassurance that the condition is benign is often not helpful, and patients may find relief only after undergoing a negative battery of tests, including electromyography (EMG) and sometimes MRI of the brain. Symptoms improve by decreasing caffeine intake, reducing stress, and limiting heavy exercise. If these lifestyle modifications are not effective, treat benign fasciculations with carbamazepine (200–800 mg bid), gabapentin (300–1200 mg tid), or clonazepam (0.5–1 mg bid).

Twisting and cramping

Chorea and athetosis

Chorea is an irregular, purposeless, jerking movement that results from basal ganglia dysfunction. Often, a patient with chorea attempts to incorporate the movement into an intended movement in order to mask the abnormality (parakinesia). Athetosis is a slow, purposeless, writhing movement. Because these two abnormal movements frequently accompany each other, they may be discussed together under the blanket term "choreoathetosis." Choreoathetoid movements involve the limbs, face, eyelids, lips, and tongue, and are often quite disabling. The following are common causes.

Huntington's disease

Huntington's disease (HD) is an autosomal-dominant neurodegenerative disorder that usually presents in young adulthood or early middle age. Symptoms usually begin with mild clumsiness or fidgetiness, which evolves over time into full-blown chorea. Some patients present with dementia or with behavioral changes such as impulsivity and irritability. There may be a family history of psychiatric disease or poorly understood early institutionalization and death. As the disease progresses, chorea becomes less prominent, and rigidity and bradykinesia dominate the clinical picture. In the absence of a suggestive family history, the diagnosis of HD is made by finding CAG repeat expansion in the huntingtin gene. Striatal atrophy on MRI may

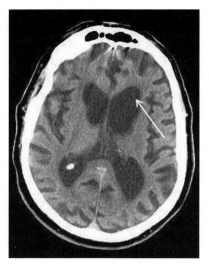

Figure 14.1 CT scan of the brain in a patient with Huntington's disease. Note *hydrocephalus ex vacuo*, involving particularly the caudate nucleus (arrow).

support the diagnosis (Figure 14.1). Unfortunately, HD is a relentlessly progressive disease, and symptomatic therapy is the mainstay of treatment. Tetrabenazine, clonazepam, or neuroleptics may help to control the chorea, but, as the disease progresses, patients require around-the-clock care, often in a nursing home setting.

Benign familial chorea

Benign familial chorea is largely a pediatric disorder in which chorea is not associated with evidence of another movement disorder or neurodegenerative disease. Make this diagnosis cautiously, as most patients who initially appear to have benign familial chorea will actually prove to have a different, usually not so benign disorder.[11]

Chorea gravidarum

Chorea may develop during the first or second trimesters of pregnancy. In many cases, an underlying cause such as Sydenham's chorea, hyperthyroidism, or the antiphospholipid antibody syndrome may be identified. In other patients, however, there is no identifiable cause, and the term chorea gravidarum is used. Although this condition usually resolves spontaneously after several weeks, neuroleptics such as haloperidol may be needed to help control disabling symptoms.

Other causes of chorea

Medications including dopamine-blocking agents, anticonvulsants, and oral contraceptives may also produce chorea. Sydenham's chorea is an autoimmune disorder that occurs in children with rheumatic fever. In rare cases, it may occur for the first time or recur in adults. Other autoimmune disorders that may be associated with chorea include systemic lupus erythematosus and antiphospholipid antibody syndrome. Hyperthyroidism and AIDS are rare causes of chorea.

Dystonia

Dystonia is an abnormal movement characterized by sustained, simultaneous contraction of muscle agonists and antagonists. Dystonia produces torsion or fixation of a body part in a consistent direction, unlike choreoathetoid movements, which are in multiple directions and vary from moment to moment. Dystonic movements are often associated with local pain and spasm, and sometimes with a superimposed tremor. They are worsened by stress and resolve during sleep. Many patients have sensory tricks in which touching or stroking a body part affected by the dystonic muscle relieves the contraction briefly. Dystonias may be focal (affecting one body part), segmental (affecting several adjacent body parts), or generalized in distribution. Focal dystonias are the most common types in adults. I will not discuss generalized dystonias in great detail: although they usually persist into adulthood, they are mainly diseases of childhood and adolescence.

Most dystonic disorders are primary, meaning that there are no nervous system abnormalities beyond the dystonia and possibly a mild tremor. Secondary dystonias are those that are caused by another neurological disorder or by a structural or metabolic abnormality. Suspect a secondary dystonia in patients with accompanying neurological symptoms such as weakness, ataxia, or severe tremor. Although there are many causes of secondary dystonia, focused evaluation including a careful medical history, medication review, MRI of the brain (to look for strokes and mass lesions affecting the basal ganglia), and assessment for Wilson's disease and HD are high-yield investigations. A comprehensive discussion of dystonia evaluation is beyond the scope of this text, and the interested reader is referred to the review by Geyer and Bressman.[12]

Cervical dystonia

This is the most common focal dystonia in adults. The head may be twisted in any direction: turned to the side (torticollis), twisted laterally so that the ear approaches or touches the shoulder (laterocollis), bent forward (anterocollis), or bent backward (retrocollis). Simultaneous torsion of the head in more than one direction is common. The severity of cervical dystonia ranges from subtle rotation of the head that is not obvious to even friends and family members to fixation of the head in one position with unbearable pain and spasm. Although agents such as benzodiazepines and baclofen may help slightly, botulinum toxin injections are the most effective treatments. Deep brain stimulation of the bilateral globus pallidus may help patients with symptoms that are refractory to botulinum toxin.[13]

Task-specific (occupational) dystonias

Dystonia, as a rule, is worse with movement. Task-specific or occupational dystonias emerge exclusively when the patient attempts to perform a specific action. Writer's cramp is the most common task-specific dystonia: patients with this condition find that their hand twists or postures when they attempt to write with a pen or pencil. Writing becomes slow, effortful, and painful, and patients resort to using larger and larger pens, writing with their other hand, or typing. The contralateral hand may be affected by milder dystonic movements. Typing, playing musical instruments, and golfing are other tasks associated with dystonia. Some patients may obtain modest symptom relief with trihexyphenidyl, but local botulinum toxin injection is the most effective treatment for task-specific dystonias.

Cramps

Cramps are characterized by strong, painful, involuntary muscle contractions. Although patients perceive cramps as being muscular pains, they are actually generated by excessive discharges of the peripheral nerves. Nocturnal cramps, particularly of the calves and foot muscles, are the most common variety. Heavy exercise, dehydration, and electrolyte imbalances may also precipitate cramps. In some cases, cramps are a manifestation of a neurogenic disease such as polyneuropathy or ALS. When evaluating patients with isolated fasciculations, check thyroid function, potassium, magnesium, and calcium, and correct as needed. Stretching the affected body part usually improves symptoms. Quinine is a very effective treatment for cramps, but is unfortunately not available due to its potential to cause arrhythmias. Options for treating cramps include clonazepam (0.5–1 mg qhs), verapamil (80–120 mg qhs), diphenhydramine (25–50 mg qhs), gabapentin (300–600 mg qhs), and B-complex vitamins.

Stiff-person syndrome

Stiff-person syndrome is an uncommon condition characterized by chronically progressive stiffness of the muscles of the trunk and limbs. The axial muscles, particularly the paraspinal muscles, are usually affected most severely, and may cause the patient to adopt an exaggerated lordotic posture, leading to opisthotonos in severe cases. Other patients first develop asymmetric symptoms in one leg or foot. Approximately 70% of patients with stiff-person syndrome will have antibodies to glutamic acid decarboxylase.[14] There is a less frequent association with antibodies to amphiphysin in women with breast cancer.[15] Patients with stiff-person syndrome often have other autoimmune disorders such as diabetes or pernicious anemia. The most effective treatments for stiff person syndrome include oral and intravenous diazepam titrated to effect and baclofen given orally (40 mg bid) or, in some cases, via an intrathecal pump. Periodic intravenous immunoglobulin infusions help some patients.[16]

Myotonia

Myotonia is the impaired relaxation of a muscle after voluntary contraction or percussion. A patient with myotonia may complain of disabling muscle stiffness with exercise or cold. Other patients, however, have very mild myotonia and are not bothered by it. There are several ways to elicit myotonia on examination. Observe for hand grip myotonia by asking the patient to shake your hand vigorously and then attempt to release their grip. Elicit myotonia of the orbicularis oculi by asking the patient to forcibly and rapidly open and close their eyes. Look for percussion myotonia by striking the thenar eminence, long finger extensors in the forearm, deltoid, or tongue briskly with a reflex hammer. If physical examination fails to reveal myotonia, it may be demonstrated electromyographically, especially upon muscle cooling.

Myotonic dystrophy

Myotonic dystrophy is an autosomal-dominant, multisystem disorder characterized by myotonia and muscle weakness. Cardiac conduction block, insulin resistance, and cataracts are common systemic features that are often more important than the neurological aspects of the disease. Patients with DM1 have predominantly distal weakness (involving preferentially the finger flexors), while those with DM2 have predominantly proximal weakness. A patient with myotonic dystrophy characteristically has a long face, frontal baldness, temporal wasting, and ptosis. Myotonic dystrophy may be divided into DM1 and DM2. Genetic testing is available to confirm both DM1 and DM2. Phenytoin (100 mg tid) or mexiletine (200–400 mg tid) may be used for patients with problematic myotonia, but, in general, the myotonia of myotonic dystrophy does not require treatment. Monitoring patients for cardiac and ophthalmological problems is an essential part of caring for the patient with myotonic dystrophy.

Myotonia congenita

Myotonia congenita is an inherited disorder characterized by myotonia in the first few seconds or minutes of exercise or movement that improves with continued activity. Muscle stiffness usually improves after warming up. Myotonia congenita is inherited by both autosomal-dominant (Thomsen's disease) and -recessive (Becker's disease) mechanisms. The recessive form may be associated with mild muscle weakness. Mexiletine (200–400 mg tid) is often helpful, but must be used cautiously as it may lead to arrhythmias. Phenytoin and carbamazepine may be useful for patients who do not respond to or do not tolerate mexiletine.

Abnormal facial movements

Myokymia

Myokymia is a rippling, undulating movement of the muscles, which is physiologically composed of spontaneous, rhythmic or semirhythmic motor unit discharges. Although it may manifest itself in the limb muscles (usually in association with neuropathic disorders and especially in the setting of radiation-induced brachial or lumbosacral plexopathies), it is most commonly observed in the face. Facial myokymia is usually secondary to an ipsilateral pontine tegmental lesion, particularly multiple sclerosis. Patients with disabling, persistent symptoms may benefit from botulinum toxin injections, carbamazepine, or phenytoin.[17]

Oromandibular dystonia

Oromandibular dystonia is characterized by a variety of abnormal facial movements including jaw clenching, mouth opening, and facial grimacing. In severe cases, these movements impair speech and swallowing. Oromandibular dystonia frequently involves adjacent body parts including the orbicularis oculi (in which case the combination is called Meige's syndrome) and the adjacent neck and shoulder muscles. Similar to other focal dystonias, oromandibular dystonia responds to directed botulinum toxin injections.

Tics

Tics are stereotyped movements of a muscle or group of muscles. They may be brief or sustained, and may involve the face, limbs, or voice. Because tic disorders are largely pediatric diseases that rarely begin in adulthood, I will not discuss them in further detail.[18]

Hemifacial spasm

Hemifacial spasm is the intermittent unilateral twitching of both the upper and lower halves of the face. It may be present at rest, but is more often triggered by facial movements. The cause of hemifacial spasm is believed to be microvascular compression of the facial nerve as it emerges from the brainstem. Brain MRI with thin cuts through the brainstem should be performed to exclude any responsible structural lesions. Treatment with anticonvulsants such as carbamazepine may help slightly, but most patients require botulinum toxin injections. In some refractory cases, surgical decompression of the facial nerve is necessary, although the procedure places the patient at risk for facial palsy.

Tardive dyskinesia

Tardive dyskinesia refers to a group of abnormal movements resulting from treatment with antipsychotics or the antiemetic metoclopramide. Symptoms develop in as little as 6 months (or even less) of exposure to these dopamine-receptor blockers, often after a dose reduction or switch from a high-potency to a low-potency agent. Common dyskinesias include tics, chorea, athetosis, and dystonia. Orofacial dyskinesias such as chewing, puckering, grimacing, and repetitive eye closure are among the most easily recognizable varieties. Tardive dyskinesia may also affect the limbs, neck, trunk, and even the diaphragm. They are sometimes present continuously and may be very disabling. Tardive dyskinesia is more likely to result from treatment with older antipsychotics such as haloperidol or fluphenazine than with one of the newer agents such as risperidone or olanzapine. The risk with the newer antipsychotics, however, is not zero. Tardive dyskinesia is often difficult to treat. The

first step is to taper or discontinue the responsible medication, if possible. For patients who are taking one of the older antipsychotics, it may be helpful to switch to a newer agent such as clozapine or quetiapine. In patients for whom changing or discontinuing antipsychotics does not work, clonazepam (0.5–2 mg bid) may reduce tardive dyskinesia symptoms. The dopamine-depleting agent tetrabenazine is not currently approved for tardive dyskinesia treatment in the USA, but may be useful in patients with debilitating symptoms. In some cases, resuming high-potency antipsychotics may paradoxically improve tardive dyskinesia.

References

1. Roberts EA, Schilsky ML. Diagnosis and treatment of Wilson disease: an update. *Hepatology* 2008;**47**: 2089–2111.

2. Hughes AJ, Ben-Shlomo Y, Daniel SE, Lees AJ. What features improve the accuracy of clinical diagnosis in Parkinson's disease: a clinicopathologic study. *Neurology* 1992;**42**:1142–1146.

3. Pollak P, Fraix V, Krack P, et al. Treatment results: Parkinson's disease. *Mov Disord* 2002;**17**:S75–S83.

4. Deuschl G, Raethjen J, Lindemann M, Krack P. The pathophysiology of tremor. *Muscle Nerve* 2001;**24**: 716–735.

5. Wijdicks EFM, Parisi JE, Sharbrough FW. Prognosis value of myoclonus status in comatose survivors of cardiac arrest. *Ann Neurol* 1994;**35**:239–243.

6. Caviness JN, Forsyth PA, Layton DD, McPhee TJ. The movement disorder of adult opsoclonus. *Mov Disord* 1995;**10**:22–27.

7. Jankovic J, Pardo R. Segmental myoclonus. Clinical and pharmacologic study. *Arch Neurol* 1986;**43**: 1025–1031.

8. Quinn N. Essential myoclonus and myoclonic dystonia. *Mov Disord* 1996;**11**:119–124.

9. Vidakovic A, Dragasevic N, Kostic VS. Hemiballism: report of 25 cases. *J Neurol Neurosurg Psychiatry* 1994;**57**:945–949.

10. Tahmoush AJ, Alonso RJ, Tahmoush GP, Heiman-Patterson TD. Cramp-fasciculation syndrome: a treatable hyperexcitable peripheral nerve disorder. *Neurology* 1991;**41**:1021–1024.

11. Schrag A, Quinn NP, Bhatia KP, Marsden CD. Benign hereditary chorea – entity or syndrome? *Mov Disord* 2000;**15**:280–288.

12. Geyer HL, Bressman SB. The diagnosis of dystonia. *Lancet Neurol* 2006;**5**:780–790.

13. Hung SW, Hamani C, Lozano AM, et al. Long-term outcome of bilateral pallidal deep brain stimulation for primary cervical dystonia. *Neurology* 2007;**68**: 457–459.

14. Meinck HM, Thompson PD. Stiff man syndrome and related conditions. *Mov Disord* 2002;**17**:853–866.

15. Murinson BB, Guarnaccia JB. Stiff-person syndrome with amphiphysin antibodies. *Neurology* 2008;**71**:1955–1958.

16. Dalakas MC, Fujii M, Li M, et al. High dose intravenous immune globulin for stiff person syndrome. *N Engl J Med* 2001;**345**:1870–1876.

17. Sedano MJ, Trejo JM, Macarron JL, et al. Continuous facial myokymia in multiple sclerosis: treatment with botulinum toxin. *Eur Neurol* 2000;**43**:137–140.

18. Chouinard S, Ford B. Adult onset tic disorders. *J Neurol Neurosurg Psychiatry* 2000;**68**:738–743.

Chapter

15

Distal and generalized sensory symptoms

Overview of sensory symptoms

Pain is the sensory symptom that most frequently brings a patient to neurological attention. The first step in evaluating pain is to determine its character. Neuropathic pain has sharp, burning, or electrical qualities. Nociceptive pain, by comparison, has dull and aching qualities. While cold or freezing sensations may be due to neuropathic processes, these sensations are more often the result of vascular insufficiency. In general, pain may be divided into focal (Chapter 16) and generalized or distal-predominant (this chapter) in distribution. Because patients may report only the most prominent location of symptoms, when taking the history, you must inquire specifically about pain involving the face, scalp, trunk, back, arms, hands, groin, legs, and feet.

Numbness is the second important symptom of sensory dysfunction. When patients use the term numbness, they may mean one of several different sensations: a lack of feeling or deadness, a sensation that the affected body part is covered by something such as a glove, sock, or extra layer of skin, or a sensation that the body part is asleep. Some patients will report that they feel as if their socks are bunched up around their feet, that they are walking on sponges, or that their hands or feet are buried in cement. Be aware that some patients with limb weakness will erroneously describe numbness rather than recognizing that a motor deficit is responsible for their abnormal sensation.

Paresthesia is a sense of tingling, pins and needles, abnormal vibration, or a feeling that a body part is asleep. Some patients with paresthesia may describe it initially as pain or numbness, and an accurate description of the problem may be obtained only by specifically asking about a perception of pins and needles. Paresthesia is highly specific for neurological dysfunction.

There are several abnormal sensations that are actually due to motor dysfunction. The most common of these are cramps, twitching (fasciculations), and restlessness.

Because sensory symptoms are entirely subjective, they can be feigned or exaggerated quite easily. Important clues to factitious sensory symptoms include a large number and variety of symptoms, requests for narcotic medications or completion of disability paperwork at an initial office visit, and a lack of a plausible anatomical distribution of symptoms.

Sensory system anatomy

Pain and temperature sensations from the limbs and trunk are mediated by small-diameter nerve fibers. These fibers travel through the nerves and nerve roots, reaching their cell bodies in the dorsal root ganglia. After entering the spinal cord, pain and temperature fibers ascend one or two segments before decussating in the ventral white commissure. They ascend through the spinal cord in the spinothalamic tract, eventually reaching the ventroposterolateral nucleus of the thalamus. These fibers from the thalamus project to the insula.

Vibratory and proprioceptive sensations are mediated by large-diameter nerve fibers. These fibers also travel through the nerves and nerve roots to reach cell bodies in the dorsal root ganglia and enter the spinal cord. Within the cord, fibers from the lower extremity travel through the gracile fasciculus, while those from the upper extremity travel through the cuneate fasciculus. These fibers reach the gracile and cuneate nuclei in the medulla and decussate in the medial lemniscus. Lemniscal fibers synapse in the ventroposterolateral nucleus of the thalamus and project to the primary sensory cortex of the postcentral gyrus.

Sensory examination

Sensory examination should include tests of pinprick, vibration, position sense, and cortical modalities.

Pinprick and temperature sensation

Pinprick examination of every square inch of the skin is time-consuming and leads to a great deal of extraneous

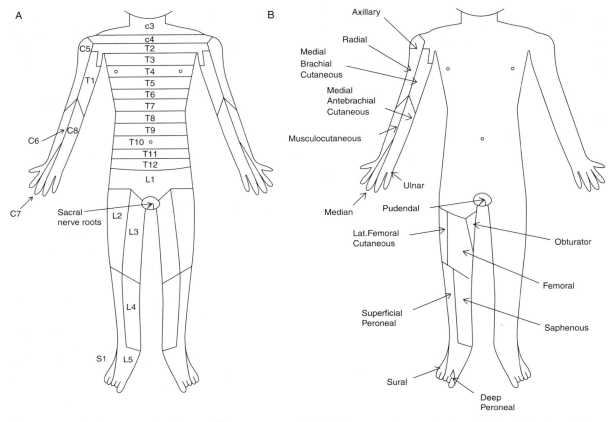

Figure 15.1 Cutaneous sensory distributions of the nerve roots and individual nerves on the ventral surface of the body. Note in particular the T2 (axilla), T4 (areolae), and T10 (umbilicus) dermatomes. See Chapter 16, Figure 16.1 for additional details on the innervation of the hand.

and sometimes misleading information. There are several strategies that improve both the diagnostic yield and efficiency of this portion of the sensory examination. First, take a thorough history in order to gain a sense of the likely distribution of sensory deficits. The examination of a patient with a probable length-dependent polyneuropathy requires a different strategy from the examination of a patient with a mononeuropathy or monoradiculopathy. It is often quite helpful to ask the patient to trace the area of cutaneous sensory loss before initiating the sensory examination. When testing pinprick, begin by examining a completely normal area to establish that the patient can perceive the sharp sensation of a pinprick accurately. Next, test an area that is possibly abnormal based on the information gained from the history, and march the pin from the abnormal area back into the normal area. For example, in a patient with a length-dependent polyneuropathy, begin distally at the toes to see whether the patient can detect the pinprick, and then march the pin proximally, determining where the patient first perceives the

sensation properly. More subtle deficits require a different technique. In a patient with mild sensory abnormalities, it is helpful to use one body part as a control and compare it with the possibly abnormal part. For example, when testing a patient with a possible right L5 radiculopathy, poke the dorsum of the left foot with the pin and tell them that this sensation is 100%. Next, poke the dorsum of the right foot and ask the patient to assign a percentage to the strength of this sensation. When examining pinprick for the purposes of a screening examination, establish that sensation is preserved by testing two or three pinpricks in each dermatome and nerve distribution (Figure 15.1).

Because pinprick and temperature perception are both mediated by small-diameter nerve fibers, examining temperature usually does not add much new information to the neurological examination. False-positive results with testing of cold sensation are frequent in patients with cold extremities. In addition, it may be difficult to find standardized cold and warm stimuli. Despite these limitations, if pinprick sensation is entirely preserved and there is a high index of suspicion for small-diameter nerve fiber dysfunction, testing perception of warmth and coldness may help to disclose an important deficit. Temperature testing is also useful for patients who do not tolerate or cannot accurately report the results of the pinprick examination.

Vibratory and joint position perception

Examine vibratory sensation with a 128 Hz tuning fork. Absence of vibratory perception at the great toe is clearly abnormal. If the patient cannot appreciate vibration at the great toe, move the tuning fork to the medial or lateral malleolus, to the knee, and then to the sternum until they feel the vibration. The normal duration of tuning fork perception is not clearly defined. Some neurologists use the criterion that both patient and doctor should feel the vibratory perception for the same length of time. Others use cut-offs such as 12 or 14 seconds of vibratory perception at the great toe. My idiosyncratic (and unvalidated) technique involves striking the tuning fork vigorously so that its heads hit each other, then placing the base of the tuning fork on the interphalangeal joint of the great toe. Using this technique, the expected number of seconds of vibratory perception at the great toe may be computed by subtracting the first digit of the patient's age from 16. For example, a 49-year-old patient should have 12 seconds of vibratory perception at the great toe.

Joint position examination generally offers little more information beyond what is obtained by testing vibratory perception. To test joint position, instruct the patient to close their eyes and tell them that you will move their great toe either upward or downward. Grasp the toe by the sides (not by the top and bottom) and move it by no more than 5 mm. Normal subjects should be able to detect this movement reliably.

Cortical sensory modalities

The most commonly tested cortical sensory modalities are graphesthesia, stereognosis, and two-point discrimination. These higher-order sensory functions are considered functions of the contralateral parietal lobe. Bear in mind that these modalities may only be tested when the patient has otherwise-preserved gross touch and pinprick sensation. Test graphesthesia by instructing the patient to close their eyes and then asking them to interpret a number that you trace on their palm. Trace at least five different numbers (2, 3, 6, 7, and 8 seem to be the most straightforward ones to interpret) on one palm, and compare the results to the

other palm. Test stereognosis by asking the patient to distinguish between three different-sized coins placed in each hand. Most patients can do this easily. Finally, test two-point discrimination by placing the tips of a caliper against the patient's skin. Determine whether they can discriminate between one point and two points separated by 5–10 mm. Abnormal graphesthesia, stereognosis, and two-point discrimination point to dysfunction in the contralateral parietal lobe, but should not be judged too strictly, as false-positive test results are common.

Polyneuropathy

Length-dependent polyneuropathy

Polyneuropathy is a pathological process that, by definition, involves all the nerves in the body. It is exceedingly rare, however, for all the nerves to be clinically involved at disease onset, or indeed at any point during the course of the disorder. Polyneuropathy is most often a length-dependent process and symptoms develop in a slowly progressive, somewhat stereotyped fashion. The classic initial complaints of polyneuropathy are numbness, tingling, and pain, which begin in the toes and spread more proximally over months to years. When symptoms reach the knees, nerves of equivalent length in the fingertips and hands become involved. By the time the elbows are involved, symptoms are present in the midline of the trunk. In patients with severe neuropathy, only small patches of sensation over the vertex of the head and along the spine are preserved. Symptoms usually do not progress to this extent, and many patients have symptoms confined to the feet and distal legs for many years.

Most patients with polyneuropathy have mostly or exclusively sensory symptoms at onset. Motor symptoms may be minor and go unnoticed by patients. Imbalance, however, is often a problem at presentation (Chapter 18). To elicit a history of balance problems, ask the patient whether they feel as if they are going to fall when they close their eyes in the shower or whether it is difficult for them to keep their balance if they get up at night to use the bathroom.

Several abnormal physical examination findings may help to confirm the localization of length-dependent polyneuropathy. Careful visual inspection may disclose wasting of the intrinsic muscles of the feet, clawing of the toes with high arches and wasting of the distal legs suggestive of Charcot–Marie–Tooth disease. Bear in mind, however, that any distal-predominant polyneuropathy may cause muscle wasting. The most obvious muscle in which wasting may be detected is the extensor digitorum brevis, a small spherical muscle that is palpable over the proximal dorsolateral foot. Another sign of polyneuropathy that may be detected with simple visual inspection is reduced hair growth over the distal legs. Patients with early polyneuropathy usually have little weakness, but when it is present, it is subtle and involves toe extension and flexion. Deep-tendon reflexes may be lost or reduced. On sensory examination, patients with polyneuropathy have a combination of pinprick and vibratory loss. The term "stocking and glove" sensory loss is often used to refer to involvement of the distal before the proximal extremities. The last examination technique that is often helpful in assessing for large-fiber involvement in polyneuropathy is testing for a Romberg sign, described further in Chapter 18.

Non-length-dependent polyneuropathy

Although length-dependent sensorimotor polyneuropathy accounts for the majority of polyneuropathies in clinical practice, you will miss many diagnoses if you consider only this variety. Polyneuropathies with predominantly motor manifestations include chronic inflammatory demyelinating polyneuropathy (Chapter 10) and multifocal motor neuropathy with conduction block (Chapter 11). Rapidly progressive polyneuropathies are discussed in Chapter 12. Some uncommon causes of polyneuropathy such as Tangier disease, lead toxicity, and porphyria may produce predominantly proximal rather than distal symptoms. Neuropathies associated with prominent ataxia include vitamin E deficiency, Sjögren's syndrome, and certain variants of Charcot–Marie–Tooth disease.

Evaluation of polyneuropathy

Laboratory screening

Polyneuropathy is caused by a wide variety of medical disorders. In the absence of a relevant past medical history or clear clinical clues to the presence of one of these underlying disorders, a screening battery should consist of a restricted number of high-yield tests (Table 15.1).

Electromyography and nerve conduction studies

The purposes of electromyography (EMG) and nerve conduction studies (NCS) are to confirm the presence of a polyneuropathy, to determine its severity, and to

Table 15.1 Screening panel for common causes of polyneuropathy

Hemoglobin A$_{1c}$ % and 2-hour oral glucose tolerance test
Thyroid-stimulating hormone
B$_{12}$ levels (homocysteine and methylmalonic acid levels if B$_{12}$ level is borderline low)
Serum protein electrophoresis, immunofixation, and urine protein electrophoresis
Blood urea nitrogen and creatinine
Alanine transaminase and aspartate transaminase
HIV antibodies
Rapid plasma reagin
Erythrocyte sedimentation rate
Antinuclear antibody

distinguish between axonal and demyelinating pathologies. Although localization of sensory complaints to the peripheral nerves is often quite straightforward, diagnostic mimics including lumbosacral polyradiculopathy, cervical myelopathy, and psychogenic disorders make EMG and NCS helpful in confusing cases. While neuropathy severity is often obvious from clinical history and examination, electrodiagnostic studies may offer insight into disease severity, which becomes important when determining appropriate treatment. Distinguishing between axonal and demyelinating pathologies is perhaps the most important role of EMG and NCS. Axonal polyneuropathies are characterized by decreased response amplitudes with normal or mildly reduced conduction velocities, whereas demyelinating polyneuropathies are characterized by relatively preserved response amplitudes and severe slowing of conduction velocities. The distinction between these two types of nerve pathology is important, as demyelinating polyneuropathies often respond to immunomodulatory therapy, while axonal polyneuropathies do not. Use of EMG and NCS should be judicious, as their sensitivities and specificities are both limited. Because NCS assess only large-diameter nerve fibers, they are frequently normal when pain is the only symptom, as pain is mediated by small-diameter nerve fibers. Although many electrodiagnostic studies offer little in the way of additional diagnostic information for polyneuropathy, the following factors always prompt me to order EMG and NCS:

- asymmetric symptom onset
- proximal symptom onset
- rapid symptom progression

- patient age < 50
- foot deformities suggestive of inherited neuropathy
- prominent motor signs
- suspected demyelinating polyneuropathy

Nerve biopsy

Sural nerve biopsy may offer additional diagnostic information for several different and uncommon etiologies of polyneuropathy including vasculitis, amyloidosis, tuberculosis, and sarcoidosis. In most cases, nerve biopsy shows nonspecific axon loss, a finding that offers little diagnostic information beyond what is provided by the clinical examination and electrodiagnostic studies. Skin-nerve biopsy may help to confirm the diagnosis of a small-fiber neuropathy, but rarely offers specific information that helps in patient management.

Etiologies of polyneuropathy

A detailed discussion of the vast number of causes of polyneuropathy can fill a multivolume textbook.[1] The following is a summary of some of the most common and important causes of polyneuropathy.

Diabetes mellitus

Diabetes mellitus is the most common cause of polyneuropathy in the USA. It may take many forms, including a length-dependent sensorimotor polyneuropathy, a painful small-fiber polyneuropathy, diabetic thoracic radiculopathy (Chapter 17), diabetic amyotrophy (Chapter 16), mononeuropathy multiplex (Chapter 11), or a syndrome that resembles chronic inflammatory demyelinating polyneuropathy (Chapter 10). Although elevated blood hemoglobin A_{1c} percentages are often used to diagnose diabetic neuropathy, oral glucose-tolerance testing is more sensitive.[2] Because diabetes is so common, it is important not to wear blinders by assuming that diabetes is the only source of neuropathy in a diabetic patient: always conduct a thorough evaluation to exclude other reversible causes. Treating diabetic polyneuropathy is somewhat unsatisfying. Tight glycemic control may arrest its progression, but reverses symptoms only rarely. Strict euglycemia may lead to the unfortunate consequence of "insulin neuritis" in which symptoms worsen as blood sugar comes under better control. In most cases, agents for neuropathic pain are the mainstay of therapy. Treatment with α-lipoic acid (600 mg qd–tid) may help in some cases.[3] One additional critical aspect of diabetic neuropathy care is prevention of foot ulcers with properly fitting shoes, careful daily foot examinations, and periodic podiatric assessments.

Vitamin B_{12} deficiency

Vitamin B_{12} deficiency may affect the brain, optic nerves, spinal cord, and peripheral nerves. In a small percentage of patients, the peripheral nerves are affected in isolation. Because the spinal cord is involved in up to 90% of cases, B_{12} deficiency is discussed further in Chapter 17.[4]

Monoclonal gammopathy

Monoclonal proteins are circulating immunoglobulins formed from a single clone of plasma cells. They are especially common in the older population, and their association with multiple myeloma is well known. Monoclonal proteins may produce neuropathy by cross-reacting with peripheral nerve antigens, but in other cases the precise mechanism of neuropathy secondary to monoclonal gammopathy is not entirely clear.[5] Neuropathies associated with monoclonal gammopathies include:

- length-dependent axonal polyneuropathy in patients with monoclonal gammopathy of undetermined significance (MGUS)
- axonal neuropathy associated with multiple myeloma
- POEMS (polyneuropathy, organomegaly, endocrinopathy, monoclonal gammopathy, skin changes), a severe demyelinating polyneuropathy associated with multiple myeloma
- anti-MAG (myelin-associated glycoprotein) neuropathy, a demyelinating polyneuropathy characterized electrophysiologically by markedly prolonged distal motor latencies
- amyloidosis, a multisystem disorder that usually produces an exquisitely painful neuropathy with prominent autonomic dysfunction

In order to ensure the highest yield for detecting monoclonal gammopathy in patients with neuropathy, request not only serum protein electrophoresis, but also immunofixation and 24-hour urine collection for protein electrophoresis.[6] Patients with MGUS should undergo evaluation for multiple myeloma including skeletal survey, calcium level measurement, and hematologic referral. Neuropathy secondary to MGUS, multiple myeloma, and amyloidosis may respond to immunosuppressive and chemotherapeutic regimens, which should be designed in conjunction with a hematologist.

Vasculitis

Vasculitic neuropathies are discussed further in Chapter 11. Although mononeuropathy multiplex is the most widely known type of vasculitic neuropathy, many patients with vasculitis have length-dependent polyneuropathies or simultaneous overlapping patterns with features of both length-dependent polyneuropathy and mononeuropathy multiplex.

Ethanol

Polyneuropathy secondary to chronic heavy ethanol use (i.e. four to six drinks a day for many years) is most likely secondary to a combination of direct toxic effects from the ethanol and nutritional deficiencies. Discontinuing ethanol consumption and ensuring adequate nutrition may result in modest symptom improvement.

Charcot–Marie–Tooth disease

Charcot–Marie–Tooth (CMT) disease is the most common inherited polyneuropathy. Wasting, weakness, and areflexia in the lower extremities usually begin in childhood or adolescence. As the disease progresses, patients develop joint deformities. The most common variety is CMT1A, an autosomal-dominant inherited demyelinating polyneuropathy caused by duplication of the PMP-22 gene. There is a wide variety of other phenotypes of CMT disease, each associated with a distinct mutation.[7] CMT2 is perhaps the most important among the other types of CMT disease in adults, as it causes a length-dependent axonal polyneuropathy, which may mimic more common causes of polyneuropathy. CMT2 is usually distinguished from other axonal polyneuropathies by the presence of severe or predominantly motor symptoms or a family history of neuropathy.[8] The mainstay of treatment for CMT disease is referral to orthopedists and podiatrists for correction of foot deformities. Unfortunately, there is no specific cure for the neuropathy.

HIV

Approximately 50% of patients with HIV, usually those with advanced disease, develop a length-dependent polyneuropathy, often with prominent pain.[9] HIV may also cause a variety of other peripheral nerve problems including chronic inflammatory demyelinating polyradiculoneuropathy and mononeuropathy multiplex. Highly active anti-retroviral therapy and pain control are the mainstays of treatment.

Table 15.2 Medications that may produce polyneuropathy

Chemotherapeutic agents:
Cisplatin
Docetaxel
Paclitaxel
Suramin
Thalidomide
Vincristine
Amiodarone
Chloroquine
Colchicine
Disulfiram
Metronidazole
Phenytoin
Pyridoxine

Thyroid dysfunction

Thyroid dysfunction is an important cause of neuropathy because it is reversible. Neuropathy usually takes a length-dependent form, and occurs more commonly in patients with hypothyroidism than in those with hyperthyroidism.[10] Because thyroid dysfunction is identified so readily by primary care physicians, new diagnoses of neuropathy related to thyroid disease are actually uncommon in neurological practice.

Medication-induced neuropathies

A variety of medications may lead to polyneuropathy (Table 15.2).

Idiopathic

After extensive screening, many patients with polyneuropathy still lack an identifiable cause. Patients with idiopathic polyneuropathy tend to have mild, slowly progressive disease and do not tend to become disabled. While there is no specific treatment to reverse idiopathic polyneuropathy, patients do respond to agents for neuropathic pain.

Treatment of neuropathic symptoms

Sensory symptoms fall into two classes: positive symptoms in which there is an emergence of abnormal sensation, such as pain or paresthesias, and negative symptoms in which sensorimotor function is attenuated or lost, such as numbness or weakness. Broadly speaking, medications are available to mask positive symptoms,

Table 15.3 Medications used to treat neuropathic pain

Medication	Class	Initial dose	Typical effective dose	Side effects
Amitriptyline	Tricyclic antidepressant	25 mg qhs	50–100 mg qhs	Dry mouth, constipation, cardiac arrhythmias
Capsaicin cream	Substance P depleting agent	Topical	–	Burning at application site, effect limited to site of application
Carbamazepine	Anticonvulsant	100 mg tid	100–200 mg tid	Drowsiness, dizziness, rash, hyponatremia, agranulocytosis,
Duloxetine	Serotonin–norepinephrine reuptake inhibitor	30 mg qd	30–60 mg qd	Nausea, dizziness, drowsiness
Gabapentin[a]	Anticonvulsant	100–300 mg tid	300–1200 mg tid	Peripheral edema
Lidocaine patch	Sodium-channel blocker	5% patch tid	5% patch tid	Effect limited to site of application
Methadone[b]	Long-acting opioid	5 mg tid	5–20 mg tid	Addiction potential, constipation, tolerance
Nortriptyline[a]	Tricyclic antidepressant	25 mg qhs	50–100 mg qhs	Dry mouth, constipation, cardiac arrhythmias
Pregabalin	Anticonvulsant	50 mg bid	50–300 mg bid	Nausea, weight gain, fatigue
Topiramate	Anticonvulsant	25 mg qhs	50–200 mg qhs	Acral paresthesias, word-finding difficulties, nephrolithiasis
Tramadol	Weak opioid agonist	50 mg bid	50–150 mg bid	May interact with selective serotonin reuptake inhibitors

[a] Preferred initial agent
[b] Should be reserved for patients with refractory symptoms

but unless a reversible cause is identified, there are few treatments for negative neuropathic symptoms. A wide variety of agents is available to treat neuropathic pain and paresthesias (Table 15.3). Because these medications all work by reducing the firing of neural impulses in both the peripheral and central nervous systems, all but the topically applied agents may lead to sedation.

Other causes of distal sensory symptoms

Spine disease

Both lumbosacral polyradiculopathy and cervical myelopathy may produce lower-extremity symptoms that mimic length-dependent polyneuropathy. Compression of the L5 and S1 nerve roots may lead to pain, numbness, and tingling in the feet unaccompanied by back pain. Examination usually shows signs of asymmetry that help to make the distinction, but, in some cases, NCS and needle EMG are required to make the diagnosis.

Cervical myelopathy may also produce distal paresthesias and numbness, and should be considered when the hands are more involved than the feet, when pain is absent, or when hyperreflexia and spasticity are present on examination. Both medical and surgical causes of cervical myelopathy may produce a pseudopolyneuropathic presentation. Further evaluation of patients with cervical myelopathy is discussed in Chapter 17.

Plantar fasciitis

Inflammation of the plantar fascia is a source of foot pain that may mimic polyneuropathy when it is bilateral. Wear and tear damage to the plantar fascia is common in obese people and in runners, and leads to pain that is most severe with the first steps in the morning. Pain is most often centered at the medial calcaneus, but may involve the entirety of the sole. On physical examination, the pain of plantar fasciitis may be reproduced by dorsiflexing the toes and palpating the plantar fascia. Treat plantar fasciitis with nonsteroidal anti-inflammatory medications, gentle physical therapy, and, in refractory cases, local steroid injections. Although patients should avoid activities that precipitate pain, it is usually impractical for patients to comply with instructions to stay off of their feet.

Tarsal tunnel syndrome

The tarsal tunnel is formed by connective tissue posterior to the medial malleolus. The tibial nerve passes through the tarsal tunnel in order to reach and innervate the sole. Compression of the tibial nerve within the tarsal tunnel may therefore lead to pain and paresthesias in the bottom of the foot. Tarsal tunnel syndrome could be considered the lower-extremity analog of carpal tunnel syndrome (Chapter 16), but it is actually quite uncommon and occurs almost always in the setting of ankle trauma rather than as a gradual-onset process secondary to overuse. Polyneuropathy and plantar fasciitis are more likely explanations for symptoms in patients referred for tarsal tunnel syndrome. Signs on examination include numbness in the sole of the foot and paresthesias reproduced by percussing the tibial nerve just posterior to the medial malleolus. Be aware that sensation over the sole is frequently decreased due simply to the thickness of the overlying skin rather than to any specific neuropathology, so pinprick examination must be interpreted cautiously. Electrodiagnostic studies show slowing of tibial NCS across the ankle, but are frequently challenging and uninformative in patients with tarsal tunnel syndrome, particularly in patients with underlying polyneuropathy. Surgical release of the tibial nerve at the tarsal tunnel is curative, although seldom performed due to the rarity of the condition.

Morton's neuroma

Morton's neuroma is a benign tumor of the plantar nerve. Patients characteristically develop pain and paresthesias in the plantar surfaces of two adjacent toes (e.g. lateral half of digit three and medial half of digit four), which worsen with pressure and wearing shoes. Symptoms may be reproduced by applying pressure directly to the plantar nerve. Morton's neuroma should be evaluated and treated by an orthopedist or podiatrist.

Cramps

Cramps are characterized by a squeezing pain, which occurs most commonly in the calves and feet and has a tendency to be worse at night. They are discussed in greater detail in Chapter 14.

Restless legs syndrome

Restless legs syndrome (RLS) is a syndrome of unclear etiology characterized by a sensation of discomfort in the lower extremities that occurs at rest, particularly in the early evening when relaxing or while trying to fall asleep. Patients with RLS describe abnormal crawling, itching, or pulling below the knees, and feel that they need to move their legs or walk around in order to get relief. There is often a family history of RLS, and women tend to be affected more often than men. The diagnosis is easily established from the clinical history alone. Although a variety of medical conditions may be associated with RLS, iron-deficiency anemia is the most common identifiable cause. Patients with ferritin levels <50 µg/l should be treated with iron supplementation.[11] Caffeine and nicotine exacerbate RLS and should be avoided before bedtime. Dopamine agonists such as pramipexole (initiated at 0.125 mg qd, increased by 0.125 mg qd every 2–3 days up to 0.75 mg qd as needed) or ropinirole (0.25 mg qd, increased by 0.25 mg qd every 2–3 days up to 2 mg qd as needed) given approximately 2 hours prior to anticipated symptom onset are the first-line treatments for RLS. In patients who do not benefit from one of the dopamine agonists, gabapentin (100–600 mg before bedtime) is usually the next choice. Other medications that may be effective for RLS include levodopa, benzodiazepines, carbamazepine, diphenhydramine, and even low doses of mild narcotics. Dopamine agonists and levodopa are associated with the augmentation phenomenon, in which symptoms appear progressively earlier and earlier in the day. For patients with augmentation, problems only worsen when agents such as pramipexole or ropinirole are administered in anticipation of symptoms. Replacing dopaminergic agents with nondopaminergic ones is the most effective strategy for treating this problem.

Raynaud's phenomenon

Raynaud's phenomenon is a very common condition caused by low blood flow to the tips of the fingers and toes. It is diagnosed when the skin of the tips of the digits undergo a biphasic color change (at least two of pallor, erythema, and cyanosis).[12] Although these color changes are the defining features of Raynaud's phenomenon, patients may be referred for evaluation of neuropathy when the most prominent complaints are tingling, burning pain, or numbness. The first step in treating Raynaud's phenomenon is to counsel the patient to avoid the cold as much as possible or to wear gloves or socks when exposed to the cold. Obviously, most patients have tried these techniques before consulting with a neurologist. The rationale for using calcium-channel blockers (e.g. nifedipine 30–180 mg qd) and topical nitroglycerin is that they presumably produce vasodilation. Unfortunately, these agents provide only marginal symptom relief.

Generalized pain disorders

Patients with generalized, whole-body pain are often referred for evaluation of possible neuropathy, but rarely have a neurological disorder. The conditions that result in generalized body pain are usually psychiatric or rheumatological in origin. Psychiatric conditions that may produce whole-body pain include depression, anxiety, adjustment disorders, malingering, and conversion disorders. The difficult task in treating these patients is to help them to recognize the psychiatric component of their illness, to not feel insulted by the diagnosis, and to facilitate contact with a physician who will be better suited to treat their problems.

Fibromyalgia

Although not a neurological disease, many patients with fibromyalgia end up being evaluated by neurologists. This disease of uncertain etiology affects mostly younger and middle-aged women and is characterized by aching pain involving the neck, mid-back, lower back, arms, legs, and chest wall. Patients with fibromyalgia may also describe burning, tingling, and lancinating pains. Weakness is a subjective complaint, although none is demonstrable on examination. Neurocognitive symptoms include forgetfulness, impaired concentration, and fatigue. Research diagnostic criteria include the presence of chronic widespread pain and tenderness to palpation of 11 of 18 specific points.[13] By the time a patient with fibromyalgia is referred to a neurologist, an extensive battery of tests to exclude other diagnoses is usually available for interpretation. These should include complete blood count, erythrocyte sedimentation rate, thyroid function tests, and creatine kinase levels. Treatment of fibromyalgia is frequently challenging. A straightforward discussion of the diagnosis reduces accumulation of disability, whereas evasiveness and unnecessary protracted evaluations do more harm than good.[14] Patients with fibromyalgia may show a modest response to antidepressants. Nonsteroidal anti-inflammatory drugs are usually not effective and narcotics should be avoided. Encourage patients to pursue alternative therapies, as conventional medical treatment is frequently disappointing. In some cases, referral to a rheumatologist (preferably one with an interest in the condition) may be helpful.

References

1. Dyck PJ, Thomas PK, Griffin JW, Low PA, Poduslo J (eds). *Peripheral Neuropathy*. Philadelphia: W. B. Saunders; 1993.

2. Sumner CJ, Sheth S, Griffin JW, Cornblath DR, Polydefkis M. The spectrum of neuropathy in diabetes and impaired glucose tolerance. *Neurology* 2003;**14**:108–111.

3. Ziegler D, Ametov A, Barinov A, et al. Oral treatment with α-lipoic acid improves symptomatic diabetic polyneuropathy: the SYDNEY 2 trial. *Diabetes Care* 2006;**29**:2365–2370.

4. Puri V, Chaudhry N, Goel S, et al. Vitamin B12 deficiency: a clinical and electrophysiological profile. *Electromyogr Clin Neurophysiol* 2005;**45**:273–284.

5. Ramchandren S, Lewis RA. Monoclonal gammopathy and neuropathy. *Curr Opin Neurol* 2009;**22**:480–485.

6. Keren DF. Procedures for the evaluation of monoclonal immunoglobulins. *Arch Pathol Lab Med* 1999;**123**:126–132.

7. Boerkoel CF, Takashima H, Garcia CA, et al. Charcot–Marie–Tooth disease and related neuropathies: mutation distribution and genotype-phenotype correlation. *Ann Neurol* 2002;**51**:190–201.

8. Teunissen LL, Notermans NC, Franssen H, et al. Differences between hereditary motor and sensory neuropathy type 2 and chronic idiopathic axonal neuropathy. A clinical and electrophysiological study. *Brain* 1997;**120**:955–962.

9. Robinson-Papp J, Simpson DM. Neuromuscular diseases associated with HIV-1 infection. *Muscle Nerve* 2009;**40**:1043–1053.

10. Duyff RF, Van den Bosch J, Laman DM, van Loon BJ, Linssen WH. Neuromuscular findings in thyroid dysfunction: a prospective clinical and electrodiagnostic study. *J Neurol Neurosurg Psychiatry* 2000;**68**:750–755.

11. Sun ER, Chen CA, Ho G, Earley CJ, Allen RP. Iron and the restless legs syndrome. *Sleep* 1998;**21**:381–387.

12. Brennan P, Silman A, Black C, et al. Validity and reliability of three methods used in the diagnosis of Raynaud's phenomenon. *Br J Rheumatol* 1993;**32**:357–361.

13. Wolfe F, Smythe HA, Yunus MB, et al. The American College of Rheumatology 1990 criteria for the classification of fibromyalgia. Report of the Multicenter Criteria Committee. *Arthritis Rheum* 1990;**33**:160–172.

14. White KP, Nielson WR, Harth M, Ostbye T, Speechley M. Does the label "fibromyalgia" alter health status, function, and health service utilization? A prospective, within-group comparison in a community cohort of adults with chronic widespread pain. *Arthritis Rheum* 2002;**47**:260–265.

Chapter 16

Focal pain syndromes of the extremities

Introduction

It is easy to assume that all patients referred to a neurologist for the evaluation of limb pain have neurological problems such as radiculopathies, compression neuropathies, or plexopathies, and that more common musculoskeletal problems have been excluded prior to referral. In practice, this is far from true, and a neurologist, therefore, must have a thorough grasp of both the neurological and nonneurological causes of pain and the modalities available for their treatment. This chapter attempts to address these issues and is organized into three sections:

- Common neurological sources of limb pain and the musculoskeletal conditions that most commonly mimic them (Table 16.1).
- Treatment of nociceptive pain.
- Controversial localized pain syndromes.

Shoulder and proximal arm pain

C5 radiculopathy

C5 radiculopathy is characterized by neck pain and paresthesias that radiate into the shoulder and upper arm. On occasion, arm pain may be present without any neck pain. Weakness of the deltoid, biceps, and infraspinatus is usually less prominent than sensory dysfunction.

Brachial plexopathy

Only a small percentage of patients referred to a neurologist for the question of brachial plexopathy will actually have a plexus lesion. The three most important etiologies of brachial plexopathy are trauma, cancer, and idiopathic brachial neuritis, each of which has a distinctive presentation.

Trauma

Trauma may affect the brachial plexus at any level. The best-known traumatic plexopathy is Erb's palsy,

caused by damage to the upper trunk of the plexus, usually from downward pressure on the shoulder with forceful separation of the shoulder from the head. In addition to pain, there is weakness of the deltoid, biceps, supraspinatus, and infraspinatus. Sensation is decreased over the lateral upper arm and sometimes the lateral forearm. Electromyography (EMG) should be performed at least 3 weeks after suspected trauma to provide the most accurate information concerning localization and prognosis. In many cases, it is necessary to image the brachial plexus and cervical spine to differentiate traumatic brachial plexopathy from cervical polyradiculopathy.

Cancer

Neoplastic infiltration of the brachial plexus results in exquisite pain in the suprascapular and supraclavicular regions that radiates into the shoulder and arm, and persists or is worse at night. Weakness and wasting of the arm and hand muscles follows the pain by several weeks. The most common cancers that infiltrate the brachial plexus are breast and lung carcinomas. Unfortunately, patients with infiltrative brachial plexopathies have a poor prognosis, and usually do not survive long enough to make a neurological recovery. Local radiation and pain relief with narcotics and agents for neuropathic pain are used to palliate symptoms.

Radiation-induced brachial plexopathy develops months to years after local radiotherapy for breast or lung cancer. The challenge in diagnosing radiation-induced plexopathy is to differentiate it from direct infiltration by tumor recurrence. Clinically, radiation-induced plexopathy is less likely to be painful or to be associated with Horner's syndrome. Electrophysiologically, radiation-induced plexopathy can be diagnosed by finding myokymia. MRI of the brachial plexus helps to differentiate between the two conditions: nodular enhancement and mass lesions are more frequent in patients with neoplastic infiltration.[1] Because radiation-induced plexopathy is secondary to

Table 16.1 Common neurological and musculoskeletal causes of limb pain

Location	Neurological conditions	Musculoskeletal conditions
Shoulder and proximal arm	• C5 radiculopathy • Upper trunk brachial plexopathy	• Rotator cuff tendonitis
Lateral forearm	• C6 radiculopathy	• Lateral epicondylitis
Medial hand and forearm	• Ulnar neuropathy • C8 radiculopathy • Lower trunk brachial plexopathy	• Medial epicondylitis
Lateral hand including thumb	• Carpal tunnel syndrome	• De Quervain's tenosynovitis • Carpometacarpal joint arthritis
Hip and proximal leg	• L2–3 radiculopathy • Meralgia paresthetica • Lumbosacral plexopathy	• Osteoarthritis of the hip • Trochanteric bursitis
Knee	• L3 radiculopathy • Gonyalgia paresthetica	• Osteoarthritis of the knee
Foot (Chapter 15)	• Polyneuropathy • Tarsal tunnel syndrome	• Plantar fasciitis

ischemic damage and fibrosis, it is frequently refractory to all treatments.

Idiopathic brachial neuritis

Idiopathic brachial neuritis (also known as brachial plexitis or Parsonage–Turner syndrome) has a fairly characteristic presentation, which includes intense local neck or shoulder pain followed several days to weeks later by arm weakness. Most patients report a viral prodrome or vaccination several weeks before the plexopathy develops. The mainstay of treatment of idiopathic brachial neuritis is pain control with agents for neuropathic symptoms. In some cases, the pain is so severe that narcotics are required. Although idiopathic brachial neuritis is a self-limited condition, it usually improves only after several months from onset.

Rotator cuff tendonitis

Inflammation of the tendons of the rotator cuff causes pain localized to the lateral shoulder, which is reproduced by repetitive overhead reaching or by lying on the affected side. On examination, patients have point tenderness over the lateral acromion or supraspinatus or infraspinatus tendons, and pain with passive abduction at the shoulder. The weakness perceived by the patient and often found on examination is due to guarding, tendon instability, and disuse atrophy, rather than to true neurological dysfunction. The cornerstones of treatment include ice, nonsteroidal anti-inflammatory drugs (NSAIDs), and avoidance of activities that exacerbate the pain. For patients who do not respond to conservative measures, local steroid injections are helpful, with surgery reserved for patients with refractory pain or rotator cuff tears.

Lateral arm pain

C6 radiculopathy

C6 radiculopathy is characterized by pain and paresthesias that radiate from the neck into the lateral arm and hand, including the thumb. Weakness may involve the biceps, triceps, and wrist flexors.

Lateral epicondylitis

Lateral epicondylitis (tennis elbow) is produced by inflammation of the extensor carpi radialis longus and brevis tendons. Pain secondary to lateral epicondylitis is elicited by palpating the painful area while the patient resists wrist extension. Treatment includes rest, ice, and NSAIDs, with corticosteroid injections reserved for patients with refractory symptoms.

Medial hand and arm pain

Ulnar neuropathy

The most common symptoms of ulnar neuropathy are paresthesias and numbness in the palmar surface of the fifth and medial half of the fourth digits. Ulnar (a)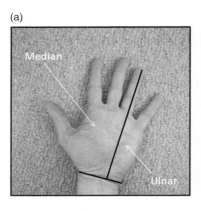

(b)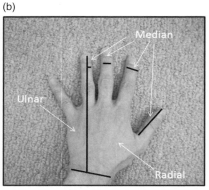

Figure 16.1 The sensory innervation of the hand.

neuropathy is most often the result of repetitive micro-trauma to the nerve as it passes around the elbow. Less common sites of ulnar neuropathy include the fore-arm and hand. Precipitants include resting the elbows on a table or lying flat on the back while the arms are supinated. On examination, weakness involves finger abduction and flexion of the distal interphalangeal joints of digits four and five. The thenar eminence and first dorsal interosseous may become atrophic. Sensory loss is found over both the palmar and dorsal surfaces of the fifth and medial half of the fourth digits and palm (Figure 16.1). Severe ulnar neuropathy produces a claw hand in which hyperextension at the fourth and fifth metacarpophalangeal joints is accompanied by flex-ion of the interphalangeal joints. To elicit Tinel's sign for ulnar neuropathy, percuss the nerve at the elbow as it runs between the olecranon process and medial epicondyle, and ask the patient if paresthesias develop in digits four and five. Ulnar neuropathy may be con-firmed electrophysiologically with nerve conduction studies. Conservative treatment of ulnar neuropathy includes avoiding precipitating activities and wearing a padded elbow sleeve to prevent further microtrauma to the nerve. Consider surgical decompression and transposition of the nerve should conservative meas-ures fail.

C8 radiculopathy

Expected complaints of C8 radiculopathy are neck pain and paresthesias radiating into the medial hand and forearm. Numbness in these distributions may accompany weakness of the intrinsic muscles of the hand. Because structural radiculopathies at the C8 lev-els are relatively uncommon, carefully consider more common possibilities such as ulnar neuropathy at the elbow before making the diagnosis.

Lower trunk brachial plexopathy

The lower trunk of the brachial plexus is comprised of nerve fibers derived from the C8–T1 roots, and damage at this site may cause pain and other sensory complaints in the medial hand, forearm, and arm. The lower trunk of the plexus, like the upper trunk, may be damaged by trauma, cancer (especially in patients with infiltrative apical lung cancer), or idiopathic inflammatory conditions. Because the lower trunk lies in proximity to the oculosympathetic chain, it may be associated with Horner's syndrome (Chapter 7). One cause of lower trunk brachial plexopathy deserves spe-cial mention because of its rarity: thoracic outlet syn-drome. This diagnosis is usually incorrect, and often is given to patients with arm pain of unclear etiology. True neurogenic thoracic outlet syndrome, however, is a legitimate diagnosis caused by compression of the lower trunk of the brachial plexus by a cervical rib or accessory band of connective tissue.[2] It requires rigorous investigation including EMG and thoracic imaging to confirm the presence of a responsible struc-tural abnormality.

Medial epicondylitis

Medial epicondylitis (golf elbow) is produced by inflammation of the flexor carpi radialis tendon, usu-ally resulting from repetitive gripping movements and wrist flexion. Pain is localized to the medial elbow and, because of the well-known course of the ulnar nerve around the elbow, patients with medial epicondylitis are often referred to neurologists for evaluation of ulnar neuropathy. Pain secondary to medial epicondylitis is elicited by palpating the painful area while the patient resists wrist flexion. Imaging studies should be obtained only to exclude alternative diagnoses. Treatment for medial epicondylitis involves rest, ice, and NSAIDs. Corticosteroid injections and gradual introduction of grip-strengthening exercises may also help.

Lateral hand pain

Carpal tunnel syndrome

Compression of the median nerve at the wrist results in carpal tunnel syndrome (CTS). In the early stages of the disorder, patients describe pain and paresthesias in the hand, mostly in the first three digits and the radial half of the fourth digit. It is also common for patients to report symptoms in the entire hand or extending proximally into the forearm and upper arm, even though these areas are outside the sensory distribution of the median nerve. Hand overuse, particularly typing, mouse use, and assembly work, precipitate or exacerbate the symptoms. Nocturnal symptoms are common, and patients may shake out their hands to relieve the paresthesias. Motor problems are not prominent early in CTS, but as the disorder progresses, the hand and fingers may become weak and grip strength may be reduced. On examination, look for weakness of thumb abduction and flattening of the thenar eminence. The sensory loss in CTS affects the palmar surfaces of the first three digits and the lateral half of the fourth digit (Figure 16.1). Because the palmar sensory branch does not pass through the carpal tunnel, sensation over the palm is spared. Tinel's and Phalen's signs support the diagnosis. To elicit Tinel's sign (Figure 16.2), tap the volar aspect of the wrist briskly with a reflex hammer and inquire about paresthesias in the first three fingers. To elicit Phalen's sign (Figure 16.3), instruct the patient to appose the dorsal surfaces of the hands to each other while the wrists are flexed for 1 minute: in patients with CTS, paresthesias should develop in the palmar surfaces of the first three fingers. Physical examination abnormalities may be limited in early CTS, and nerve conduction studies may be necessary to make the diagnosis. Patients with mild disease may improve with wrist braces and activity restriction. Local corticosteroid injections are a temporizing measure that may reduce sensory symptoms. Carpal tunnel release surgery is the definitive treatment for patients with more severe CTS.

De Quervain's tenosynovitis

This condition, caused by inflammation of the tendons of the extensor pollicis brevis and abductor

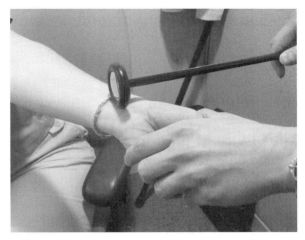

Figure 16.2 Tinel's sign. Tap the distal volar aspect of the wrist briskly with a reflex hammer. The sign is positive when the patient reports paresthesias in the palmar surfaces of digits one to three.

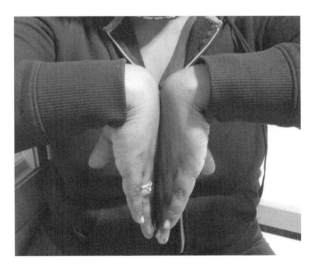

Figure 16.3 Phalen's sign. Instruct the patient to appose the dorsal surfaces of the hands for 1 minute. Patients with carpal tunnel syndrome will report paresthesias in the palmar surfaces of digits one to three.

pollicis longus, may lead to referral for CTS or superficial radial neuropathy, a rare compression neuropathy. Patients with de Quervain's tenosynovitis describe pain in the thumb and radial styloid, especially with pinching maneuvers. On examination, the radial styloid is tender to palpation. The Finkelstein test is a provocative maneuver for de Quervain's tenosynovitis in which pain is reproduced by enclosing the thumb inside the fist and deviating the wrist in the ulnar direction (Figure 16.4). Treat de Quervain's tenosynovitis with rest, NSAIDS, and immobilization of the thumb using (a)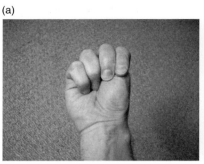

(b)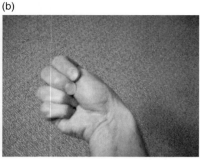

Figure 16.4 The Finkelstein maneuver. Instruct the patient to enclose their thumb inside their fingers (A) and deviate the hand in the ulnar direction (B). Patients with de Quervain's tenosynovitis will note pain in the lateral aspect of the thumb.

a thumb spica splint. Refractory cases may require corticosteroid injection and possibly surgical referral.

Carpometacarpal joint arthritis

Osteoarthritis of the carpometacarpal (CMC) joint is present in the majority of people over 65 and is characterized by pain at the base of the thumb and radial aspect of the wrist, and sometimes by grip weakness. This condition often leads to neurological consultation for evaluation of CTS. Carpometacarpal joint arthritis is diagnosed on physical examination by demonstrating tenderness to compression at the CMC joint (Figure 16.5). Plain radiographs, although usually not necessary, confirm the diagnosis. Treatment involves immobilization, NSAIDs, and heat application.

Thigh and hip pain

L2 and L3 radiculopathy

While intervertebral disc herniations usually spare the upper lumbar nerve roots, spinal stenosis is a common cause of upper lumbar radiculopathy in older patients (see Chapter 17). Pain and paresthesias may radiate from the back into the lateral (L2) or medial (L3) thigh. Weakness of hip flexion, hip adduction, and knee extension may accompany an upper lumbar radiculopathy. The patellar reflex may be reduced or absent. Because it may be challenging to differentiate among upper lumbar radiculopathy, lumbosacral plexopathy, and femoral neuropathy by history and physical examination, nerve conduction studies and EMG are often required.

Meralgia paresthetica

Entrapment of the lateral femoral cutaneous nerve, usually at the inguinal ligament, leads to meralgia paresthetica. Pain and paresthesias, often quite severe, involve the lateral thigh and sometimes radiate into the knee.

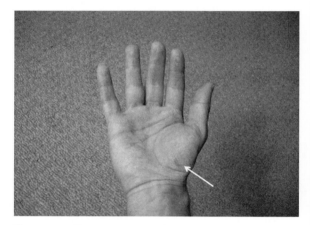

Figure 16.5 The carpometacarpal joint.

Because this nerve has no motor distribution, there is no muscle weakness: any muscle weakness on examination is due to guarding or to an unrelated condition. Meralgia paresthetica usually develops in obese patients or in those who have recently lost a large amount of weight. Nerve conduction studies are frequently unhelpful in establishing the diagnosis, as a sensory response from the lateral femoral cutaneous nerve is difficult to obtain, even in normal subjects. Meralgia paresthetica may improve with weight loss and avoidance of restrictive clothing such as tight belts. Most patients, however, do not improve with these conservative measures and require local steroid injections at the inguinal ligament.[3] Surgery is necessary only on rare occasions.

Lumbosacral plexopathy

Many of the general rules described above for brachial plexopathy also apply to lumbosacral plexopathy. Although etiologies common to both brachial and lumbosacral plexopathies include trauma, cancer, and idiopathic lumbosacral plexitis, there are several distinct pathologies that affect the lumbosacral plexus.

Trauma

Traumatic lumbosacral plexopathy results from severe hip trauma (usually involving a fracture) or pelvic surgery. Depending on the site of trauma, sensorimotor symptoms may involve the entire leg or just a restricted part of it. Electromyography helps to localize and quantify the deficits. Lumbosacral plexopathy related to pregnancy is a specific traumatic etiology that is discussed further in Chapter 11.

Retroperitoneal hematoma

Retroperitoneal hematoma, usually related to anticoagulation, a bleeding diathesis, or a procedure involving femoral catheterization, is an important cause of lumbosacral plexopathy. Rapid identification of the problem and correction of any contributing coagulation abnormalities may prevent life-threatening exsanguination. Plexopathy related to hematoma tends to resolve as the blood is reabsorbed.

Cancer

Neoplasm-related lumbosacral plexopathies, like those that involve the upper extremities, may be divided into infiltrative and radiation-induced plexopathies, and are evaluated in a fashion similar to those that affect the brachial plexus. The most common tumors that infiltrate the lumbosacral plexus are colon and ovarian cancers.

Diabetic amyotrophy

Most patients who develop this disorder of the lumbosacral nerve roots and plexus have mild type 2 diabetes at symptom onset. Weight loss, fevers, and night sweats frequently precede or accompany the lumbosacral plexopathy. Diabetic amyotrophy begins with exquisite pain, usually in the hip and thigh, which often spreads to involve the lower leg and, in many cases, the contralateral leg. Leg weakness, often profound, develops several days later. Patients with diabetic amyotrophy require pain control with agents for neuropathic pain and sometimes with narcotics. Physical therapy may help restore mobility. Immunomodulatory therapy including intravenous methylprednisolone and intravenous immunoglobulin is effective on an anecdotal basis.[4] Unfortunately, recovery takes many months to years and is often incomplete.

Idiopathic lumbosacral plexitis

Idiopathic lumbosacral plexitis, although similarly named, should not be considered the lower extremity counterpart of idiopathic brachial neuritis, as it is generally a more severe disorder. Idiopathic lumbosacral plexitis is essentially the same condition as diabetic amyotrophy, except that it occurs in patients without diabetes.[5]

Trochanteric bursitis

Trochanteric bursitis is caused by the breakdown of the bursa surrounding the greater trochanter of the femur. It often accompanies or is confused with meralgia paresthetica or upper lumbar radiculopathy. Pain is located in the lateral hip, and becomes worse when the patient moves the hip or lies on it. Trochanteric bursitis is diagnosed clinically by finding tenderness to palpation of the trochanteric bursa. Conservative treatment includes a combination of NSAIDs, heat, and physical therapy. Local steroid injections may benefit patients who do not respond to these measures.

Osteoarthritis of the hip and occult hip fracture

Osteoarthritis, almost universal in the elderly population, is a common cause of hip pain. Because pain may radiate into the groin, back, or knee, it may lead to evaluation for lumbosacral radiculopathy. Patients typically report groin pain with attempted internal rotation. Treatment with NSAIDs may help, but patients often require orthopedic referral. Severe anterior or lateral hip pain with difficulty bearing weight suggests the possibility of hip fracture and should prompt plain films of the hip and orthopedic referral.

Knee pain

Isolated knee pain results so rarely from a neurological process that more common orthopedic conditions should be evaluated exhaustively before undertaking any neurological investigation. L3 radiculopathy is a possible source of knee pain, but is almost always accompanied by back pain that radiates into the leg. Gonyalgia paresthetica is an even less common cause of knee pain and results from entrapment of the infrapatellar branch of the saphenous nerve.

General principles of nociceptive pain treatment

In an ideal world, neurologists would treat pain that was exclusively of neuropathic origin. The musculoskeletal pain syndromes described in this chapter, however, produce nociceptive rather than neuropathic pain and therefore require a different strategy. The standard approach to nociceptive pain management involves escalating from weaker doses of medications with few side effects, to stronger medications that may have more side effects, to multidisciplinary pain treatment, and finally to alternative therapies:

- Although most nociceptive pain responds to over-the-counter medications such as acetaminophen, aspirin, ibuprofen, and naproxen, patients who respond to one of these treatments usually do not reach neurological attention.
- Prescription NSAIDs are effective for some patients who do not respond to over-the counter analgesics. Common prescription-strength NSAIDs include oxaprozin (600–1200 mg qd), ketorolac (10 mg qid for up to 5 consecutive days), and diclofenac (100 mg bid). Side effects of these medications include gastrointestinal hemorrhage and nephrotoxicity.
- Physical therapy, ice, heat, and massage are effective treatments for some patients with musculoskeletal pain.
- The opioid agonist tramadol (50–100 mg bid) has a lower rate of side effects than the true narcotic medications, and may be used to treat a variety of musculoskeletal complaints refractory to acetaminophen or NSAIDs.
- Narcotic analgesics should be avoided if possible, as these medications have addictive properties, are sedating, and have a thriving black market for resale. Avoid rapid-onset, short-acting narcotics such as hydrocodone, oxycodone, hydromorphone, meperidine, and short-acting morphine, as their brief durations of action lead to frequent spikes in pain. Longer-acting narcotic options include fentanyl patches or methadone, which should still be prescribed sparingly.
- Local anesthetic or steroid injections may be helpful for patients with herniated intervertebral discs, bursitis, and other musculoskeletal conditions that do not respond to oral medications.
- Many pain syndromes are difficult to treat due to the severity of the underlying condition or to superimposed or preexisting psychological factors. Tricyclic antidepressants, selective serotonin reuptake inhibitors, and newer agents such as

duloxetine and pregabalin may help patients with refractory chronic pain and comorbid depression.
- Psychological counseling, biofeedback, and alternative treatments such as acupuncture and homeopathic treatments may be effective in treating severe pain.

Controversial localized pain syndromes

Complex regional pain syndrome

Complex regional pain syndrome (CRPS), alternatively known as reflex sympathetic dystrophy or causalgia, is characterized by pain, edema, trophic skin changes, and a decreased range of motion in an extremity. In the early stages, however, pain may be unaccompanied by other signs and symptoms. The condition is divided into CRPS type I in which there is no definable nerve lesion and CRPS type II in which there is a history of a preceding nerve injury. The mechanism by which CRPS develops is unclear, and the diagnosis is, in itself, a controversial one. Many patients with limb pain of uncertain etiology are told that they have CRPS when no clear source for their pain can be identified. However, I have never made this diagnosis or seen a convincing case. There are staunch advocates for[6] and against[7] the existence of CRPS. While I tend to agree with the latter school, I maintain an open mind.

Myofascial pain syndrome

Myofascial pain syndrome is the name that is often assigned to any focal musculoskeletal pain of unclear etiology despite thorough investigation. Problems such as depression, fatigue, and forgetfulness frequently accompany the pain. Myofascial pain syndrome may represent a restricted form of fibromyalgia, and responds (or fails to respond) to the same treatments as that disorder (Chapter 15).

References

1. Thyagarajan D, Cascino T, Harms G. Magnetic resonance imaging in brachial plexopathy of cancer. *Neurology* 1995;**45**:421–427.
2. Cuetter AC, Bartoszek DM. The thoracic outlet syndrome: controversies, overdiagnosis, overtreatment, and recommendations for management. *Muscle Nerve* 1989;**12**:410–419.

3. Harney D, Patijn J. Meralgia paresthetica: diagnosis and management strategies. *Pain Med* 2007;**8**:669–677.

4. Chan YC, Lo YL, Chan ESY. Immunotherapy for diabetic amyotrophy. *Cochrane Database Syst Rev* 2009; (3): CD006521.

5. Dyck PJB, Windebank AJ. Diabetic and nondiabetic lumbosacral radiculoplexus neuropathies: new insights into pathophysiology and treatment. *Muscle Nerve* 2002;**25**:477–491.

6. Schwartzman RJ, Popescu A. Reflex sympathetic dystrophy. *Curr Rheum Rep* 2002;**4**:165–169.

7. Ochoa JL. Truths, errors, and lies around "reflex sympathetic dystrophy" and "complex regional pain syndrome". *J Neurol* 1999;**246**:875–879.

Chapter 17

Back pain, radiculopathy, and myelopathy

Definitions, history, and examination

Although back and neck pain is commonly managed by primary care physicians, it may come to neurological attention when it is refractory to treatment or when it is accompanied by signs or symptoms of radiculopathy, myelopathy, or cauda equina syndrome.

Radiculopathy

Radiculopathy is the clinical syndrome caused by pathology at the level of what neurologists call the nerve root, a structure that, strictly speaking, is a mixed spinal nerve containing both sensory and motor fibers. The classic history for radiculopathy is back or neck pain that radiates into the arm or leg in a band-like distribution. The pain should have a sharp, burning, or stabbing character, and is often accompanied by paresthesias. Although monoradiculopathy may produce weakness, this is often mild because most muscles are innervated by more than one nerve root (Table 17.1). Sensory loss due to radiculopathy follows a dermatomal distribution, and may also be mild or incomplete due to the overlapping distributions of the cutaneous sensory nerves (Table 17.2 and Chapter 15, Figure 15.1). Patients with radiculopathy may have focal weakness (Chapter 11) or sensory disturbances (Chapter 16) in the extremities without accompanying back pain. The two most useful provocative tests for radiculopathy are the straight leg raise test for lumbosacral root lesions and Spurling's test for cervical root lesions. To perform the straight leg raise test, instruct the patient to lie supine with their leg extended. Leg pain with passive flexion of the hip between 30 and 70° suggests the presence of a herniated disc secondary to L5 or S1 root compression. Anterior thigh pain with passive extension of the hip while the patient is prone suggests L2 or L3 root compression. To perform Spurling's test, instruct the patient to tip their head to the symptomatic side. The test is positive for cervical radiculopathy if compressing the head from above in that position causes pain and paresthesias to radiate into the symptomatic arm.

Myelopathy

Myelopathy is the pattern of sensorimotor deficits produced by damage to the spinal cord. An understanding of spinal cord neuroanatomy is necessary to determine the level of myelopathic deficits. For the purposes of clinical localization, the spinal cord consists of (Figure 17.1):

- The dorsal columns, which contain ascending sensory fibers mediating vibration and proprioception. Dorsal column lesions produce sensory deficits below the level of the lesion on the same side of the body.
- The lateral spinothalamic tracts, which contain ascending sensory fibers mediating pain and temperature. Spinothalamic tract lesions produce sensory deficits in all dermatomes beginning one to two levels below the level of the lesion on the opposite side of the body.
- The lateral corticospinal tracts, which contain descending motor fibers. Corticospinal tract lesions produce weakness and spasticity below the level of the lesion on the same side of the body.
- The dorsal horns, which relay all sensory information from the dorsal root ganglia to the dorsal columns and lateral spinothalamic tracts. Dorsal horn lesions produce loss of all sensory modalities at the level of the lesion on the same side of the body.
- The anterior horns, which contain the lower motor neurons. Anterior horn cell lesions produce flaccid paralysis at the level of the lesion on the same side of the body.
- The ventral white commissure, which contains decussating sensory fibers connecting the pain and temperature information in the dorsal horns to the contralateral spinothalamic tracts. Commissural lesions produce sensory loss one or two levels below the lesion both ipsilaterally and contralaterally.

Table 17.1 Muscle weakness organized by myotomes

Root level	Weak muscles
C5 + C6	Deltoid, biceps, supraspinatus
C6 + C7	Triceps, wrist extensors, wrist flexors
C8 + T1	Abductor pollicis brevis, abductor digiti minimi, extensor indicis proprius
L2 + L3	Iliopsoas, adductor longus, quadriceps
L4	Tibialis anterior, quadriceps
L5	Tibialis anterior, tibialis posterior, peroneus longus, gluteus medius
S1	Gastrocnemius, hamstrings, gluteus maximus

See Chapter 10 for additional details of testing.

Table 17.2 Sensory loss organized by dermatomes

Root level	Distribution of sensory symptoms
C5	Lateral upper arm
C6	Lateral forearm, thumb and index finger
C7	Midline of forearm, middle finger
C8	Medial forearm, ring and pinky finger
T1	Medial upper arm
L2	Lateral thigh
L3	Medial thigh
L4	Medial leg
L5	Lateral leg and dorsum of foot
S1	Lateral foot, sole, and Achilles tendon
Lower sacral roots	Perineum, scrotum

See also Chapter 15, Figure 15.1

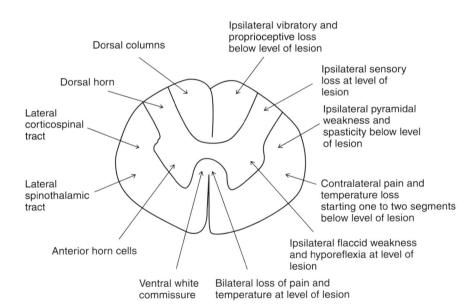

Figure 17.1 Cross-sectional diagram of the spinal cord showing locations of the clinically important structures on the left and expected clinical deficits on the right.

A complete myelopathy therefore produces sensorimotor loss at myotomes and dermatomes caudal to the level of the lesion, hyperreflexia, and upgoing toes. In addition, cord lesions lead to urgency of both bowel and bladder. Many patients have incomplete lesions, which may lead to patchy sensorimotor problems. In these patients, the distribution of weakness is most helpful in defining the presence of myelopathy.

In the acute stage, weakness from a severe spinal cord lesion is usually flaccid, and does not become spastic for several days to a few weeks following the injury. While severe lesions may produce complete plegia of the limbs, milder paresis with disproportionately greater weakness of the "upper motor neuron" muscles (see Chapter 10, Table 10.1) is more common. Be aware, though, that upper motor neuron weakness is a guideline rather than a hard and fast rule, and that many patients with spinal cord lesions do not conform strictly to this pattern.

Cauda equina syndrome

The lumbar and sacral nerve roots emerge from the spinal column to form the cauda equina. Compression or infiltration of the cauda equina produces a distinctive lumbosacral polyradiculopathy characterized by weakness and sensory loss in the lower extremities, sphincter weakness with incontinence of both bowel and bladder, and sensory loss in the perineum. Sphincter tone may be reduced and an anal wink may be absent in patients with cauda equina syndrome. Anal sphincter tone is established by placing the finger inside the anus and asking the patient to bear down. An anal wink is tested by stroking the perianal skin and observing for contraction of the anal sphincter. Cauda equina syndrome is a true neurological emergency, and should be evaluated and treated as quickly as possible. In most cases, it is secondary to a large posterior intervertebral disc herniation or spinal stenosis. Important inflammatory causes of cauda equina syndrome include neoplastic invasion and cytomegalovirus infection.

Back pain due to neurological disease

Red flags

When evaluating back and neck pain, it is critical to seek red flags that point to dangerous conditions such as malignancy, epidural abscess, cord compression, and cauda equina syndrome. Any patient with a history of cancer, fevers, bowel or bladder dysfunction, or rapidly progressive weakness requires urgent imaging of the clinically involved area of the spine, preferentially MRI with and without contrast. Also consider urgent MRI for patients with thoracic-level signs or symptoms, as malignant processes such as epidural cord compression and epidural abscess have a propensity to involve this level of the spine.

Herniated nucleus pulposus

The intervertebral discs lie between the vertebral bodies, provide the spine with structural stability, and allow joint mobility. The discs consist of a tough fibrous annulus fibrosus surrounding a softer, more gelatinous nucleus pulposus. Posterior herniation of the nucleus pulposus is the most common cause of radiculopathy and myelopathy in people between the ages of 30 and 50. Although the precise mechanisms by which disc herniations produce symptoms are not entirely clear, it is likely that the herniated disc incites an inflammatory reaction leading to pain, while physical compression of the nerve root within the neural foramen or the

spinal cord within the central canal is mechanistically more important in generating weakness and sensory loss. Trauma or excessive stretching or exercise may immediately precede symptoms, but clear precipitants of intervertebral disc herniation are often absent. Disc herniations are most common at the C5–6, C6–7, L4–5, and L5–S1 levels, and are distinctly uncommon in the thoracic spine. Discs may herniate posteriorly, posterolaterally, or far laterally, compressing different structures in each case. Table 17.3 summarizes the deficits expected with disc herniation at each of the four most common spinal levels.

If there are no red flags, treat patients with suspected herniated intervertebral discs conservatively and defer neuroimaging studies. Because resuming normal activity ultimately should be the goal of patients with intervertebral disc herniation, I usually recommend that patients continue their normal routines rather than beginning programs of bed rest or aggressive "boot camp" physical therapy. Instruct patients with cervical disc disease to wear a soft cervical collar at night, while using a computer, and while driving. Prescribe mild pain relievers including ibuprofen and acetaminophen as the first line of analgesia. Stronger medications including tramadol (50–100 mg bid) and long-acting narcotics (sustained-release oxycodone 10–20 mg bid) may be prescribed cautiously for patients with severe symptoms. Because back pain is often chronic, it is best to delay initiating narcotics for as long as possible. A short trial of corticosteroids (e.g. prednisone 60 mg × 3 days, 40 mg × 3 days, 20 mg × 3 days) is frequently very helpful in reducing the inflammation produced by a herniated disc. Agents for neuropathic pain such as gabapentin and nortriptyline do little for patients with intervertebral disc herniations except make them sleepy.

If conservative therapy does not improve symptoms after 6 weeks, more aggressive evaluation and treatment is indicated. MRI of the clinically involved level of the spine should be used to confirm the diagnosis, and possibly to plan surgery. Electromyography may be considered, but rarely offers any additional helpful information. Epidural steroid injections may provide short-term relief of pain, but do little to nothing for motor deficits and lack long-term efficacy.[1] Surgical referral is indicated for patients with pain that persists despite 6 weeks of conservative therapy, progressive motor deficits, or incontinence of the bowel or bladder.

Table 17.3 Common intervertebral disc herniation syndromes

Direction of herniation	Herniation at C5–6	Herniation at C6–7	Herniation at L4–5	Herniation at L5–S1
Posterior	Spinal cord	Spinal cord	L5 nerve root, possibly cauda equina	S1 nerve root, possibly cauda equina
Posterolateral	C6 nerve root	C7 nerve root	L5 nerve root	S1 nerve root
Far lateral	C6 nerve root	C7 nerve root	L4 nerve root	L5 nerve root

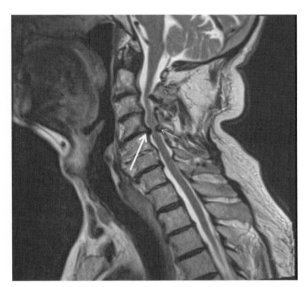

Figure 17.2 Sagittal T2-weighted MRI showing a herniated intervertebral disc (thick arrow) and hypertrophic ligamentum flavum (thin arrow) in a patient with spinal stenosis. Note the disappearance of the hyperintense CSF signal at the greatest level of stenosis. The faint hyperintense signal change in the spinal cord indicates significant cord compression.

Spinal stenosis

As people age, the intervertebral discs desiccate, and a greater portion of the axial load must be assumed by the facet joints and ligamentum flavum. The combination of disc herniation, facet joint and ligament hypertrophy, and bony spur formation leads to osteoarthritic narrowing of the central spinal canal and neural foramina (Figure 17.2). Like intervertebral disc herniation, spinal stenosis may produce back pain, radiculopathy, myelopathy, or a cauda equina syndrome. Unlike symptoms from disc herniation, those from spinal stenosis typically develop in a subacute to chronic fashion. Spinal stenosis may also be distinguished from disc herniation by its greater tendency to involve the upper lumbar levels.

Neurogenic claudication is a well-known manifestation of spinal stenosis characterized by pain in the back and legs, with fatigue that develops with standing or walking and is relieved by rest and bending over. Neurogenic claudication is often difficult to differentiate from vascular claudication of the lower extremities (Table 17.4). In many older patients, both disorders exist simultaneously. If there is any doubt as to the source of claudication symptoms, referral to a vascular specialist may help to reach the correct diagnosis.

Conservative therapy of spinal stenosis is similar to that described for intervertebral disc herniation. Abnormal neuroimaging findings in patients with spinal stenosis must be interpreted cautiously, as many asymptomatic older people have radiographic evidence of degenerative arthritis. Electromyography is unhelpful in diagnosing spinal stenosis or in planning its treatment. Unfortunately, most patients with spinal stenosis do not improve markedly with physical therapy, medications, or epidural steroid injections. Consider surgery for patients with intractable pain, sphincter dysfunction, progressive weakness, or disabling exercise intolerance. Many spine surgeons are understandably reluctant to perform operations for older patients with spinal stenosis, as these patients frequently require multilevel operations, have medical comorbidities that make them poor surgical risks, and improve modestly at best with surgery.

Neoplasm

Neoplastic epidural cord compression, most commonly caused by metastasis, represents a neurological emergency. The most common tumors that produce cord compression are those of the breast, lung, prostate, and lymphoreticular system.[2] The most common site of epidural cord compression is the thoracic spine due to both its relatively rich vascular supply and to the greater number of thoracic vertebrae. Back pain, sometimes accompanied by radiculopathic symptoms, is usually the first sign of metastasis, and may go unnoticed for several months, especially in patients with undiagnosed cancer. As cord compression progresses,

Table 17.4 Differentiating between neurogenic and vascular claudication

Clinical feature	Neurogenic claudication	Vascular claudication
Pain improves with flexion (e.g. leaning over a shopping cart)	Yes	No
Pain relief after rest	After several minutes	Almost immediately
Peripheral pulses	Normal	Reduced
Leg weakness	May be present	Should be absent

weakness develops in a myelopathic pattern and the patient becomes incontinent of bowel and bladder.

Any patient with known cancer who develops back pain should have MRI with and without contrast to look for cord compression. Time is of the essence in diagnosing and treating this condition, as the likelihood of maintaining ambulation and continence of the bowel and bladder is related to the severity of the deficits when treatment begins. Initiate corticosteroids as soon as cord compression is suspected: treat patients with severe weakness with 100 mg dexamethasone orally followed by 24 mg q6h, tapering the dose by 50% every 2–3 days.[2] Definitive therapy of metastatic cord compression is determined by the patient's overall prognosis and the type of primary tumor. Treat patients who are expected to survive for at least 3 months with a combination of surgical decompression and radiotherapy.[3] Radiation without surgery is indicated for patients with radiosensitive tumors such as leukemia, lymphoma, and germ cell tumors, or those with otherwise poor prognosis. In patients without a known cancer history who present with epidural cord compression, evaluate for a primary tumor with a torso CT, mammogram for women, and testicular examination and prostate-specific antigen level for men. If these tests do not disclose a primary neoplasm, biopsy of the lesion may aid in diagnosis. Although the overall prognosis of patients who develop metastatic cord compression is poor, the probability of maintaining ambulation is excellent if appropriate measures are taken immediately.

Epidural abscess

Bacterial infection of the epidural space occurs either by hematogenous spread from a distant infectious source or by extension of a local infection. The most common organism responsible for epidural abscess is *Staphylococcus aureus*. Other frequently encountered organisms include *Staphylococcus epidermidis*, *Escherichia coli*, and *Pseudomonas aeruginosa*. The well-known clinical triad of back pain, fever, and

neurological deficits referable to the spine is present in only a minority of patients, and the diagnosis is most often missed when the triad is incomplete. Failure to detect and treat epidural abscess leads to potentially irreversible weakness, sphincter dysfunction, and distant spread of the infection. MRI of the spine with and without contrast is the diagnostic study of choice in patients with suspected epidural abscess. Unless there are clear signs that the abscess is restricted to a particular vertebral level, the best practice is to image the entire length of the spine in order to detect all possible foci of infection. Patients with epidural abscess and neurological dysfunction require surgical drainage plus a 6-week course of vancomycin (1 g IV bid), ceftriaxone (2 g IV bid), and metronidazole (500 mg IV q8h).

Inflammatory radiculopathies (radiculitis)

The majority of radiculopathies are caused by structural disease of the spine. Inflammatory radiculopathy and polyradiculopathy are less common but important, as they frequently reflect serious and reversible underlying medical conditions. In general, radiculitis should be considered in patients with radiculopathy and normal imaging studies or imaging studies that show inflammation of the nerve roots without obvious structural spinal disease. Spinal fluid analysis is essential to the evaluation of patients with suspected radiculitis. Common causes of inflammatory radiculopathy include Lyme disease, diabetes (especially at the thoracic levels), sarcoidosis, malignant nerve root invasion, and viral infections (most commonly herpes zoster, cytomegalovirus, and herpes simplex).

Musculoskeletal back pain

A wide variety of musculoskeletal conditions may produce back and neck pain. Although such pain is generally self-limited, it may also be chronically disabling and lead to missed work and financial hardship.

In addition, because there are no reliable diagnostic tests for musculoskeletal back pain, it is fertile ground for malingerers. Patients with refractory musculoskeletal back pain are frequently referred to neurologists to "rule out a neurological cause." Thus, it is essential to be able to differentiate between neurological sources of back pain and nonneurological ones. Typical characteristics of nonneurological back pain include tightness, aching, swelling, point tenderness, and a lack of symptom radiation into the extremities. Paresthesias and true motor dysfunction (not give-way weakness, which is frequently the result of pain or poor effort) should be absent. Although most patients with musculoskeletal pain cannot be given a precise diagnosis, the following are some of the exceptions that should be familiar to all neurologists.

Strains and sprains

Muscle strains and ligament sprains are the most common nonneurological causes of back pain. The patient usually describes a history of injury such as lifting a heavy suitcase or moving a piece of furniture, which is followed several hours to a few days later by nonradiating, dull, aching pain. Strains and sprains are usually identified and treated by primary care physicians, but, in some cases, atypical symptoms such as tingling or burning may lead to neurological referral. A combination of rest, ice, and nonsteroidal anti-inflammatory drugs (NSAIDs) generally improves symptoms in a few days.

Spinal fractures

Osteoporosis, trauma, and metastasis are the most important causes of spinal fractures. Fractures due to metastasis are more likely to involve the thoracic levels. Obviously, unstable fractures are a medical emergency and need to be treated with immobilization and possibly with surgical stabilization. Acute compression fractures without compromise of the cord may be treated with immobilization and pain relievers. Vertebroplasty is commonly performed for osteoporotic fractures, but offers no real advantage compared with that provided by conservative measures.[4,5]

Sacroiliac joint dysfunction

Pain derived from the sacroiliac joints is possibly among the most common causes of lower back pain, but may be unrecognized because it is not a well-defined clinical entity. Patients complain of back pain, which may mimic radiculopathy because it radiates into the groin, hip, thigh, or leg. The mainstay of treatment is NSAIDs and gentle physical therapy. Focal injections are reserved for patients with refractory symptoms.

Coccygodynia

Pain in the coccygeal region may mimic sacral radiculopathy or lead to evaluation for cauda equina syndrome. Although there may be a history of trauma, coccygodynia may be the result of nothing more than prolonged sitting. The diagnosis is confirmed by finding tenderness with direct manipulation of the coccyx. Treat patients with coccygodynia with cushioned seating and local steroid injections.

Painless myelopathy

A variety of processes, most of which are intrinsic to the cord, lead to painless subacute or chronic myelopathy.

Transverse myelitis and multiple sclerosis

These are two of the most common causes of myelopathy caused by intrinsic cord disease, and are discussed further in Chapter 22.

Vitamin B_{12} deficiency

Vitamin B_{12} deficiency may affect the myelin of the cerebrum, optic nerves, spinal cord, or peripheral nerves. The most common presentation is subacute-to-chronic myelopathy with prominent numbness and paresthesias in the hands and feet. Causes of vitamin B_{12} deficiency include vegetarianism, pernicious anemia, and gastric bypass. The diagnosis is straightforward when the serum B_{12} level is low. If the B_{12} level is more than the laboratory-defined lower limit of normal but still relatively low (e.g. <500 pg/ml), look for elevated levels of homocysteine and methylmalonic acid to diagnose subtle B_{12} deficiency.[6] Although high-dose oral and intramuscular formulations are presumably equivalent, most patients with myelopathy secondary to B_{12} deficiency should be treated with intramuscular B_{12}, starting at 1 mg daily for 1 week, 1 mg weekly for 1 month, and then 1 mg monthly thereafter.

Adrenoleukodystrophy

Adrenoleukodystrophy (ALD) is an X-linked disorder that usually causes cognitive decline, blindness, and quadriparesis in young boys. Both men and women between their second and fourth decades may develop adrenomyeloneuropathy (AMN), a milder form of the disease characterized principally by myelopathy.[7] The majority of these patients have adrenal dysfunction, and some also have cerebral involvement, which preferentially involves the parietal and occipital lobes. Nerve conduction studies characteristically show slow nerve conduction velocities reflective of demyelination. The diagnosis is established by finding elevated levels of very long chain fatty acids in the plasma. There is no cure for ALD, but affected patients may be referred for a clinical trial of Lorenzo's oil.

Metachromatic leukodystrophy

Metachromatic leukodystrophy (MLD) is an autosomal recessive disorder that presents uncommonly in adults as a painless myelopathy, spastic paraparesis, or a neuropsychiatric disorder.[8] Brain MRI usually shows symmetric, periventricular cerebral white matter changes that spare the subcortical U-fibers. Nerve conduction studies characteristically show nerve conduction velocities in the demyelinating range. The disorder is diagnosed by finding low levels of leukocyte arylsulfatase A. Unfortunately, there is no cure for MLD.

Tropical spastic paraparesis

Human T-cell leukemia virus (HTLV) is endemic to the Caribbean, Japan, and Africa. It is transmitted through sexual contact, blood transfusion, or intravenous drug use. However, fewer than 5% of patients infected with the virus develop tropical spastic paraparesis.[9] This disorder is a slowly progressive, painless myelopathy characterized by gait instability, hyperreflexia, and sphincter dysfunction. All myelopathic patients from endemic regions or with risk factors for infection with the virus should undergo serum HTLV polymerase chain reaction (PCR) testing. Although treatment of tropical spastic paraparesis is of limited benefit, diagnosis and counseling are important to prevent further transmission of the virus.

Dural arteriovenous fistula

Dural arteriovenous fistula (AVF) is an uncommon but important cause of slowly progressive, usually painless myelopathy. In general, the presentation is identical to that of other chronic myelopathies, although some patients may report that their symptoms characteristically worsen with exercise. The diagnosis is often elusive, and symptoms may progress for years before the condition is identified correctly. If dural AVF is suspected, MRI and magnetic resonance angiography (MRA) of the spine should be performed first, as they help to guide conventional angiography. Embolization of the fistula cures a minority of patients, and most will ultimately require surgical treatment.[10]

Copper-deficiency myelopathy

Copper-deficiency myelopathy, identified only recently, is characterized by slowly progressive lower extremity weakness and spasticity.[11] Patients who use excessive amounts of zinc-containing denture cream or zinc supplements (zinc competes with copper for intestinal absorption) are at risk of developing the disorder. The diagnosis is established by finding low serum copper levels. Copper supplementation may help patients with copper-deficiency myelopathy, but the response is usually modest.

Hereditary spastic paraplegia

Hereditary spastic paraplegia (HSP) is a heterogeneous group of conditions causing lower extremity weakness, spasticity and hyperreflexia.[12] It may be inherited in any fashion, although autosomal dominant forms are the most common. The diagnosis of HSP may be straightforward in patients with a suggestive family history. Simple HSP is characterized by spastic paraparesis, while complicated HSP includes additional dysfunction of other parts of the nervous system.

Spinal cord infarction

Spinal cord infarction is much less common than cerebral infarction. The two main varieties of spinal cord infarction are the anterior spinal artery syndrome and transverse spinal cord infarction. Both varieties tend to affect the mid-thoracic spine, as this is the vascular watershed territory between the upper thoracic arteries and the artery of Adamkiewicz (which enters the cord from T10–L1 and supplies the lower thoracic and lumbar regions). The typical clinical history of spinal cord infarction is sudden-onset back pain (although pain may be absent in many patients) followed by weakness and sensory loss in the trunk and legs. Because the anterior spinal artery supplies the ventral two-thirds of the cord, patients with anterior spinal artery syndrome lose motor and spinothalamic function below the level of the lesion while maintaining dorsal column sensibilities. Transverse cord infarction produces a state of spinal shock characterized by flaccid weakness, areflexia, and sphincter dysfunction.

Etiologies of spinal cord stroke include emboli that result from cardiac or aortic surgery, spinal vascular malformations, and vasculitis. Unfortunately, imaging of spinal cord stroke is not as reliable as is imaging of cerebral stroke: diffusion-weighted imaging protocols for the spine are not yet solidified, and the characteristic MRI changes (T2 hyperintensity within the cord with T1 showing evidence of cord edema) are usually not visible for several days. Treatment options for spinal cord stroke are somewhat limited. In addition to supportive care and modification of risk factors for vascular disease, the mainstays of therapy include steroids and CSF drainage. Unfortunately, there are few rigorous data to recommend any particular medical therapy.

References

1. Koes BW, Scholten RJ, Mens JM, Bouter LM. Efficacy of epidural steroid injections for low back pain and sciatica: a systematic review of randomized clinical trials. *Pain* 1995;**63**:279–288.

2. DeAngelis LM, Posner JB. *Neurologic Complications of Cancer*. Oxford: Oxford University Press; 2009.

3. Patchell RA, Tibbs PA, Regine WF, et al. Direct decompressive surgical resection in the treatment of spinal cord compression caused by metastatic cancer: a randomised trial. *Lancet* 2005;**366**:643–648.

4. Kallmes DF, Comstock BA, Heagerty PJ, et al. A randomized trial of vertebroplasty for osteoporotic spine fractures. *N Engl J Med* 2009;**361**: 569–579.

5. Buchbinder R, Osborne RH, Ebeling PR, et al. A randomized trial of vertebroplasty for painful osteoporotic vertebral fractures. *N Engl J Med* 2009; **361**:557–568.

6. Savage DG, Lindenbaum J, Stabler SP, Allen RH. Sensitivity of serum methylmalonic acid and total homocysteine determinations for diagnosing cobalamin and folate deficiencies. *Am J Med* 1994;**96**:239–246.

7. Moser HW. Adrenoleukodystrophy: phenotype, genetics, pathogenesis and therapy. *Brain* 1997; **120**:1485–1508.

8. Rauschka H, Colsch B, Baumann N, et al. Late-onset metachromatic leukodystrophy. Genotype strongly influences phenotype. *Neurology* 2006;**67**:859–863.

9. Orland JR, Engstrom J, Fridey J, et al. Prevalence and clinical features of HTLV neurologic disease in the HTLV Outcomes Study. *Neurology* 2003;**61**:1588–1594.

10. van Dijk JMC, TerBrugge KG, Willinsky RA, Farb, RI, Wallace, MC. Multidisciplinary management of spinal dural arteriovenous fistulas: clinical presentation and long-term follow-up in 49 patients. *Stroke* 2002; **33**:1578–1583.

11. Kumar N, Gross JB, Ahlskog JE. Myelopathy due to copper deficiency. *Neurology* 2003;**61**:273–274.

12. Salinas S, Proukakis C, Crosby A, Warner TT. Hereditary spastic paraplegia: clinical features and pathogenetic mechanisms. *Lancet Neurol* 2008; 7: 1127–1138.

Chapter 18

Gait disorders

Introduction

Gait disorders and falls are common in the elderly population and frequently lead to injury or hospitalization. Because gait dysfunction may be the result of pathology at any level of the neuraxis, evaluation may be quite challenging. Unlike most neurological problems, the history is usually unhelpful: the patient may say that their legs are weak, that their legs give out on them, that they feel off balance, or simply that they fall and do not know why. The examination is usually more powerful than the history in making the diagnosis. Often, you will be able to make a very accurate guess as to the cause of gait dysfunction by watching the patient walk from the waiting area to the examining room. When this is not the case, formal gait analysis, testing provocative maneuvers, and a thorough neurological examination will allow you to localize the problem.

Natural gait

Examine natural gait by having the patient walk up and down a long hallway. Everyone can identify a normal gait intuitively, but what is less intuitive is how to describe that gait in words. Formal gait analysis is a distinct field of biomechanics and neurophysiology, but for clinical purposes, examining the following seven components is sufficient to accurately characterize normal and pathological gaits:

- Posture. Does the patient stand up straight or are they hunched over? Is the patient hyperextended at the waist and neck?
- Base. Does the patient stand with their feet close together or is their base abnormally widened? When they walk, are the medial edges of their feet separated by >6 inches?
- Initiation. When they start to walk, do they do so quickly or is there some delay?
- Stride length. Does the patient appear to be taking normal-length strides or are their strides shortened?

- Stride appearance. Do the patient's feet elevate appropriately or do they just barely clear the ground? Does the patient land normally or awkwardly? Do they shuffle or slap the ground with their feet? Is there any posturing of the arms?
- Stability. Does the patient appear stable on their feet or do they constantly seem to be at risk of falling?
- Turns. Does the patient require more than two or three steps to turn 180°?

Over time, familiarity with abnormal gait patterns will become second nature (see "Abnormal gait patterns" below), but in unclear cases, breaking up gait into these seven components is an essential part of defining the problem.

Provocative maneuvers

Provocative maneuvers may be instrumental in revealing subtle abnormalities that are not detected by examination of natural gait.

Trendelenburg's sign and Gowers' sign

These are two signs of proximal muscle weakness. To test for Trendelenburg's sign, observe the patient from behind as they stand on one foot: in patients with weakness of hip stabilization, the trunk will sink to the side of the elevated leg. Gowers' sign is present when a patient needs to use their arms to rise from a seated position on the floor. It is usually sought in children with suspected muscular dystrophy. Normal healthy adults have greater difficulty performing this task, and similar information about proximal weakness may be obtained by finding that the patient is unable to rise from a chair while their arms are folded across their chest.

Heel and toe walking

Distal lower extremity weakness is an important source of gait difficulty. Walking on the toes requires integrity of the gastrocnemius–soleus complex and its innervation from the tibial nerve and S1 nerve root. Walking on the heels relies on the tibialis anterior innervated by the peroneal nerve and the L4–5 nerve roots. Due to the relatively greater length of the peroneal compared with the tibial nerve, heel walking tends to be impaired earlier than toe walking in patients with polyneuropathies.

Tandem gait

Although any cause of gait impairment may lead to difficulty with tandem gait, an inability to tandem walk is most often associated with an ataxic gait. To test tandem gait, instruct the patient to "walk a tightrope" or do the "drunk test" by placing one foot in front of the other, taking each step with the heel directly in front of the toe. Bear in mind that both older and obese patients who are otherwise neurologically normal perform this task poorly.

Stress gait

This test may be instrumental in establishing a diagnosis of early Parkinson's disease. To test stress gait, ask the patient to walk on the sides of their feet. While they are doing this, observe their hands and arms for subtle tremor or posturing indicative of extrapyramidal dysfunction.

Pull test

This test is commonly performed when an extrapyramidal disorder is suspected. Because this test poses a serious possibility of injury, perform it with caution. Instruct the patient to stand with their feet spread slightly apart and their arms abducted approximately 15° away from the trunk. Stand behind them and tell them that you will pull them and that they will need to maintain their balance. Prepare to catch the patient should they fall, and then briskly pull them backwards by the shoulders. They should require at most one step backwards to correct their balance. Sufficiently advanced Parkinson's disease may cause postural instability, and the patient will require multiple steps to correct their balance or may even fall backwards into your arms.

Romberg's sign

Rombergism reflects disorders of the proprioceptive or vestibulocerebellar systems. To test for Romberg's sign, first ask the patient to stand with their feet placed together, and make sure that they can keep their balance. Next, instruct them to close their eyes. Most patients with mild proprioceptive deficits will sway when their eyes are closed. The strict definition of a positive Romberg's sign, however, requires that the patient actually falls when this test is performed.

General neurological examination

Confirm all abnormalities detected by gait observation with a thorough neurological examination. In some cases, the general examination will disclose an explanation for gait impairment that was not uncovered by gait analysis or provocative maneuvers. Prior to concluding that the source of a patient's gait abnormality is neurological, perform musculoskeletal, ophthalmological, and peripheral vascular examinations to look for evidence of dysfunction in other organ systems that may lead to instability and falls.

Abnormal gait patterns

Frontal gait

A patient with a frontal gait disorder initiates walking with difficulty, elevates their feet minimally, and takes small, short steps. Sometimes this pattern of gait is labeled as "apraxic," a term that is more properly reserved for disorders of *learned* movement. Frontal gait disorder is often accompanied by dementia. Common causes of frontal gait disorder include the multi-infarct state and normal pressure hydrocephalus (Chapter 4).

Spastic gait

Chronic corticospinal tract lesions result in a spastic gait in which the affected leg is stiff and hyperextended. The leg is circumducted (swung out from the hip in an arc) rather than moved back and forth in the sagittal plane. Corticospinal tract lesions within the brain such as stroke, demyelinating disease, or brain tumor produce contralateral spasticity that also involves the arm. Lesions of the frontal convexity may affect the leg in isolation. Spastic gait is also the characteristic abnormality of patients with myelopathy (Chapter 15), in which case the two legs tend to be involved relatively symmetrically.

Parkinsonian gait

In early Parkinson's disease (PD), gait may be affected minimally or not at all (Chapter 13). The earliest abnormalities may be slightly reduced arm swing or asymmetric hand posturing or tremor that appear upon stress gait testing. Patients with fully developed PD are hunched over, initiate slowly, and take short strides. They turn slowly and require multiple steps to do so. Postural instability may be elicited by performing the pull test. Advanced PD may be associated with festination and freezing. Festination is a distinctive gait abnormality characterized by tiny steps, which progressively increase in velocity to the point that the patient appears to be running in place. Freezing, as its name suggests, occurs when a patient comes to a complete stop while walking and cannot seem to reinitiate their gait.

Progressive supranuclear palsy gait

Gait difficulty and frequent falls are early features of progressive supranuclear palsy (PSP) (Chapter 13). Although the natural gait is often somewhat nonspecific in its appearance, patients with PSP are classically hyperextended at the neck and trunk and fall backwards.

Ataxic gait

Gait ataxia is characterized by veering from side to side with over- and understepping of the target. Falls and injury are perhaps less frequent than might be expected, often because ataxic patients quickly realize their instability and avoid walking altogether. Gait ataxia is classically associated with peripheral and central lesions of the vestibulocerebellar system. However, patients with dorsal column or large-fiber peripheral nerve disorders account for the majority of patients with gait ataxia in clinical practice.

Waddling gait

Disorders affecting the proximal musculature, especially the hip flexors and trunk stabilizers, lead to waddling (Chapter 10). The patient is not able to elevate their legs sufficiently to clear the ground, and as a result, must shift their weight from side to side and rotate the trunk in order to make forward progress. Signs of proximal weakness that accompany waddling include Trendelenburg's sign and Gowers' sign. Common localizations of proximal muscle weakness include the muscle, neuromuscular junction, and motor neurons.

Steppage gait

Foot drop is most commonly the consequence of lesions of the motor neurons, L4 or L5 nerve roots, or peroneal nerve (Chapter 11). In order for the foot to clear the ground, a patient with dorsiflexion weakness lifts their hip and knee in an exaggerated fashion, leading to the high step that lends this gait abnormality its name. The foot strikes the ground heavily and sometimes it is the slapping sound as the patient walks rather than the appearance of foot drop that is most helpful in making the diagnosis. Steppage may be corrected with an ankle foot orthosis to stabilize the ankle joint and allow normal foot elevation.

Antalgic gait

Any cause of lower extremity pain may produce an antalgic gait in which the patient steps gingerly on the affected side while placing the bulk of their weight on the unaffected leg. Careful musculoskeletal and neurological assessment is needed to separate an antalgic gait from one caused by neurological dysfunction. Antalgic gait improves if the source of pain is identified and treated appropriately.

Psychogenic gait

Gait dysfunction may be the sole manifestation of malingering or conversion disorder. While the veering, unsteady, often bizarre gait seen in many patients with psychogenic gait disorders most closely resembles ataxia, psychogenic gait may mimic any abnormal pattern. Clues to the presence of a psychogenic gait disorder include the absence of injury during falls, fluctuating severity and semiology over time, and normal ambulation when the patient thinks that they are not being observed. The diagnosis of a psychogenic gait disorder may be made, however, only after organic disease is exhaustively excluded. Tactful psychiatric evaluation and treatment is the most effective treatment for psychogenic gait disorders.

Multifactorial gait disorder

It may be difficult or impossible to isolate the source of gait dysfunction to a single site in the nervous system. Patients with more than one contributor, by definition, have a multifactorial gait disorder. This condition is particularly common in the elderly, in whom osteoarthritis, parkinsonism, cervical myelopathy, and polyneuropathy are common and frequently coexist. For patients with multifactorial gait disorder, examination of the individual components of the nervous system is generally more helpful than gait analysis. Although they may derive modest benefit from physical therapy, many patients with multifactorial gait disorder require canes, walkers, or motorized scooters.

General recommendations for patients with frequent falls

Obviously, any reversible neurological causes of frequent falls should be identified and treated. In many cases this is not possible, and preventive therapy becomes the mainstay of treatment. Appropriate pain treatment and correction of orthopedic infirmities may eliminate some falls or help restore normal ambulation. Counsel patients to wear sensible shoes and avoid long pant legs and dresses, which may lead to tripping. Home safety evaluation is invaluable in reducing the risk of falls, as it often uncovers easily correctable fall precipitants including excessive clutter, poorly placed rugs, slippery surfaces, and uneven floors. Many patients ultimately require walking sticks, canes, walkers, or wheelchairs to avoid frequent falls. These should be prescribed in conjunction with a physical therapist or physiatrist.

Chapter 19

Headache and facial pain

History

Headache is among the most common complaints evaluated by primary care physicians and neurologists. Although all neurological diagnoses are ultimately established through a carefully taken history, this is true for no condition more than headache. A thorough review of the following factors usually helps to establish the diagnosis.

Epidemiology

Patient age, gender, and medical history may suggest specific headache etiologies in some instances. While the description of the actual events is more important than any single epidemiological factor, the following associations between patient population and headache etiology are clinically useful:

- Patients older than 55 are at risk for temporal arteritis.
- Young women are the population that is most likely to have migraines.
- Middle-aged men are susceptible to cluster headaches.
- Obese young and middle-aged women are the patients most likely to have pseudotumor cerebri.
- Puerperal women and those with hypercoagulable states are at greatest risk for cerebral venous sinus thrombosis.

Location

Because most headaches are frontal or holocranial, location may not be particularly helpful in establishing headache etiology. Temporal and parietal headaches are also fairly nonspecific. Occipital or nuchal headaches are most commonly tension headaches or occipital neuralgia. Common causes of unilateral retro-orbital headaches include migraine, cluster headaches, and indomethacin-responsive headaches.

Character

Headache character is frequently the most helpful factor in classifying it. Dullness and squeezing are typical features of tension headaches, but are also common in many other headache types, including those caused by dangerous conditions such as brain tumors, temporal arteritis, and pseudotumor cerebri. Throbbing and pulsation are the typical qualities of migraines and other vascular headaches. Sharp, stabbing pain is most typical of cluster headaches and indomethacin-responsive headaches.

Rapidity of onset

Most headaches develop over minutes to hours. Sudden-onset, severe headaches require immediate attention, as they often represent life-threatening neurological emergencies such as subarachnoid hemorrhage, carotid artery dissection, and pituitary apoplexy.

Duration

Headache duration often has limited value in establishing a diagnosis, as most headaches can last for half an hour at a time or for days on end. Important exceptions to this rule include cluster headaches and indomethacin-responsive headaches, which are very brief, usually lasting from just a few seconds to several minutes at a time. Occipital neuralgia may last for only seconds at a time. Although it may not help to classify the type of headache, duration is often important to establish headache severity and to determine the need for treatment.

Diurnal variation

Most headaches, including tension headaches and migraines, develop in the late morning or early afternoon. Exceptions include cluster headaches and headaches caused by increased intracranial pressure, which are usually worse at night and may awaken a patient from sleep.

Associated symptoms

Aura

Symptoms that accompany headaches are often the ones that help to clinch the diagnosis. This is perhaps most true for migraines, in which the headache itself may be somewhat nonspecific, and the diagnosis rests on the presence of an aura or other accompanying features. An aura is a neurological symptom that begins several minutes prior to migraine onset and most commonly takes the form of visual hallucinations of flashing lights, lightning strikes, starburst patterns, or distortions in size such as micropsia and macropsia. Auras are not restricted to vision, and may have sensorimotor manifestations including tingling, weakness, and numbness. Aura symptoms characteristically spread over 15–20 minutes, which distinguishes them from stroke (sudden-onset symptoms) and seizure (symptoms that develop over seconds).

Other neurological symptoms

Sudden unilateral or sequential visual loss is a worrisome symptom that suggests temporal arteritis. Seizures or other rapidly developing, fixed neurological signs point to serious pathologies including intracranial hemorrhage, mass lesions, venous sinus thrombosis, encephalitis, or hypertensive encephalopathy.

Systemic symptoms

Nausea, vomiting, photophobia, and phonophobia frequently accompany migraine. Conjunctival injection, lacrimation, and rhinorrhea are features of both cluster and indomethacin-responsive headaches. Visual loss, scalp tenderness, jaw claudication (pain with chewing), low-grade fever, and proximal muscle tenderness are all well-known systemic symptoms of temporal arteritis.

Exacerbating factors

High stress levels worsen almost all headaches. Actions that strain the neck including excessive head turning, staring at a computer screen for prolonged periods, and even sleeping in the wrong position tend to precipitate tension headaches. Not eating, poor sleep, excessive caffeine or caffeine withdrawal, the menstrual period, chocolate, cheese, and red wine all exacerbate migraine headaches. Lying flat and sleeping worsen headaches due to increased intracranial pressure, while standing precipitates or worsens low-pressure headaches secondary to spontaneous intracranial hypotension or lumbar puncture.

Alleviating factors

Other than medications, patients describe a variety of different factors that help to alleviate their headaches. Rest in a quiet, dark room improves migraines. Loosening a tight necktie, massage, or applying heat often helps tension headaches. Lying down improves low-pressure headaches, while standing up improves headaches due to increased intracranial pressure.

Frequency

With the exception of cluster headache in which multiple episodes of headache occur within a span of a few weeks or months, headache frequency is not very helpful in establishing a specific diagnosis. It may, however, be important in determining which patients require only symptomatic treatment and which will need prophylactic treatment. If there is any doubt about the actual headache frequency, instruct the patient to keep a headache diary.

Severity and disability level

While severity and disability level do not help to classify headaches accurately, they are important to determine appropriate treatment. Although grading headache severity on a scale of 1 to 10 is often used in practice, this rating system is frequently unhelpful, as each patient has their own pain "nocistat" that reflects numerous psychosocial factors. One rule of thumb is that a patient who reports that they have a high pain tolerance almost never does. While I do not want to dismiss numeric rating scales completely, the best way to establish pain severity is to ask the patient whether they ever miss work or school because of their headaches. Frequent interference with daily commitments essentially mandates treatment.

Prior evaluation and treatment

Many patients undergo neuroimaging or other laboratory studies prior to neurological consultation, and it is obviously necessary to review these studies before determining the need for additional ones. Patients usually try to treat their headaches with over-the-counter medications such as acetaminophen, ibuprofen, and naproxen. Primary care physicians often prescribe triptans for migraine patients before obtaining a neurologist's assistance, and some even feel comfortable prescribing a prophylactic agent such as propranolol, amitriptyline, or topiramate. Because many patients who seek neurological attention for headache management have refractory headaches, it is important to keep an updated log containing a patient's response to and tolerance of all medications.

Dangerous headaches

Although most headaches are benign and may be managed safely in the outpatient setting, some headaches reflect dangerous and sometimes life-threatening conditions. Headache red flags include sudden onset, fixed neurological symptoms, seizures, and change in headache character. Headaches in patients with known cancer or immunosuppression are also worrisome. Patients older than 55 with new-onset headache are at risk for temporal arteritis. Dangerous headaches may be divided into sudden-onset or "thunderclap" headaches and chronic headaches.

Sudden-onset dangerous headache syndromes

Subarachnoid hemorrhage

Subarachnoid hemorrhage (SAH) due to aneurysmal rupture is among the most serious of neurological emergencies. The concept that "the worst headache of my life" and SAH headache are synonymous is widely known but slightly misleading. Every person will eventually have the worst headache of their life, and SAH will be the cause in only a small fraction.[1] While SAH headaches are usually extremely severe, it is their rapid onset rather than their intensity that defines them. Subarachnoid hemorrhage headache builds to a climax in just a few seconds, and is sufficiently jarring to stop the patient in their tracks. Vomiting and stiff neck often accompany the headache, and in many cases, seizure and loss of consciousness occur at onset. Some patients may have a sentinel headache due to leakage of a small amount of blood from the responsible aneurysm and preceding the SAH by up to 2 weeks. The exact incidence of sentinel headache is unknown, but may be as high as 40%.[2]

Urgent and thorough evaluation is necessary for all patients with suspected SAH. Noncontrast head CT, the first diagnostic test in evaluating potential SAH, is extremely powerful in detecting acute subarachnoid blood (Figure 19.1), but the likelihood of finding subarachnoid blood after SAH decreases with time[3,4]:

- 95% between 0 and 1 days after rupture
- 90% between 1 and 2 days after rupture

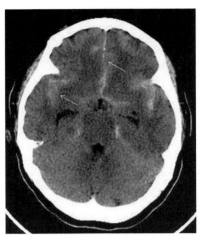

Figure 19.1 Noncontrast head CT demonstrating subarachnoid hemorrhage (arrows).

- 85% at 5 days after rupture
- 50% at 1 week after rupture
- 30% at 2 weeks after rupture
- almost zero at any time after 3 weeks

Although the sensitivity of a CT scan is very high in the first few hours after SAH, the penalty for missing the diagnosis is extreme. Thus, all patients with suspected SAH and negative CT scans should undergo lumbar puncture to look for subarachnoid blood. Visual inspection of the CSF may be sufficient to diagnose SAH, but in some cases, it may be difficult to differentiate between blood due to a traumatic lumbar puncture and SAH. The best way to distinguish between SAH and a traumatic tap is by using spectrophotometry to find bilirubin reflective of hemolysis within the CSF.[5]

Any patient with evidence of aneurysmal SAH should undergo conventional angiography, as both magnetic resonance angiography (MRA) and computed tomography angiography (CTA) have limited sensitivities to detect aneurysms smaller than 5 mm.[6] Patients with confirmed subarachnoid hemorrhage should be evaluated by a neurosurgeon for possible surgical clipping or endovascular coiling of the responsible aneurysm. Because aneurysmal SAH is principally a neurosurgical disease, it will not be discussed further here. The interested reader is referred to the American Heart Association's article on *Guidelines for the management of aneurysmal subarachnoid hemorrhage*.[6]

Box 19.1 Unruptured intracranial aneurysms

Intracranial aneurysms most commonly come to clinical attention when they rupture, resulting in SAH. Unruptured aneurysms are almost always asymptomatic and are noted when neuroimaging is performed to evaluate headache, memory loss, or another vague neurological complaint. The first step to determine the best course of action is to understand the chance of aneurysmal rupture. The two main factors that determine this probability are the size and location of the aneurysm. Data on the 5-year risk for aneurysmal rupture from the International Study of Unruptured Intracranial Aneurysms (ISUIA) are shown below.[7]

This risk for aneurysmal rupture must be weighed against the risk for surgical or endovascular interventions. Based again on data from the ISUIA, the 1-year risk for death or poor neurological outcome is approximately 13% in patients undergoing open surgical clipping and 9% in patients undergoing endovascular coiling.[7] As might be predicted, older age, larger aneurysm size, and posterior circulation location are all associated with a greater likelihood of poor outcome. Ultimately the decision to intervene on an unruptured intracranial aneurysm must be made on an individual basis after careful discussion with the patient and neurosurgeon. The patients with the most obvious benefit from intervention are younger patients with aneurysms between 7 and 24 mm in diameter. Patients with aneurysms smaller than 7 mm in diameter or asymptomatic intracavernous aneurysms should not undergo intervention.

Aneurysm location	<7 mm in diameter	7–12 mm in diameter	13–24 mm in diameter	>24 mm in diameter
Anterior (carotid) circulation	0%	2.6%	14.5%	40%
Posterior (vertebrobasilar) circulation	2.5%	14.5%	18.4%	50%
Intracavernous carotid artery	0%	0%	3.0%	6.4%

Carotid artery dissection

Dissection of the cervical carotid artery may produce a sudden-onset, severe headache. Trauma, especially that caused by vigorous exercise, yoga, or chiropractic manipulation, is commonly identified as the precipitant. The headache of carotid dissection is typically unilateral, throbbing, and retrobulbar, and may therefore be misdiagnosed as migraine. When accompanied by ipsilateral Horner's syndrome (due to involvement of the oculosympathetic fibers, which ascend into the skull with the internal carotid artery), it may be misdiagnosed as cluster headache. The diagnosis is confirmed with CTA or MRA of the neck. The most important problem posed by carotid artery dissection is obviously not the headache, but rather the possibility of embolic stroke: thrombus at the dissection site is fertile ground for small clots, which are thrown distally into the anterior circulation. Treatment therefore must focus on preventing such emboli. Although there is no clear difference in stroke prevention between anticoagulation or antiplatelet therapy (meta-analysis of multiple nonrandomized studies showed an approximate embolic stroke risk with either therapy of 2%), most stroke specialists choose short-term anticoagulation to prevent distal embolization.[8]

Pituitary apoplexy

Pituitary apoplexy occurs most often when a rapidly growing pituitary adenoma outstrips its vascular supply, leading to infarction of the pituitary gland. The headache of pituitary apoplexy is sudden in onset and resembles that of SAH. Neurological signs that accompany pituitary apoplexy include bitemporal hemianopsia due to compression of the optic chiasm and ophthalmoplegia due to involvement of the ocular motor nerves in the adjacent cavernous sinus. The most urgent problem facing a patient with pituitary apoplexy, however, is hypotension, which results from the acute loss of adrenocorticotropic hormone. Treat patients with suspected pituitary apoplexy with dexamethasone (4 mg IV) to prevent adrenal insufficiency, and intravenous fluid boluses to maintain adequate blood pressure. Definitive management of pituitary apoplexy requires the assistance of an endocrinologist and possibly a neurosurgeon.

Migraine

Of the sudden-onset, severe headaches that bring patients to the emergency room, at most 25% are actually secondary to subarachnoid hemorrhage.[9] Although migraine likely accounts for the majority of sudden-onset, severe headaches, it should be considered a diagnosis of exclusion.

Subacute and chronic dangerous headache syndromes

Temporal arteritis

The headache of temporal arteritis may have fairly nonspecific features, and therefore masquerade as a more benign disorder such as migraine or tension headache. Temporal arteritis is exclusively a disease of patients older than 55. Despite its name, the headaches do not occur exclusively in a temporal distribution. Clues to the diagnosis include monocular visual loss, jaw claudication, scalp tenderness, and fever. Polymyalgia rheumatica, characterized by pain in the shoulders and hips, frequently accompanies temporal arteritis. Firmness, tenderness, and induration of the superficial temporal arteries are classical but not universal physical examination findings. Because visual loss is the principal danger of temporal arteritis, it is discussed further in Chapter 5.

Cerebral venous sinus thrombosis

Cerebral venous sinus thrombosis (CVST) produces a variety of signs and symptoms including headache, seizures, encephalopathy, and venous strokes. The condition often takes several weeks to develop, and in its earliest stages, a nonspecific headache that resembles migraine or tension headache may be the only problem. Women in the puerperium and those who use oral contraceptives are at increased risk for cerebral venous sinus thrombosis. Sepsis, malignancy, dehydration and hypercoagulable states are other important risk factors. Neurological examination may be entirely normal, may show an encephalopathy, or may show focal signs that reflect a venous stroke. Contralateral leg weakness due to superior sagittal sinus thrombosis is particularly suggestive of stroke due to CVST. Neuroimaging of CVST shows a wide variety of abnormalities. The best known (although often absent) of these is the positive delta sign on contrast-enhanced CT scan, which indicates collateral channels surrounding a torcular thrombus. A CT scan may also show hemorrhagic infarction or cerebral edema. In milder cases, the diagnosis is made only with the aid of magnetic resonance venography (MRV). Although the quality of the evidence guiding CVST treatment is limited, anticoagulation likely reduces morbidity and mortality.[10] My preference is to treat patients with heparin to achieve a goal

partial thromboplastin time (PTT) of 60–80 seconds in the acute setting, and transition to warfarin with a goal international normalized ratio (INR) of 2–3 for 3–6 months after diagnosis. Serious neurological problems that may result from CVST include increased intracranial pressure (Chapter 2), seizure (Chapter 20), and stroke (Chapter 21).

Meningitis

Bacterial and viral meningitis are potentially serious neurological emergencies characterized by fever and sometimes by headache and stiff neck. Headache may be the most prominent or a solitary symptom in immunocompromised patients. Further evaluation and treatment of meningitis is discussed in Chapter 1.

Headache secondary to mass lesions

Headaches from intracranial masses are classically worse while recumbent, may awaken the patient in the middle of the night, and may be associated with focal neurological signs or seizures. In clinical practice, however, these features are actually uncommon, as most patients with brain tumors (and other mass lesions) have headaches that resemble tension headaches.[11] Evaluation of intracranial mass lesions is discussed further in Chapter 23.

Pseudotumor cerebri (idiopathic intracranial hypertension)

Pseudotumor cerebri is a syndrome of uncertain etiology characterized by headache and visual loss. Because it is widely known that young, obese women are the most commonly affected population, the diagnosis is often missed in other groups. Precipitants of pseudotumor other than obesity include excess vitamin A, lithium, tetracyclines, and both steroid administration and withdrawal. The headaches of pseudotumor cerebri are fairly nonspecific and often resemble tension headaches. In the earliest stages of disease, visual symptoms may be limited to occasional blurriness or transient orthostatic visual loss. As pseudotumor cerebri progresses, visual symptoms become more constant, and blindness may occur if increased intracranial pressure goes untreated. Four diagnostic studies help to confirm the presence of pseudotumor cerebri:

1. CT scan or MRI of the brain to exclude the possibility of true tumor or another cause of increased intracranial pressure.
2. Lumbar puncture showing an opening pressure of at least 20 cmH$_2$O.

3. Dilated funduscopic examination to look for papilledema.
4. Formal perimetry to determine the exact extent of visual field loss.

Obviously, the first step in treating pseudotumor cerebri is to discontinue any potentially responsible medications. Although weight loss may help reverse many of the symptoms of pseudotumor, most patients are not able to lose the weight necessary to result in a meaningful improvement. The mainstay of medical treatment is acetazolamide, administered at doses ranging from 250 mg bid to 1000 mg bid. Perioral and acral paresthesias may be dose-limiting side effects of this medication. If acetazolamide is not effective, the next line of treatment is serial lumbar punctures, which are obviously impractical for doctor and patient alike. If serial lumbar punctures provide consistent relief, then consider ventriculoperitoneal shunting as a more permanent method to remove CSF and lower intracranial pressure. Patients with rapidly progressive visual loss may need optic nerve sheath defenestration to prevent complete blindness.

Hypertensive encephalopathy

Despite popular belief, essential hypertension does not lead to headaches. Hypertensive encephalopathy (a cause of posterior reversible encephalopathy syndrome or PRES, Chapter 1), however, occurs in patients with either very high blood pressure or rapid increases in blood pressure. In addition to headaches, patients with hypertensive encephalopathy may be confused, seize, lose their vision, or have essentially any focal neurological finding. Hypertensive encephalopathy is frequently accompanied by other problems related to malignant hypertension including angina, pulmonary edema, and renal failure. It is imperative to rapidly lower the blood pressure in patients with hypertensive encephalopathy in order to prevent irreversible neurological and systemic damage.

"Benign" headaches

Migraine headache

Many patients describe any severe headache as a migraine, even if they actually have tension or cluster headaches. It is, therefore, essential to ask the patient what they mean by migraine and ensure that their self-diagnosis is correct. In its most typical form, migraine is characterized by a throbbing, unilateral headache

associated with nausea, vomiting, photophobia, and phonophobia. It is common but not universal for migraineurs to describe a variety of aura symptoms including visual loss, scintillating scotoma, tingling in the extremities, and even weakness resembling stroke. Most patients with migraine experience their first attacks during their teens or early 20s. The disorder is three times as common in women as it is in men. Migraines do not usually begin in patients over the age of 50, and other causes of headache should be excluded in this patient population before attributing their headaches to migraines. The diagnosis is ultimately made on clinical grounds, with neuroimaging studies being used mainly to exclude other more serious conditions.

The first step in treating migraines is lifestyle modification. Ask the patient about migraine precipitants such as sleep deprivation, stress, not eating, menstruation, and foods such as chocolate, cheese, caffeine, and red wine. A headache diary is often helpful to keep track of these exposures and the consequent migraine frequency. Lifestyle modifications may reduce headache frequency considerably or even cure the headaches in a very small minority. Most patients with migraines respond to an over-the-counter abortive medication such as acetaminophen, ibuprofen, or naproxen, and never come to the attention of a neurologist. The usual first-line agent in patients who do not respond to one of these medications is a triptan (serotonin 1B/1D agonist). These agents are effective in aborting migraines if given early enough in the course of an attack: ideally, a patient should take the triptan within 30 minutes of developing a headache, but they may still benefit up to 3 hours after headache onset. The main side effects of triptans include chest pain, flushing, nausea, and grogginess. These medications should be avoided in patients with cardiovascular or cerebrovascular disease and in those who are taking monoamine oxidase inhibitors. Table 19.1 gives a brief summary of the triptans. There is no convincing evidence that one triptan is superior to another. Sumatriptan (20 mg) and zolmitriptan (5 mg) are both available in inhaled formats, which makes them particularly useful for patients with disabling nausea. Sumatriptan is also available in an injectable (6 mg) formulation. It is important to monitor triptan use, as excessive intake may precipitate chronic daily headaches.

Some patients will have migraines of such frequency and severity that they will require prophylactic medication. In general, consider prophylactic medications for patients with more than three migraines a month or

Table 19.1 Triptans

Triptan	Starting dose	Maximum daily dose
Almotriptan	6.25 mg	25 mg
Eletriptan	20 mg	80 mg
Frovatriptan	2.5 mg	7.5 mg
Naratriptan	2.5 mg	5 mg
Rizatriptan	5 mg	30 mg
Sumatriptan	25 mg	200 mg
Zolmitriptan	2.5 mg	10 mg

Table 19.2 Migraine prophylactic agents

Agent	Starting dose	Side effects
Amitryptiline	10 mg qhs	Fatigue, dry mouth, cardiac arrhythmia
Gabapentin	100 mg tid	Minimal beyond sedation and sometimes dizziness
Mirtazapine	30 mg	Weight gain
Propranolol	40 mg qd	Orthostatic hypotension, bradycardia, fatigue, depression
Riboflavin	400 mg qd	Urinary discoloration
Topiramate	25 mg qhs	Weight loss, anomia, nephrolithiasis, acral paresthesias
Valproic acid	250 mg bid	Tremor, thrombocytopenia, pancreatitis, hyperammonemia, weight gain, hair loss
Verapamil	120 mg qd	Bradycardia, hypotension

for patients with attacks that interfere with the patient's ability to work or to attend school. Table 19.2 contains a summary of some of the commonly used migraine prophylactic agents.

Tension headache

Tension headaches are the most common type of headache. They are characterized by bifrontal, holocranial, nuchal, or occipital squeezing or tightness. Severe tension headaches may be accompanied by nausea and vomiting, symptoms that are more typical of migraines. Precipitants include neck strain, sitting still for a prolonged time, and sleeping in an awkward position. While most tension headaches respond to treatment with mild analgesics such as acetaminophen or ibuprofen, those that are severe enough to cause a patient to seek neurological attention are usually refractory to these medications. Heat application and stretching exercises may help. Muscle relaxants such as diazepam (2–5 mg tid), metaxalone (400–800 mg bid), baclofen (10–40 mg bid), or cyclobenzaprine (5–10 mg tid) are also often helpful. For patients with refractory tension headaches, trigger point injections in the cervical paraspinal muscles, occipital muscles, and trapezii may relieve pain.

Cluster headaches

The typical cluster headache patient is a middle-aged man who is awakened from sleep by a severe, retrobulbar headache. The headache lasts for seconds to minutes at a time and is associated with conjunctival injection, tearing, and rhinorrhea. Ipsilateral Horner's syndrome is a frequent finding. Cluster headaches derive their name from the fact that they occur in clusters that occur night after night for several weeks. The differential diagnosis of cluster headaches includes carotid artery dissection, chronic paroxysmal hemicrania, and sometimes subarachnoid or intraparenchymal hemorrhage. In most cases, the diagnosis may be made by the clinical features alone. Acute treatment options for cluster headaches include inhaled 100% oxygen, triptans (see above), or intranasal lidocaine (1 ml 4% solution). The two main prophylactic agents are verapamil (120–240 mg qd) and lithium (300 mg bid, titrated to 600 mg bid with a goal plasma level between 0.6 and 1.2 mmol/l). Be cautious when prescribing lithium, as it produces a number of side effects including tremor, ataxia, hyperthyroidism and renal failure.

Chronic paroxysmal hemicrania

Chronic paroxysmal hemicrania (CPH) is characterized by brief, episodic unilateral headaches, which are accompanied by conjunctival injection, tearing, and rhinorrhea. It is most frequent in young women, and is sometimes confused with migraine or cluster headaches. It is distinguished from other forms of headache by its exquisite sensitivity to indomethacin at doses of 25–100 mg bid–tid.

Visual strain headaches

Most headaches due to disease of the eye and its supporting structures come to the attention of ophthalmologists rather than neurologists. Visual strain headaches are mentioned here because they are exceedingly common and may be confused with primary headache disorders. Following excessive reading, television watching, or computer work, patients note an aching or burning pain behind the eyes accompanied by ocular fatigue and sometimes by conjunctival injection. The pain often radiates into the forehead or temples. Correction of refractive errors often helps to reduce the frequency and severity of these headaches.

Medication-related headache

Headache is listed as a side effect in the product inserts of almost every medication. Common offenders include beta-blockers, cyclosporine, dipyridamole, isotretinoin, and vasodilators such as nitroglycerin. It is often difficult to distinguish between headaches caused by medication and those that are caused by a primary headache disorder. A brief trial of withdrawing the presumed precipitant may be warranted.

Postlumbar puncture headaches

Severe headaches affect approximately 20–30% of patients following lumbar puncture, and are caused by persistent leakage of CSF through the puncture site. The headaches characteristically develop between 1 and 2 days after the lumbar puncture is performed, involve the frontal or occipital regions bilaterally, appear within seconds of assuming an upright position, and are relieved (often completely) by lying flat. The first step in treating these headaches is to instruct the patient to lie flat for 24 hours and drink caffeinated, carbonated beverages. If symptoms do not resolve, try the combination of caffeine/butalbital/acetaminophen for no more than 72 hours, as chronic use of this medication may actually worsen headaches. For patients who do not respond to conservative therapy, an epidural blood patch, which promotes sealing of the dural tear, is almost always effective.

Spontaneous intracranial hypotension

Spontaneous intracranial hypotension (SIH) is caused, in most cases, by a traumatic dural tear with resulting spinal fluid leakage.[12] The characteristic holocranial or occipital headache develops suddenly and occurs when the patient is upright, and improves or resolves

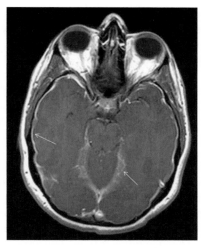

Figure 19.2 Axial fluid attenuation inversion recovery (FLAIR) MRI showing diffuse meningeal enhancement in a patient with spontaneous intracranial hypotension (arrows).

completely when they lie flat. The patient may report vertigo and diplopia, and some patients develop sixth-nerve palsies. Neuroimaging findings include sagging of the cerebellar tonsils and diffuse pachymeningeal enhancement (Figure 19.2). Treatment of SIH includes aggressive hydration, caffeine, and epidural blood patches. In some cases, multiple epidural blood patches are needed. Patients with refractory symptoms should undergo CT myelography for the purpose of localizing the leak and planning surgical closure.

Occipital neuralgia

Occipital neuralgia is an uncommon disorder characterized by brief, intermittent, stabbing pains that radiate from the nuchal region into the occipital region. Attacks are generally unilateral, may occur many times per day, and may be quite disabling. Physical examination is usually normal, and the diagnosis rests on the clinical history. Occipital nerve blocks may be used for both diagnostic and therapeutic purposes.[13] Medications used for trigeminal neuralgia (see below) may help in some cases. MRI of the upper cervical spine (sensory fibers over the occiput are derived from the C2 and C3 nerve roots) and brain is indicated for patients who do not improve with nerve blocks, who have continuous rather than intermittent symptoms, and who have fixed sensory loss.

Headache in pregnancy

Pregnant women may develop headaches that range in severity from entirely benign to malignant and life-threatening. Uncommon but dangerous causes of headache that may develop during pregnancy include cerebral venous sinus thrombosis (see above), eclampsia (Chapter 20), and pituitary apoplexy (see above). As a rule of thumb, any woman without a prior history of headaches should undergo MRI of the brain, especially if the headaches are associated with neurological findings. The two most common headache types in pregnancy are migraines (which tend to improve in frequency and severity during pregnancy) and tension headaches (which often worsen during pregnancy). In general, it is best to avoid medications as much as possible during pregnancy. Acetaminophen (650–1000 mg) or local ice pack application are the most benign treatments, and should be tried first. For women who do not respond to these conservative approaches, use low doses of codeine (30–60 mg) or short courses of NSAIDs. Avoid NSAIDs in the late part of the third trimester, as they may lead to premature closure of the ductus arteriosus. Stronger opioids should be used sparingly, as they pose a risk for neonatal withdrawal. Avoid triptans and dihydroergotamine altogether, as these medications may cause placental vasoconstriction. Consider propranolol or nortryptiline for women who require migraine prophylaxis.

Status migrainosus

Status migrainosus is defined as migraine that lasts continuously for >72 hours.[14] It seldom occurs as the first manifestation of migraine, and it usually does not affect patients with mild, infrequent headaches. Precipitants include noncompliance with prophylactic medications, stress, poor sleep, and head trauma. Treating status migrainosus is often a difficult task, and it is important to be patient when approaching this problem. Depending on the severity of symptoms, some or all of the following interventions may be necessary:

1. Basic supportive care. Place the patient in a dark, quiet room and obtain intravenous access to administer medications and replace fluids. Because patients with status migrainosus are usually bed bound, provide prophylaxis against deep venous thrombosis as needed.
2. Antiemetic agents. It is important to control the severe nausea and vomiting that often accompany status migrainosus. Commonly prescribed antiemetics include:
   - Promethazine 25–50 mg IV q6h
   - Prochlorperazine 5–10 mg IV q6h or 25 mg PR q6h
   - Ondansetron 4–8 mg IV q6h

3. Acute pain control.
   - Ketorolac (15–30 mg IV q6–8h) is a powerful nonsteroidal anti-inflammatory drug (NSAID) that is often effective in patients with status migrainosus. It may be used safely for only 48–72 hours because prolonged use frequently leads to gastrointestinal ulceration.
   - Intravenous narcotics are another option for acute pain treatment. Battles between migraineur and doctor over narcotic selection and dosage are unfortunately frequent. Fast-acting, short-lasting agents such as morphine, oxycodone, and hydromorphone must be used sparingly in favor of longer-acting formulations. Patient-controlled anesthesia may be necessary in patients in whom oral sustained-release morphine or oxycodone prove ineffective or intolerable.
4. Migraine abortive agents. Triptans are ineffective by the time a patient meets the operational definition for status migrainosus. Dihydroergotamine (1 mg IV), however, is a vasoconstrictor and serotonin 1B/1D agonist that may help abort migraine symptoms, even after 72 hours of symptoms.
5. Sleep aids. In many cases, the best way to break an acute migraine attack is with sleep. Diazepam (5–10 mg PO or IV) is often effective as a sleep aid and in helping to resolve status migrainosus.
6. Steroids. Short courses of prednisone (60 mg PO qd) or dexamethasone (10 mg IV) are often employed for status migrainosus, although there is little evidence to suggest that they are effective.
7. Other therapies. Conventional medical treatment often fails to resolve status migrainosus completely. Additional options for this scenario include trigger point injections, lidocaine or ketamine infusions, biofeedback, acupuncture, and psychiatric evaluation.

Once an attack of status migrainosus is under control, the patient must be transitioned to a regimen that is appropriate for outpatient use. Switch to long-acting orally administered pain relievers and discontinue antiemetics, narcotics, and sleeping aids as tolerated. Prophylactic regimens must be augmented to prevent recurrence of status migrainosus.

Chronic daily headache

Chronic daily headache (CDH) is a syndrome characterized by headaches that occur at least 15 days/

month and last for at least 4 hours/day.[15] The headaches in patients with CDH are usually a mix of migraines and tension headaches. Medication overuse, especially of narcotics, caffeine-containing medications, barbiturates, and triptans, plays an important role in the development of CDH. Psychiatric factors including depression, personality disorders, and malingering are other important contributors. Unfortunately, treating CDH is extremely challenging, and any approach that I offer is better in theory than in practice. First, limit habit-forming analgesics as much as possible, as these only worsen symptoms over time. Use NSAIDs, or, if absolutely required, longer-acting narcotics such as methadone or fentanyl for pain relief. Periodic lidocaine or ketamine infusions may also help. Although changing migraine and tension headache prophylactic regimens is usually of limited benefit, do not discard it as a futile approach. Alternative therapies including biofeedback, acupuncture, and massage are effective for some patients. Finally, it is essential to address any important psychosocial factors such as depression, domestic abuse, and malingering. Although curing CDH is rare, a multidisciplinary approach may help to restore the patient back to a reasonable functional level.

Facial pain

Trigeminal neuralgia

Trigeminal neuralgia, as its name suggests, is characterized by pain in the distribution of the trigeminal nerve, most commonly in its maxillary and mandibular divisions. Patients describe sudden attacks of intense burning or electrical pain that shoot into the face and last for a few seconds at a time. In between the attacks of neuralgia, patients may note a residual aching pain in the trigeminal distribution. Almost all patients have multiple attacks per day. Patients with trigeminal neuralgia are characteristically able to trigger their pain by touching the cheek or jaw, shaving, brushing their teeth, or eating.

The presumed cause of trigeminal neuralgia is microvascular compression of the trigeminal nerve as it enters the pons. Mass lesions or demyelinating lesions of the pons produce trigeminal neuropathy, which is distinguished from simple trigeminal neuralgia by accompanying sensory loss in the trigeminal nerve distribution. Patients with facial numbness, therefore, should undergo MRI with thin cuts through

the brainstem and along the course of the trigeminal nerve. It may also be worthwhile considering MRI in patients younger than 40 in order to exclude the possibility of multiple sclerosis.

Anticonvulsants and antidepressants are the mainstays of medical treatment for trigeminal neuralgia. The agent of first choice is carbamazepine, typically started at a dose of 200 mg bid and increased up to 600 mg bid as needed. Alternatives include:

- phenytoin 100 mg tid
- gabapentin 300 mg tid titrated up to 1200 mg tid
- baclofen 10 mg tid titrated up to 20 mg tid
- oxcarbazepine 300 mg bid titrated up to 900 mg bid
- pregabalin 75 mg bid titrated up to 150 mg bid

Because trigeminal neuralgia pain is intense and disabling (it may precipitate suicide attempts in rare cases), it is important to switch medications quickly if it does not appear that the first agent chosen is working. Do not hesitate to prescribe narcotics in the acute stage of trigeminal neuralgia.

Unfortunately, some patients do not respond to medical treatment. Consider radiofrequency ablation (RFA) or gamma knife radiosurgery for patients with refractory symptoms. The appropriate choice and optimal timing of referral for one of these procedures depends somewhat on personal experience, and it is not clear whether there is any real difference between them.[16] My practice is to refer patients for RFA or gamma knife radiosurgery after unsuccessful trials of two first-line medications. I reserve microvascular decompression for patients with persistent symptoms after failing one of the less invasive procedures. For patients who do not respond to even microvascular decompression, peripheral neurectomy of the affected branch of the trigeminal nerve is an option of last resort, as it results in permanent facial numbness and may do little to improve symptoms.

Glossopharyngeal neuralgia

Glossopharyngeal neuralgia is characterized by lancinating pain affecting the larynx, tonsil, tongue, and ear. Pain is often triggered by chewing, swallowing, touching the ear, or yawning. Physical examination is usually normal, although the gag reflex and palatal elevation may be reduced ipsilateral to the lesion. All patients with glossopharyngeal neuralgia should undergo MRI with thin cuts through the brainstem to look for a responsible lesion in the lower pons or medulla, a mass lesion at the jugular foramen, or compression of the nerve in its course through the neck. The medical treatment of glossopharyngeal neuralgia is similar to that employed for trigeminal neuralgia. In most cases, neurosurgical evaluation is not required, but microvascular decompression of the glossopharyngeal nerve may help patients with refractory symptoms.

Sinus headache

Inflammation of the nasal mucosa and sinuses commonly produces a sensation of facial pressure rather than frank pain. Patients with sinusitis describe fullness or aching in the cheeks, the bridge of the nose, and the upper jaw. Nasal discharge and blockage usually accompany the pressure. Finding tenderness to percussion of the sinuses or maxilla helps to make the diagnosis, but a CT scan of the sinuses may be required in unclear cases. Be aware that radiographic evidence of sinus congestion is frequent in otherwise healthy people, and that many patients who are diagnosed with sinus headaches by their primary care physicians actually have migraines. Treat sinus headache patients with decongestants, and refer patients with refractory symptoms to an otorhinolaryngologist.

Temporomandibular joint disease

Temporomandibular joint (TMJ) disease is a relatively common myofascial pain syndrome that consists of preauricular aching, limitation of mandibular motion, and crepitus with jaw movement. The exact etiology of the syndrome is unclear, but includes both biological and psychosocial factors.[17] The pain is usually unilateral and is often present with or without chewing. Jaw locking is a common symptom. Occasionally, TMJ disease presents to a neurologist as a primary headache localized to the temple, vertex, or occiput. Pain with palpation of the TMJ and crepitus with jaw movement suggest the diagnosis. Panoramic radiographs are the most useful screening study. Heat, muscle relaxants, NSAIDs, and tricyclic antidepressants may improve symptoms. Refer patients with refractory disease to a dentist with a specific interest in TMJ disease for fitting of an intra-oral occlusive orthotic device (bite plate) or possibly for surgical correction of the problem.

Herpes zoster and postherpetic neuralgia

Varicella zoster infection may lie dormant in the trigeminal sensory ganglia for years, being reactivated by stress or illness. Symptoms typically begin with paresthesias or lancinating pains, which are followed in a few days by a vesicular rash in one of the divisions of the trigeminal nerve. The rash may be painful and after it heals, the patient may continue to complain of exquisite pain in the affected dermatome (postherpetic neuralgia). Treat herpes zoster with valacyclovir (1000 mg tid for 7 days). Use gabapentin (300–1200 mg tid) for acute pain or postherpetic neuralgia. Some patients benefit from capsaicin cream, which should obviously be used cautiously in patients with herpes zoster ophthalmicus.

Atypical facial pain syndrome

Atypical facial pain is characterized by unilateral or bilateral facial pain, which usually has a dull, aching quality. Patients often undergo evaluation and treatment for years before the diagnosis is made. The etiology of atypical facial pain is unclear, but the condition often overlaps with myofascial pain syndromes and fibromyalgia. Atypical facial pain should be considered only after other sources of facial pain are excluded by careful clinical history, examination, and neuroimaging studies. The mainstays of treatment include selective serotonin reuptake inhibitors and tricyclic agents. Patients with atypical facial pain who are evaluated by neurologists frequently have refractory symptoms, and a multidisciplinary approach including alternative therapies is often required.

Primary headache disorders presenting with facial pain

Tension, migraine, and cluster headaches may present as facial pain rather than as headache. The diagnosis may be fairly straightforward when the typical headaches accompany the facial pain. However, when facial pain occurs as the sole manifestation of a primary headache disorder, the diagnosis is more challenging. A trial of empiric treatment is often the only way to establish that a primary headache disorder is the source of facial pain.

References

1. Edlow JA, Caplan LR. Avoiding pitfalls in the diagnosis of subarachnoid hemorrhage. *N Engl J Med* 2000;**342**:29–36.

2. Polmear A. Sentinel headaches in aneurysmal subarachnoid hemorrhage: what is the true incidence? A systematic review. *Cephalalgia* 2003;**23**:935–941.

3. Adams HP, Kassell NF, Torner JC, Sahs AL. CT and clinical correlations in recent aneurysmal subarachnoid hemorrhage: a preliminary report of the Cooperative Aneurysm Study. *Neurology* 1983;**33**: 981–988.

4. van Gijn J, van Dongen KJ. The time course of aneurysmal haemorrhage on computed tomograms. *Neuroradiology* 1982;**23**:153–156.

5. UK National External Quality Assessment Scheme for Immunochemistry Working Group. National guidelines for analysis of cerebrospinal fluid for bilirubin in suspected subarachnoid hemorrhage. *Ann Clin Biochem* 2003;**40**: 481–488.

6. Bederson JB, Connolly S, Batjer HH, et al. Guidelines for the management of aneurysmal subarachnoid hemorrhage. *Stroke* 2009;**40**: 994–1025.

7. Wiebers DO, Whisnant JP, Huston J, et al. Unruptured intracranial aneurysms: natural history, clinical outcome, and risks of surgical and endovascular treatment. *Lancet* 2003;**362**:103–110.

8. Menon R, Kerry S, Norris JW, Markus HS. Treatment of cervical artery dissection: a systematic review and meta-analysis. *J Neurol Neurosurg Psychiatry* 2008;**79**:1122–1127.

9. Schwedt TJ, Matharu MS, Dodick DW. Thunderclap headache. *Lancet Neurol* 2006;**5**:621–631.

10. Stam J, de Bruijn S, deVeber G. Anticoagulation for cerebral sinus thrombosis. *Cochrane Database Syst Rev* 2002;(4):CD002005.

11. Forsyth PA, Posner JB. Headaches in patients with brain tumors: a study of 111 patients. *Neurology* 1993;**43**:1678–1683.

12. Mokri B. Low cerebrospinal fluid pressure syndromes. *Neurol Clin N Am* 2004;**22**:55–74.

13. Kuhn WF, Kuhn SC, Gilberstadt H. Occipital neuralgias: clinical recognition of a complicated headache. A case series and literature review. *J Orofacial Pain* 1997;**11**:158–165.

14. Headache Classification Subcommittee of the International Headache Society. The international classification of headache disorders: 2nd edition. *Cephalalgia* 2004;**24**:S24–S136.

15. Silberstein SD, Lipton RB. Chronic daily headache, including transformed migraine, chronic tension-type headache, and medication overuse. In: Silberstein SD, Lipton RB, Dalessio DJ, eds. *Wolff's Headache and Other Head Pain*. New York: Oxford University Press; 2001; 247–282.

16. Gronseth G, Cruccu G, Alksne J, et al. Practice parameter: the diagnostic evaluation and treatment of trigeminal neuralgia (an evidence based review). *Neurology* 2008;**71**:1183–1190.

17. Scrivani SJ, Keith DA, Kaban LB. Temporomandibular disorders. *N Engl J Med* 2008;**359**:2693–2705.

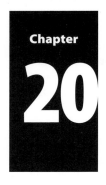

Seizures and epilepsy

The first seizure

An epileptic seizure is a transient occurrence of signs and/or symptoms due to abnormal, excessive, synchronous neuronal activity in the brain.[1] According to a large epidemiologic study conducted at the Mayo Clinic, the annual incidence of seizures is approximately 61 in 100 000 with people at the extremes of age being at the greatest risk.[2] An organized five-step approach is helpful in evaluating patients with a first-time seizure:

1. Get the best account of the seizure manifestation (ictal semiology) from a firsthand observer.
2. Determine whether the event was actually a seizure.
3. If it was a seizure, determine whether it was the first one.
4. Define the etiology of the seizure.
5. Determine whether treatment is needed, and if so, what agents are appropriate.

Ictal semiology

Generalized tonic–clonic seizures

The generalized tonic–clonic seizure (GTCS) is the most easily recognized type of seizure, and the one that most frequently leads to emergency room consultations. Because a GTCS is usually quite alarming, eyewitness accounts are often unreliable, even when provided by a physician or nurse. Sometimes, the only available information is that the patient passed out and shook. Although there is considerable heterogeneity, a GTCS in an adult generally lasts for an average of about a minute and may consist of some or all of the following phases[3]:

1. Partial seizure. A GTCS may be generalized from onset, or it may arise from a partial seizure (see below) in a process known as secondary generalization. If this partial seizure is a simple partial seizure, the patient may remember it after the seizure has finished. However, patients will not be able to remember a GTCS that is generalized from onset or that develops from a complex partial seizure.

2. Onset of generalization. After the partial seizure ends, secondary generalization is usually heralded by a forced head movement to one side (versive movement) or by a brief vocalization.

3. Pretonic clonic phase. In approximately half of patients, generalization begins with irregular, asymmetric clonic jerking of the extremities.

4. Tonic phase. This is a generalized and sustained contraction of all the muscles in the body, and may be accompanied by some clonic jerking.

5. Tremulous phase. This phase is characterized by fast muscle shaking, but is too rapid to be classified as clonus.

6. Clonic phase. This is the final phase of the seizure itself, characterized by slower muscle jerking, which eventually decreases in frequency before stopping.

7. Postictal state. After a GTCS, the patient lies limp, in a deep sleep. After several minutes, he awakens and is confused and may have a headache and muscle pain from the seizure.

Partial seizures

Partial seizures begin in a focal area of the brain and are the most common seizure type in adults. Because they may arise from any area of the cerebral cortex, partial seizures produce a vast array of motor, sensory, perceptual, and behavioral manifestations. Partial seizures may be divided into simple partial seizures (SPSs, also called auras) in which consciousness is preserved, and which therefore can be described by the patient, and complex partial seizures (CPSs), which are associated with an impairment of consciousness.

Simple partial seizures

Motor seizures

Simple partial seizures (SPSs) arising from the motor cortex may take the form of forced head deviation to one side, speech arrest or vocalizations, stereotyped limb or facial movements such as twitching or jerking, or coordinated, almost purposeful-appearing movements. When a motor seizure remains restricted to one area of the cortex, it produces only a single manifestation. If the electrical activity spreads to adjacent areas of the motor cortex, a Jacksonian march in which there is sequential spread of the seizure into the ipsilateral face, arm, and leg occurs over seconds. Focal motor seizures may be followed by Todd's paralysis in which muscle weakness persists for several minutes to hours.

Sensory seizures

Simple partial seizures may affect any sensory modality. Common sensory auras include visual (seeing spots, stars, or bright lights), auditory (ringing, buzzing, or musical sounds), somesthetic (tingling, numbness, or electrical sensations), olfactory (the smell of burning rubber or other foul odors), gustatory (acidic, bitter, or sweet tastes), vestibular (vertigo), or epigastric (the sensation of rising in the abdomen, descending a rollercoaster, or having butterflies in the stomach). Auras that involve the primary sensory cortex are generally unformed and primitive, whereas those that involve the higher-level association cortex or mesial temporal structures are more detailed.

Behavioral and psychic seizures

Simple partial seizures may also produce a wide variety of behavioral or psychic phenomena. *Déjà vu* is the sensation of visual familiarity whereas *déjà entendu* is the sensation of auditory familiarity. *Jamais vu* and *jamais entendu* are feelings of unfamiliarity in the visual and auditory realms, respectively. Patients with temporal lobe SPS may also describe a dreamlike or disconnected state, or a sense that they are watching themselves (autoscopy). Depersonalization, fear, pleasure, religious ecstasy, and forced thinking are also well-described psychic auras that arise from the temporal lobes.

Complex partial seizures

Complex partial seizures (CPSs) are partial seizures that are characterized by impairment of consciousness. They frequently arise from SPSs, and may progress to GTCSs. Complex partial seizures are often accompanied by automatic, repetitive, stereotyped behaviors known as automatisms. Automatisms arising from the temporal lobe tend to be simple and include lip smacking, chewing, swallowing, grasping, fumbling, blinking, and eye fluttering. Automatisms arising from the frontal lobe are usually more complex and often appear purposeful. Orbitofrontal automatisms may have bizarre characteristics including bicycling movements of the legs, pelvic thrusting, and sexual activity mimicry.

Absence seizures

Absence seizures begin in childhood or adolescence. In some cases, they are misdiagnosed as CPSs and the correct diagnosis is not made until adulthood. Typical absence seizures last for just a few seconds, and are characterized by unresponsiveness, a fixed blank stare, eye fluttering, and facial twitching.[4] Accompanying seizure manifestations may include increases or decreases in postural tone, brief clonic movements, and automatisms that resemble those of patients with CPSs. Patients with absence seizures may or may not be aware of the attack, and resume preictal activities as soon as the seizure is completed.

Myoclonic seizures

Myoclonus is a sudden, involuntary, brief jerk of a muscle or group of muscles which is discussed in further detail in Chapter 14. Although myoclonic seizures tend to occur in children, they may also begin in adolescents or young adults as part of juvenile myoclonic epilepsy (see below). The progressive myoclonic epilepsies are a group of uncommon degenerative disorders, which include adult-onset neuronal ceroid lipofuscinosis, Lafora body disease, Unverricht–Lundborg disease, and myoclonic epilepsy with ragged red fibers (MERRF).

Atonic seizures

Atonic seizures are associated with mental retardation and Lennox–Gastaut syndrome (see below). They are sudden drop attacks in which the patient suddenly loses tone and falls to the ground. They are frequently included in the differential diagnosis of falls and syncope, but should be omitted because they *do not occur in cognitively normal adults*.

The differential diagnosis of seizures

Syncope

The main condition that is confused with GTCS is syncope, a sudden, brief loss of consciousness that results from reduced cerebral blood flow (Chapter 9). It is usually preceded by lightheadedness, diaphoresis,

Table 20.1 Factors that help differentiate between seizure and syncope

Seizure	Syncope
Tongue biting (particularly lateral tongue)	Lightheadedness
Urinary incontinence	History of cardiovascular disease
Head turning	Chest pain
Posturing	Diaphoresis
Amnesia for the event	Facial flushing
Postictal confusion	Lasts for a few seconds
Lasts for 1–2 minutes	

and anxiety. Syncope may be confused with seizure because it is accompanied by multifocal jerking movements in 50–90% of patients.[5] These myoclonic movements usually last for only 3–10 seconds, and are brainstem release phenomena rather than abnormal, synchronous cortical discharges. Syncopal patients regain consciousness and coherence within a few seconds, often in response to elevation of their feet, which restores cerebral blood flow. Patients with GTCSs require minutes to hours to recover from an event. Features that help to differentiate between seizures and syncope are found in Table 20.1. The most reliable of these is the presence of a postictal state, which strongly favors seizure.

Migraine and transient ischemic attack

Simple and complex partial seizures have a broader differential diagnosis than GTCSs. Among neurological conditions, the two that are often difficult to distinguish from partial seizures are migraine aura and transient ischemic attack (TIA). Prior history of migraine or risk factors for cerebrovascular disease may help to differentiate among the three conditions. In the absence of a relevant past medical history, the time course with which symptoms develop is the most important piece of information: with some exceptions, seizures develop over seconds, migraine auras develop over several minutes, and TIA symptoms are maximal at onset.

Movement disorders

Motor seizures may be confused with movement disorders, especially myoclonus and hemiballismus (Chapter 12). With the rare exception of epilepsia partialis continua in which partial seizures occur continuously, movement disorder symptoms tend to be relatively continuous activities while seizures are usually discrete events that are spaced widely apart in time. For example, intermittent flinging of the arm that lasts for days on end is more likely to be hemiballismus than a focal motor seizure. The most important exception to this rule is paroxysmal kinesigenic dyskinesia, a condition that is often misdiagnosed as a seizure disorder. Paroxysmal kinesigenic dyskinesia is characterized by sudden and episodic choreoathetotic or dystonic movements that last from seconds to minutes at a time, are precipitated by movement, and are often preceded by an aura. They tend to respond to treatment with carbamazepine.

Sensory symptoms

The differential diagnosis of sensory seizures depends, obviously, on the affected sensory modality. In all cases, think carefully about dysfunction of the sensory end organ (e.g. the eye in patients with visual symptoms) before concluding that the problem is coming from the brain. Patients with olfactory or gustatory phenomena, for example, may have primary otorhinolaryngological disorders or exposure to some toxin or medication that leads to their abnormal smells or tastes. Auditory hallucinations usually occur in the context of psychotic disorders. Somatosensory deficits secondary to seizures should not be fixed, unlike disorders such as radiculopathy, compression neuropathy, and multiple sclerosis.

Psychiatric disorders

Psychic and affective partial seizures must be differentiated from psychosis and depression, a task that usually requires the assistance of a psychiatrist. Malingering and conversion disorders (see below) are relevant considerations in all patients with paroxysmal disorders. Despite careful history and observation, an EEG recorded during an event is often the only reliable way to determine whether a behavior or perception is a seizure.

Narcolepsy

Narcolepsy is a disorder characterized by the tetrad of excessive daytime sleepiness, cataplexy (sudden loss of body tone, often precipitated by laughter or other emotional states), hypnagogic hallucinations (those that occur upon going to sleep), and sleep paralysis. Although differentiating narcolepsy from seizures is almost always straightforward, rare patients with cataplexy as their first or only symptom may be referred to a neurologist for seizure evaluation. The diagnosis should be obvious from history alone. A multiple sleep latency test (MSLT) helps to establish the diagnosis in unclear cases. Treatment should include referral to a sleep specialist. Modafinil (200 mg qd–bid) and methylphenidate (10 mg bid) are helpful in managing excessive daytime sleepiness, while REM-suppressing medications such as extended-release venlafaxine (75–150 mg qd) or fluoxetine (20–40 mg qd) are most often used for cataplexy.

Parasomnias

Parasomnias are a group of sleep disorders characterized by unusual movements or behaviors that arise from sleep. Well-known examples of parasomnias that may be confused with seizures include:

- Somnambulism (sleepwalking). Although more common in childhood, some adults may engage in sleepwalking.
- Sleep terrors. These arousals characterized by screaming, yelling, and sometimes violent behavior are more common in children.
- Periodic limb movements of sleep. Sudden involuntary limb movements during sleep may awaken the patient, or more commonly, their bed partner.
- Rapid eye movement (REM) sleep behavior disorder. This disorder, characterized by acting out one's dreams, commonly precedes the development of a synucleinopathy such as Parkinson's disease or dementia with Lewy bodies (Chapter 13).

The diagnosis of a parasomnia is often straightforward from history alone. In confusing cases, a sleep study with video recording assists in making the diagnosis. Referral to a sleep specialist is indicated for most patients with parasomnias.

Was this really the first seizure?

Determining whether a seizure was actually a patient's first one is essential to guide further evaluation and treatment. When asking a patient about prior seizures, keep in mind that a person who has a GTCS will remember only the postictal state and not the seizure itself. Ask the patient, therefore, if they have ever awoken with a confused feeling, unexplained injuries, tongue lacerations, or loss of urine. Because most people are not familiar with seizures

other than GTCSs, when determining whether a seizure was really a patient's first, it is important to inquire directly about specific SPS and CPS phenomena, staring spells indicative of absence seizures, and myoclonic seizures.

Determining seizure etiology

Because a seizure is a symptom of brain dysfunction rather than a disease unto itself, determining its underlying cause is an essential but surprisingly overlooked part of the evaluation. Seizure etiologies may be divided broadly into two groups: those that are caused by identifiable and often reversible metabolic or structural processes, and those that have no identifiable cause and are therefore labeled idiopathic. In the search for a seizure etiology, all patients require a careful and complete medical and neurological history. Laboratory studies, neuroimaging, and EEG are also important elements of the evaluation.

Laboratory testing

Laboratory testing is very similar to that which is performed for the confused patient (Chapter 1) and should include a complete blood count, chemistry studies with calcium, magnesium, and phosphorus levels, liver function tests, a toxicology screen, and urinalysis. Although many patients with seizures have minor laboratory abnormalities, these are often not the proximate cause of the seizure. Lumbar puncture should be performed on all patients with fever, a history of immunosuppression, or other reason to suspect meningitis or encephalitis. Although GTCSs by themselves may cause CSF pleocytosis, the number of cells rarely exceeds 1–2 cells/mm^3 and any value exceeding 10 cells/mm^3 should prompt more careful evaluation for meningitis or encephalitis.[6]

Neuroimaging

All patients with a first-time seizure should undergo a neuroimaging study: approximately 10–15% of patients will have an abnormal, responsible finding.[7] In the acute setting, noncontrast head CT is sufficient to evaluate for structural lesions that require urgent attention such as brain hemorrhages, tumors, abscesses, and cysts. Slowly growing tumors, encephalitis, and ischemic stroke are seizure etiologies that may not be detected by CT scan. MRI with diffusion-weighted imaging and contrast enhancement are indicated if one of these processes is suspected.

Electroencephalography

EEG is perhaps the most valuable diagnostic tool in evaluating a patient with a first-time seizure: it helps to differentiate epileptic seizures from conditions that mimic them, to classify seizure types, and to tailor therapy. The vast majority of patients with a first-time seizure will have their EEG between seizures (an "interictal" EEG), rather than during a seizure. Abnormal interictal epileptiform discharges (Figures 20.1 and 20.2) are present in approximately 30–50% of these patients, but also in approximately 2% of normal subjects.[7,8] The yield of EEG is increased by sleep deprivation, by performing multiple studies, and by performing the study within 24–48 hours after the seizure.[9] EEG obtained with sphenoidal electrodes may offer greater sensitivity to focal seizures originating from the temporal lobes.[10]

Specific seizure etiologies

Electrolyte abnormalities

Many electrolyte abnormalities are minor and not the direct cause of seizures. The following are rough guidelines to electrolyte levels that might be expected to cause seizures:

- Hyponatremia <120 mEq/l
- Hypocalcemia <6.0 mg/dl

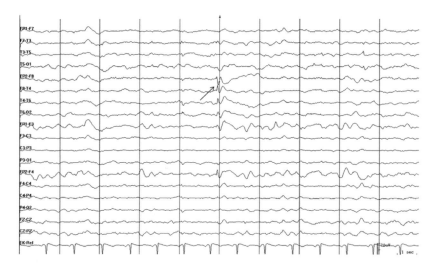

Figure 20.1 Interictal EEG in a patient with a recent partial-onset seizure. Note the sharp wave with phase reversal at the F8 lead (arrow), placing the likely seizure focus in the right anterior temporal lobe. Image courtesy of Dr. Julie Roth.

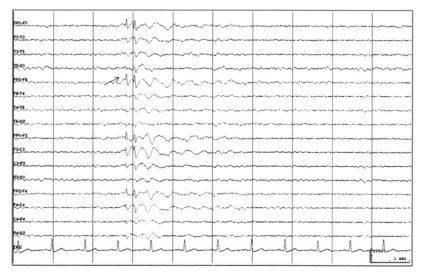

Figure 20.2 Interictal EEG in a patient with primary generalized epilepsy. Note the generalized sharp discharges (arrow) followed by slow waves. Image courtesy of Dr. Julie Roth.

- Hypomagnesemia <0.8 mg/dl
- Hypophosphatemia <1.0 mg/dl

Careful correction of these electrolyte abnormalities should reduce the chances of seizure recurrence.

Uremia and dialysis disequilibrium syndrome

Both acute and chronic renal failure leads to the accumulation of toxic metabolites and uremic encephalopathy (Chapter 1).[11] Patients with uremic encephalopathy may have both generalized and partial seizures, although GTCSs are more common. Uremic seizures are often accompanied by myoclonus. There is no single blood urea nitrogen, creatinine, or glomerular filtration rate that predicts seizures: the diagnosis must be made clinically. Dialysis is the definitive treatment of seizures secondary to uremia, but some patients with recurrent seizures require anticonvulsants, as seizures may recur even after an adequate dialysis schedule is arranged. In addition to uremia, patients in renal failure are at risk for seizures secondary to dialysis, the so-called dialysis disequilibrium syndrome (DDS), which may include encephalopathy, seizures, blurred vision, loss of consciousness, or coma. It is usually a self-limited condition that is best avoided by gentle dialysis.

Glucose imbalance

Because glucose is the brain's primary energy source, hypoglycemia is an obvious substrate for neurological dysfunction including seizures. The glucose level at which seizures occur varies from patient to patient: in diabetics, seizures may occur at relatively higher glucose levels than in healthy patients, while nondiabetics may be free of seizures and other neurological dysfunction, even at blood sugar levels of 40 mg/dl. Nonketotic hyperglycemia may also precipitate seizures (sometimes taking the form of continuous focal seizures, i.e. epilepsia partialis continua). Because ketosis raises the seizure threshold, ketotic hyperglycemia is not a direct cause of seizures.

Hepatic encephalopathy

Hepatic encephalopathy and associated seizures are discussed in greater detail in Chapter 1.

Posttraumatic seizures

Although figures vary from study to study, a rough estimate of seizure risk following head trauma is 5% for patients with closed head injuries and 50% for those with penetrating head injuries.[12] Not surprisingly, the seizure risk is greater in patients with severe injuries

than in those with mild injuries. Posttraumatic seizures may be divided into early seizures, which occur within 1 week of head injury, and late seizures, which occur more than 1 week after head injury. Because early seizures are not necessarily associated with a higher risk for developing posttraumatic epilepsy, anticonvulsants are not clearly indicated.[13,14] Neurosurgeons, however, commonly prescribe phenytoin as prophylaxis for all patients with severe head injuries in the first week after injury, as the consequences of seizures including increased intracranial pressure may be severe in this population.[12] Patients with late seizures are at increased risk for developing epilepsy, even 10 years after the injury, and should be treated with anticonvulsants.[13]

Alcohol withdrawal

Alcohol withdrawal may lead to seizures, which are almost exclusively GTCSs. Almost all seizures occur within 72 hours of the last drink, with a peak between 6 and 24 hours after alcohol discontinuation.[15] Do not assume that all seizures in a patient who is withdrawing from alcohol are due to the withdrawal itself, as comorbid conditions including head trauma, electrolyte abnormalities, and meningitis may also precipitate seizures. Unless seizures are frequent or status epilepticus ensues, patients with alcohol withdrawal seizures do not necessarily require acute treatment. Long-term prophylaxis is rarely, if ever, indicated.

Other medications and toxins

A variety of medications including certain antidepressants, antipsychotics, stimulants, anesthetics, and antibiotics may precipitate seizures. It is a good policy to review the manufacturer's prescribing information to determine whether a new medication played a role in lowering a patient's seizure threshold and then to discontinue the offending medication as necessary. Intoxication with drugs of abuse, particularly stimulants and hallucinogens, and withdrawal from benzodiazepines are also important causes of seizures.

Meningitis and encephalitis

Patients with meningitis and encephalitis are obviously at risk for seizures. Any patient with a new seizure and a fever should undergo lumbar puncture after a space-occupying lesion is excluded by head CT. Chapter 1 contains a more detailed discussion of meningitis and encephalitis.

Neurocysticercosis

Infection of the brain parenchyma by the parasite *Taenia solium* is the most common cause of seizures in many Latin American and African countries. Cysts of all stages, including calcified cysts, may precipitate seizures. Other manifestations of neurocysticercosis include headaches, focal neurological disturbances, and in some cases, hydrocephalus due to obstruction of the ventricular system. The diagnosis of neurocysticercosis is usually established by finding cysts on a neuroimaging study in a patient from an endemic part of the world (see Chapter 23). When the diagnosis is in doubt, enzyme-linked immunoelectrotransfer blot assay plays a confirmatory role. Treat patients with seizures and enhancing cysts with a combination of anticonvulsants and albendazole (15 mg/kg/day) and prednisone (60–80 kg qd) under the guidance of an infectious disease specialist.

Neoplasms

Although precise numbers are difficult to establish, between 3 and 15% of epilepsy is due to brain tumors, with middle-aged patients having the greatest chance of a neoplastic etiology.[2] Approximately 35% of patients with brain tumors will eventually have a seizure: the relative likelihood is greatest with low-grade gliomas, then with meningiomas, followed by high-grade gliomas, and is least for metastatic tumors.[16] Tumors are more likely to be the source of seizure when postictal deficits are prolonged. The study of choice to evaluate for brain tumor is MRI with and without contrast (Chapter 23). When evaluating patients with known cancer who develop seizures, it is important to keep in mind sources of seizures other than metastasis, including meningitis from immunosuppression, paraneoplastic limbic encephalitis, radiation necrosis, scarring from surgical resection sites, and hemorrhage due to coagulopathy. Because chemotherapy used to treat the tumor often decreases anticonvulsant levels, levetiracetam (which has few drug–drug interactions) is often the agent of choice for patients with brain tumors. Despite common practice, anticonvulsant prophylaxis is not required for all patients with brain tumors, unless they have already had a seizure.[17]

Stroke

Cerebrovascular disease is the most commonly identifiable source of epilepsy in adults, and is especially common in the elderly. One prospective study showed that approximately 9% of patients with a stroke will have a seizure, usually within 24 hours of the stroke.[18] In the acute setting, the likelihood of seizure is predictably greater for patients with hemorrhagic strokes than for those with ischemic strokes. Seizure risk from hemorrhage decreases considerably, however, as intracranial blood is reabsorbed, while patients with ischemic strokes remain at higher risk for seizures months to years later.[18]

Arteriovenous malformations

Arteriovenous malformations may cause a variety of symptoms including intracranial hemorrhage, stroke, and seizure. They are discussed further in Chapter 23.

Neurodegenerative diseases

Up to 15% of patients with Alzheimer's disease (AD) may have seizures, usually GTCSs.[19] It is not clear how frequently the seizures are the direct consequence of AD, but in many patients, there may be no other identifiable risk factor. Other neurodegenerative diseases including Creutzfeldt–Jakob disease and frontotemporal dementia may also produce seizures.

Eclampsia

Preeclampsia is a condition specific to pregnancy consisting of the triad of hypertension, proteinuria, and edema. It may occur at any time between week 20 of gestation and 6 weeks postpartum. The only cure for preeclampsia is delivery of the baby. Eclampsia is the occurrence of seizures in a woman with preeclampsia. These are usually GTCSs, may be severe, and may threaten both mother and baby. Multiple studies indicate that magnesium sulfate is the preferred therapy to prevent preeclampsia from developing into eclampsia and to prevent seizure recurrence in women who have already had an eclamptic seizure.[20–22] Therefore, treat women with severe preeclampsia or eclamptic seizures with 6 g IV magnesium sulfate followed by an IV drip of 2–3 g/hour. Because high levels of magnesium may cause respiratory depression, neuromuscular transmission failure, or kidney dysfunction, it is important to hold the infusion for any decline in respiratory rate, loss of deep tendon reflexes, or decrease in urinary output.

Idiopathic seizures

The majority of adults with new-onset seizures have no specifically identifiable etiology.[2] These patients presumably have an underlying genetic basis or unidentified environmental exposure that is responsible for their seizures.

Table 20.2 Anticonvulsants and specific applications

Application	Anticonvulsants of choice
Partial seizures and secondarily generalized seizures	Phenytoin, carbamazepine, oxcarbazepine, levetiracetam, lamotrigine, valproate
Primary generalized tonic–clonic seizures	Valproate, lamotrigine
Absence seizures	Valproate, lamotrigine, ethosuximide
Juvenile myoclonic epilepsy	Valproate, lamotrigine
Need to start anticonvulsant quickly at goal dose	Phenytoin, levetiracetam
Patient taking multiple medications that may potentially interact with anticonvulsants	Levetiracetam, gabapentin
Medication expense is a concern	Phenytoin, carbamazepine, valproate
Pregnancy	Lamotrigine, levetiracetam (avoid valproate if possible)
Hepatic failure	Levetiracetam, topiramate, gabapentin
Elderly patient	Lamotrigine, carbamazepine, oxcarbazepine

Treatment of the first-time seizure

Provoked seizures

Provoked seizures are those that are caused by a specific, identifiable abnormality, and which do not recur when that abnormality is corrected. Common causes of provoked seizures include electrolyte disturbances and alcohol withdrawal. By definition, provoked seizures should not be treated as they have a low likelihood of recurrence.

Benefits and risks of anticonvulsants

Choosing to prescribe anticonvulsants for a patient after a single seizure is often a difficult decision. The main benefit of prescribing anticonvulsants is greater security for both patient and doctor that seizures will be controlled. This benefit, however, must be balanced against the potential for the anticonvulsant to cause side effects such as sedation and dizziness, and the cost of the medication. While each patient must be approached individually, understanding the risk for seizure recurrence is helpful in deciding when to start anticonvulsants. For an adult with a single unprovoked seizure, the 2-year risk for seizure recurrence is approximately 50%.[23,24] The probability of seizure recurrence increases to 60–70% if there is a history of prior neurological injury, developmental abnormalities, abnormal imaging studies, or EEG with epileptiform features.[23] Although a 50% risk for seizure recurrence would seem to warrant anticonvulsant therapy, the side effects of taking these medications

must be weighed against their protective effects. Most neurologists, including myself, do not usually prescribe an anticonvulsant for a patient with a single seizure, normal EEG, and normal imaging results. Obviously, this rule must be flexible. For example, it makes sense to have a lower threshold to start an anticonvulsant in a patient whose livelihood depends on the ability to drive.

After a second seizure, the 2-year risk for further seizures increases to approximately 70%.[24] Because this risk of a second seizure is so high, I almost always prescribe anticonvulsants after a second seizure. Possible exceptions to this rule include patients with non-disabling nocturnal seizures or elderly nursing home residents who are at high risk for side effects from anticonvulsants.

Choosing an anticonvulsant

In most cases, there is little difference in efficacy among the various anticonvulsants, and the choice of agent is usually based on the anticipated side effects, interactions with other medications, cost, and speed with which the medication can be titrated to effective levels. Obviously, there is no single anticonvulsant that can be labeled as the "best" or "first choice" for all applications. Table 20.2, however, contains a summary of common applications in which certain anticonvulsants may be preferred based on expert consensus[25] and personal experience, while Table 20.3 contains a summary of the dosing and side effects of commonly used anticonvulsants.

Table 20.3 Common anticonvulsants

Anticonvulsant name	Starting dose	Titration method	Initial goal dose	Typical therapeutic levels (µg/ml)[a]	Side effects[b]
Phenobarbital	30 mg qd	Increase by 30 mg every 2 weeks	60–120 mg qd	10–40	Excessive sedation
Phenytoin	300 mg qd	See Box 20.1	See Box 20.1	10–20	Rash, pseudolymphoma, gingival hyperplasia, hirsutism, polyneuropathy, cerebellar degeneration
Carbamazepine	200 mg bid	Increase by 200 mg total every 3 days	200–400 mg bid	4–12	Rash including Stevens–Johnson syndrome, hyponatremia, agranulocytosis
Valproate	500 mg bid	Increase by 250 mg per dose each week	500–1000 mg bid	50–100	Tremor, thrombocytopenia, pancreatitis, hyperammonemia, weight gain, hair loss
Lamotrigine	25 mg qd	Increase by 25 mg each week (see Box 20.2)	100–200 mg bid		Rash including Stevens–Johnson syndrome
Gabapentin	300 mg qd	Increase by 300 mg total every 3 days	600–1200 mg tid		Minimal beyond sedation, dizziness, and ataxia
Topiramate	25 mg qd	Increase by 25 mg each week	100–200 mg bid		Weight loss, anomia, nephrolithiasis, acral paresthesias
Oxcarbazepine	150 mg bid	Increase total dose by 300 mg each week	300–600 mg bid		Hyponatremia, rash including Stevens-Johnson syndrome
Levetiracetam	500 mg bid	Increase total dose by 500 mg each week	500–1000 mg bid		Minimal beyond sedation, dizziness, and ataxia
Zonisamide	50 mg qd	Increase total dose by 50 mg each week	100–200 mg qd		Nephrolithiasis, weight loss

[a] Reference ranges are also available for the newer anticonvulsants, but are used less frequently in clinical practice.
[b] Side effects of all medications include dose-related sedation, dizziness, and ataxia.

Anticonvulsants in patients with renal dysfunction

Many hospitalized or otherwise chronically ill patients have renal dysfunction, which plays a significant role in anticonvulsant selection. In addition, patients with renal dysfunction often undergo hemodialysis, which may remove anticonvulsants entirely, partially, or not at all. Table 20.4 contains a summary of dose adjustments for common anticonvulsants in patients with renal dysfunction and in those who are undergoing hemodialysis.

Counseling after the first seizure

Patients react to a new seizure diagnosis in a variety of ways including fear, depression, nonchalance, defiance, and even rage. It is absolutely essential to address any concerns that the patient and their family might have about seizures. It is important to discuss seizure manifestations (especially for patients with partial seizures) and what to tell schools or workplaces about the seizures. It is also essential to tell family members that they should not put a spoon or other object into

Box 20.1 Phenytoin dosing and levels

The usual initial dose of phenytoin is 300 mg/day. In some patients, it is necessary to achieve a therapeutic level quickly: these patients require loading with intravenous phenytoin or fosphenytoin (20 mg/kg). Therapeutic levels of phenytoin are typically in the range of 10–20 μg/ml, although many patients achieve excellent seizure control at levels <10 μg/ml and some patients continue to seize despite levels >20 μg/ml. Because phenytoin is highly protein bound, the serum level may be misleading, and it is important to determine free phenytoin levels. If rapid measurement of free phenytoin levels is not readily available, then the true phenytoin level may be approximated by the equation:

$$\text{Corrected phenytoin level} = \frac{\text{measured phenytoin level}}{(0.2 \times \text{albumin}) + 0.1}$$

Make the following adjustments as necessary:

- For patients with total levels <5 μg/ml, reload phenytoin orally (three doses of 300 mg, each separated by 3 hours) or intravenously and increase the total daily dose by 100 mg.
- For patients with levels between 5 and 10 μg/ml, increase the total daily dose by 100 mg.
- For patients with continued seizures despite levels between 10 and 20 μg/ml, increase the total daily dose by 30–50 mg. This small increase is necessary because, at higher doses, phenytoin metabolism assumes zero-order kinetics at which point no more phenytoin is metabolized and drug levels rise precipitously into the toxic range.

Table 20.4 Anticonvulsants in patients with renal dysfunction[26]

Anticonvulsant name	Adjustment in renal failure	Supplemental dose after hemodialysis?
Phenobarbital	No	Yes
Phenytoin	No	Yes
Carbamazepine	No	No
Valproate	Frequent monitoring	Yes
Topiramate	No	Yes
Lamotrigine	No	Yes
Gabapentin	CrCl 30–60 ml/min: 300 mg bid; CrCl 10–30 ml/min: 300 mg qd; CrCl <10 ml/min: 300 mg qod	Yes
Oxcarbazepine	No	No
Levetiracetam	CrCl 50–80 ml/min: 500–1000 mg bid; CrCl 30–50 ml/min: 250–750 mg bid; CrCl <30 ml/min: 250–500 mg bid	Yes
Zonisamide	Frequent monitoring	Yes

CrCl = creatinine clearance.

a patient's mouth during a seizure: a person cannot swallow their own tongue, but they certainly can swallow a foreign body or aspirate it. Instruct family members that the safest place for a patient during a GTCS is on the floor, placed on their side to prevent aspiration. Let family members know than any GTCS that lasts >5 minutes is potentially dangerous and requires medical assistance. It is often helpful to instruct patients and their families to look at their watches as soon as a seizure begins, because seizure duration is often overestimated. It is the physician's duty to know the individual state's laws about driving restrictions for patients with seizures and to inform patients of these laws or report seizures as necessary. Lastly, it is important to instruct patients that they should only swim with a companion and should take showers rather than baths to prevent accidental drowning.

Epilepsy

Epilepsy is a disorder of the brain characterized by the occurrence of at least one epileptic seizure and an enduring predisposition to generate epileptic seizures.[1] For some patients, the diagnosis of epilepsy can be made after a single seizure and an EEG showing characteristic epileptiform discharges. For others, the diagnosis is established only after a second seizure occurs. The first job in treating a patient with epilepsy is to define the source of the epilepsy by using a combination of ictal semiology, EEG findings, and neuroimaging or laboratory studies. In general, epilepsy may be divided into symptomatic forms in which the source of the epilepsy is known, idiopathic forms in which there is no identifiable structural lesion but rather a presumed genetic source, and cryptogenic in which the epilepsy is likely symptomatic but the underlying source is not known. Defining the syndrome allows appropriate tailoring of treatment and consideration of surgical intervention for patients with seizures that are likely to be medically refractory.

Epilepsy syndromes

A variety of epilepsy syndromes produce characteristic patterns of seizures and respond to specific therapies. In adults, some of the more common epilepsy syndromes include the following.

Temporal lobe epilepsy

Temporal lobe epilepsy (TLE) commonly begins in childhood or adolescence. Typical simple partial seizures include an epigastric rising sensation, olfactory hallucinations, déjà vu, or ictal fear. Complex partial seizures are often associated with automatisms such as lip smacking, chewing, swallowing, or sniffing. Secondary generalization of partial seizures is common but not universal. Temporal lobe epilepsy may be difficult to treat medically, and is a frequent source for surgical referrals in the adult population.

Juvenile myoclonic epilepsy

Juvenile myoclonic epilepsy (JME) usually begins in adolescence, but may go undiagnosed until early adulthood. Many patients have absence seizures in youth. Myoclonic jerks in the arms, usually after awakening in the morning, are the most common initial feature in adolescence. Later in the course, GTCSs develop and are often the events that bring the patient to clinical attention. In many cases, the features of the syndrome may be identified only retrospectively by careful history. Interictal EEG characteristically shows 4–6 Hz spike-wave complexes (Figure 20.3). Although it is considered a benign form of epilepsy, most patients with JME require lifelong treatment, generally with valproate or lamotrigine, in order to prevent seizure recurrence.

Autosomal dominant nocturnal frontal lobe epilepsy

Autosomal dominant nocturnal frontal lobe epilepsy (ADNFLE) may begin in children or young adults and is inherited in an autosomal dominant fashion. It is characterized by brief motor seizures that awaken the patient from non-REM sleep. Bizarre automatisms secondary to frontal lobe involvement accompany the seizures, which often leads to this syndrome being diagnosed as a parasomnia or as a psychogenic disorder. This syndrome responds to traditional anticonvulsants.

Reflex epilepsies

Reflex epilepsies are a group of epilepsy syndromes in which sensory stimuli such as flashing lights, the voice of a specific person, or a piece of music precipitate seizures. Avoiding the stimulus is helpful in preventing seizure recurrence, but, in many cases, the

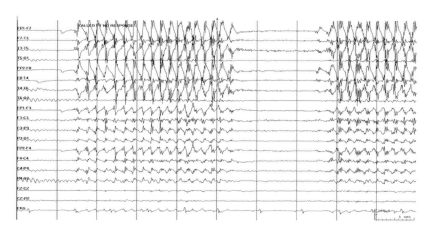

Figure 20.3 4–5 Hz generalized polyspike-wave complexes seen in a patient with juvenile myoclonic epilepsy. Image courtesy of Dr. Julie Roth.

stimulus is so frequent that the patient may require anticonvulsants.

Refractory epilepsy

Almost all adults with epilepsy are treated with medications and the first anticonvulsant leads to seizure freedom approximately 70% of the time.[27] Up to 30%, therefore, will have refractory seizures. The challenge in managing this group of patients is to determine the reason for poor seizure control. It is good practice to start from scratch by retaking the patient's history, defining ictal semiology (usually with the help of an observer), asking about precipitating factors, reviewing EEG and neuroimaging findings, and inquiring about responses to past medication trials. Usually, the explanation for refractory seizures may be divided into one of the following:

1. *Complex partial seizures are misdiagnosed and treated as absence seizures or vice versa.* This is most often a problem in children and adolescents. Carbamazepine and phenytoin are quite effective for CPSs, but may worsen absence seizures. Ethosuximide, used exclusively for patients with absence seizures, worsens CPSs. For patients with refractory staring spells, the duration of postictal confusion is the most reliable clinical way to distinguish between CPSs and absence seizures: postictal confusion lasts for minutes in CPSs and seconds (or not at all) in absence seizures. Although automatisms are more likely to be present in CPSs, they may also accompany absence seizures. EEG may differentiate between CPSs and absence seizures if any doubt remains after the history. Patients with absence seizures have characteristic 3 Hz spike-wave discharges

(Figure 20.4), often elicited by hyperventilation whereas those with CPSs are more likely to have focal spikes or sharp waves.

2. *Avoidable precipitants lower the seizure threshold.* Factors that lower the seizure threshold include excessive alcohol intake, sleep deprivation, and stress. Lifestyle modifications, easier in principle than in practice, may reduce seizure frequency.

3. *The patient is not taking their medication.* Factors that lead to medication noncompliance include frequent dosing, high monetary expense, and undesirable side effects. Some patients with large numbers of medications often skip one or more of them. Others are simply not "pill people." If you suspect medication noncompliance, ask the patient to bring his pill bottles to his appointments so that you may count his remaining medication. Checking serum drug levels may also help to establish medication noncompliance (Table 20.3).

4. *The patient may not have epileptic seizures.* The differential diagnosis of seizures, including syncope, movement disorders, and psychiatric disorders, is discussed above. Approximately 20% of patients who are referred to epilepsy centers for refractory epilepsy actually have psychogenic pseudoseizures.[28] These are most often the manifestations of conversion disorders, but in some cases may be secondary to malingering. Pseudoseizures may allow patients to miss work and family responsibilities, to avoid legal actions, and to gain attention and affection. Features that suggest pseudoseizures include gradual onset and offset of seizure activity, preserved awareness in the presence of bilateral motor activity, and development of multiple different seizure types in

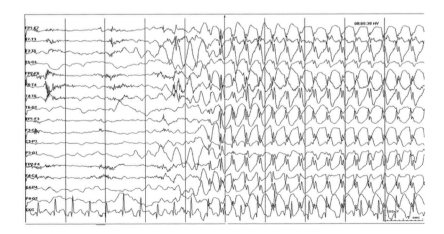

Figure 20.4 3 Hz generalized spike-wave complexes in patient with absence seizures. Image courtesy of Dr. Julie Roth.

a short time frame. Patients with pseudoseizures have events almost exclusively when there is an audience available to witness them. Elements of borderline, histrionic, and dependent personality disorders are present in many patients with pseudoseizures. These traits, however, cannot be used to make the diagnosis. Although serum prolactin levels drawn within 10–20 minutes of an event may be elevated in a patient with an epileptic seizure, they are not diagnostic of a pseudoseizure if normal.[29] The only reliable way to make the diagnosis is with video-EEG monitoring showing a lack of epileptiform changes accompanying the events. Be aware, however, that mesiofrontal and orbitofrontal seizures may appear bizarre and quite similar to pseudoseizures, and the associated electrical changes may be missed by video-EEG monitoring.[30] For patients with mesiofrontal or orbitofrontal seizures, it is the stereotyped nature of the events that usually helps to differentiate them from pseudoseizures, which often vary considerably from event to event. The presence of pseudoseizures does not exclude coexisting epilepsy, as approximately 10% of patients with a diagnosis of pseudoseizures will also have epileptic ones.[31] Treating psychogenic pseudoseizures is frequently more challenging than treating epileptic seizures because patients often resist the psychiatric treatment that will actually improve their symptoms. Patience and frank but gentle discussion about the nature of the events are more helpful than evasiveness and a string of invasive tests and ineffective or potentially toxic placebos.

5. *The patient may have seizures that are not adequately prevented by their current medical regimen.* If a patient continues to have seizures and appears to be tolerating their medication, try to increase the dose to the higher end of the therapeutic range. Measuring drug levels may be helpful to determine whether the anticonvulsant dose is adequate. If the patient does not tolerate the first medication or seizures persist despite a higher dose, try another first-line anticonvulsant (see Table 20.2). Adding a second first-line agent to the first one (polytherapy) is an alternate approach that has both merits and drawbacks (see Table 20.5 and Box 20.2). The question often arises as to the appropriate duration of an anticonvulsant trial. A good rule of thumb is that a medication should

be tried for five to ten times the average interval between seizures prior to its initiation.[32] Despite adequate medical therapy, many patients with refractory seizures may require surgical evaluation (see below).

6. *The patient has a refractory epilepsy syndrome that will respond poorly to any medical or surgical treatment.* The classic example of this is Lennox–Gastaut syndrome (LGS), characterized by a panoply of different seizure types, most commonly atypical absence, tonic, and atonic seizures. Patients with LGS are usually mentally retarded and may also have myoclonic seizures, GTCSs, and partial seizures. The interictal EEG signature of LGS is the 2–2.5 Hz spike-and-wave

---

Box 20.2 Antiepileptic drug interactions

Interactions between antiepileptic drugs may become problematic in patients receiving polytherapy. The following is a brief summary of common and important drug interactions.

The older anticonvulsants phenobarbital, phenytoin, and carbamazepine all induce hepatic P450 enzymes, which in turn decrease the levels of carbamazepine, valproate, lamotrigine, topiramate, and zonisamide. It is therefore important to monitor clinical effects and medication levels closely in patients who are receiving polytherapy with these agents. Interactions may be especially complex when two of the older medications are combined.

Carbamazepine induces its own metabolism (and therefore decreases its own level), a process that usually stabilizes 20–30 days after initiating or changing the dose.[33]

Phenobarbital, phenytoin, and carbamazepine induce the uridine glucuronyl transferases, which metabolize lamotrigine. Patients taking one of these medications may, therefore, require higher doses of lamotrigine.

Valproate inhibits the metabolism of phenobarbital, phenytoin, carbamazepine, and lamotrigine. The reduced metabolism of lamotrigine is particularly important, as it may lead to toxicity. For patients already taking valproate, lamotrigine should therefore be started at half the typical starting dose and titrated half as quickly. In addition, valproate displaces phenytoin from its protein-binding sites, leading to an increase in the free serum concentration of phenytoin.

Table 20.5 Suggested polytherapy combinations

First medication	Seizure type	Phenytoin	Carbamazepine	Valproic acid	Lamotrigine	Topiramate	Oxcarbazepine	Levetiracetam	Zonisamide
Phenytoin	Partial + secondary generalized			X	X			X	
Carbamazepine	Partial + secondary generalized			X	X			X	
Valproate	Primary generalized including myoclonic and absence				X	X			X
Lamotrigine	Partial + secondary generalized	X	X	X			X	X	
Lamotrigine	Primary generalized including myoclonic			X		X			X
Oxcarbazepine	Partial + secondary generalized	X		X	X			X	
Levetiracetam	Partial + secondary generalized	X	X	X	X		X		

complex (Figure 20.5). Although seizures develop in early childhood, patients with LGS commonly survive into adulthood and are often admitted to inpatient epilepsy monitoring units during stretches of poor seizure control. Unfortunately, seizures tend to be refractory to standard treatments, and creative combinations of medical and surgical therapy are usually required. Most patients need high doses of traditional and experimental anticonvulsants supplemented by benzodiazepines. Medications used specifically for LGS, but rarely for other indications, include felbamate and rufinamide. A variety of surgical therapies including corpus callosotomy and vagus nerve stimulation may be helpful. Some patients benefit from the ketogenic diet.

Epilepsy surgery

Because seizure control with a third anticonvulsant after two unsuccessful medication trials is unlikely, consider epilepsy surgery evaluation for patients with poorly controlled seizures despite adequate trials of two first-line anticonvulsants.[34] Presurgical evaluation is usually done by a multidisciplinary group including a neurologist, neurosurgeon, clinical psychologist, and epilepsy nurse. The evaluation of potential candidates begins with MRI of the brain to look for surgically correctable structural abnormalities and inpatient video-EEG monitoring to localize the seizure focus. If a relevant seizure focus is found,

testing proceeds with evaluation of language and memory (including a Wada test, transcranial magnetic stimulation, and neuropsychological evaluation) to minimize the chance that resection will produce adverse behavioral consequences. Surgical options include curative surgeries, which involve resection of a seizure focus (e.g. temporal lobectomy), and palliative surgeries, such as corpus callosotomy and multiple subpial transections, which are used in patients with severe refractory seizure disorders including LGS. Among curative surgeries, patients who undergo temporal lobectomy have a better long-term outcome than those who undergo occipital and parietal resections.[35] Frontal lobe resection is the least likely to be successful. While corpus callostomy and multiple subpial transections do not usually result in seizure freedom, they may decrease seizure frequency enough to have a positive impact on a patient's quality of life.

Vagus nerve stimulation

The vagus nerve stimulator (VNS) is a pacemaker-like device, which is implanted under the left clavicle. Stimulation of the vagus nerve reduces seizure frequency and aborts seizures, possibly by activating neuronal networks in the thalamus and limbic system.[36] Meta-analysis of VNS efficacy data shows that approximately 45% of patients who undergo implantation achieve a 50% reduction in seizure frequency.[36] Common side effects of VNS include hoarseness,

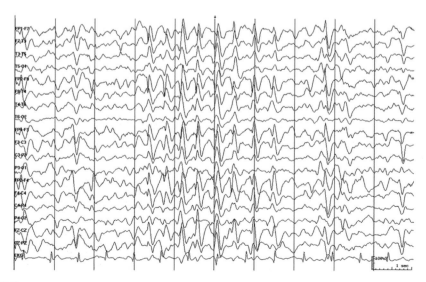

Figure 20.5 2 Hz generalized discharges characteristic of Lennox–Gastaux syndrome. Image courtesy of Dr. Julie Roth.

throat pain, and cough, all of which may be remedied by adjusting device parameters.

Withdrawing anticonvulsants

Slow anticonvulsant tapering over 2–3 months may be appropriate for patients with long periods of seizure freedom. In patients who are seizure free for at least 2 years, the chance to remain seizure free over the next 2 years is approximately 80% in patients who continue to take anticonvulsants and 60% in those who discontinue them.[37] Ideally, candidates for medication withdrawal should have normal neurological examinations, neuroimaging studies, and EEG results at the time of medication withdrawal. Factors that predict successful anticonvulsant discontinuation include longer periods of seizure freedom, use of a single anticonvulsant to achieve seizure freedom, and a lack of tonic–clonic seizures. It is important to involve the patient in the discussion about medication withdrawal: some are eager to discontinue their anticonvulsants, while others enjoy a greater peace of mind if they continue to take them.

Status epilepticus

Status epilepticus is defined as seizure activity that lasts for at least 30 minutes. This definition, however, has limited clinical utility, as seizures that last for even as little as 5 minutes are unlikely to resolve on their own and should be treated as status epilepticus.[38] Status epilepticus is divided into convulsive and nonconvulsive types. Convulsive status epilepticus (repetitive GTCSs) is a true medical emergency and will be the focus of this section. Nonconvulsive status epilepticus is discussed further in Chapter 1. Because it is easy to panic when dealing with a patient in convulsive status epilepticus, it helps to have a systematic approach to reduce uncertainty and to guide appropriate management, as follows.

Step 1: life support

Protecting the airway (with mechanical intubation if necessary) and obtaining intravenous access are the first steps in managing status epilepticus. Although some anticonvulsants may be given intramuscularly or rectally, most anticonvulsants used for status epilepticus require intravenous access. When establishing access, draw blood for laboratory studies including a complete blood count, chemistry panel, liver function tests, anticonvulsant levels, and toxicology screens.

Step 2: abort seizures

Phase 1: benzodiazepines

Intravenous lorazepam (0.1 mg/kg) will abort status epilepticus in approximately two-thirds of patients.[37] If the patient lacks intravenous access at seizure onset, alternative benzodiazepine choices include diazepam (20 mg rectally) or midazolam (10–20 mg intramuscularly).[39] Administer a second dose of lorazepam if the first dose fails to abort seizure activity within 5 minutes.

Phase 2: fosphenytoin

Treat patients who do not respond to lorazepam with intravenous fosphenytoin (20 mg/kg at a rate of 150 mg/minute). Fosphenytoin is preferred to phenytoin because it produces less local irritation at the infusion site, can be administered safely through peripheral intravenous lines, and can be infused three times faster than phenytoin.

Phase 3: intravenous anticonvulsants that require intubation

Patients with status epilepticus that is refractory to lorazepam and fosphenytoin will require transfer to an intensive care unit and stronger medications that necessitate intubation. The options at this stage of treatment are:

- phenobarbital 20 mg/kg IV
- midazolam 0.2 mg/kg loading dose followed by 0.05–2.0 mg/kg/hour continuous infusion
- propofol 1–2 mg/kg loading dose followed by 2–10 mg/kg/hour continuous infusion

Additional anticonvulsants that may be considered at this stage include intravenous valproate (30 mg/kg over 10 minutes) and intravenous levetiracetam (20 mg/kg over 14 minutes).

Phase 4: pentobarbital coma

If phenobarbital, midazolam, or propofol fail to control status epilepticus, the next line of treatment is pentobarbital coma. Patients must be attached to continuous bedside EEG telemetry, as the induced coma will suppress the motor manifestations of status epilepticus that are normally used to monitor treatment success or failure. Pentobarbital is loaded at a dose of 5 mg/kg followed by IV infusion of 1–10 mg/kg/hour, titrated gradually upwards to a burst-suppression pattern on EEG (Figure 20.6). Pentobarbital coma is typically

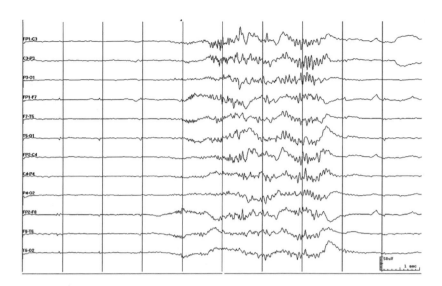

Figure 20.6 Burst suppression in a patient with status epilepticus being treated with pentobarbital coma. Image courtesy of Dr. Julie Roth.

maintained for 24 hours, at which point the medication is weaned gradually, using the EEG for guidance.

Step 3: determine the underlying etiology of status epilepticus

Once seizure control is established, focus on determining the etiology of status epilepticus. Obtain collateral history if possible, with special attention to a prior history of epilepsy and anticonvulsant use. Common precipitants of status epilepticus include medication noncompliance, infections (especially meningitis and encephalitis), metabolic disturbances, drug overdose, and cardiac arrest. If a clear cause of status epilepticus is not identified from the initial history and laboratory studies, expand the evaluation to include neuroimaging and CSF analysis.

Step 4: prevent further episodes

Correcting the proximate cause of status epilepticus is obviously the first step in preventing further episodes. Some patients with provoked seizures may not require new medications. Patients with known epilepsy need augmentation of their anticonvulsant regimens. Medication noncompliance and other seizure precipitants must be addressed if relevant.

References

1. Fisher RS, van Emde Boas W, Blume W, et al. Epileptic seizures and epilepsy: definitions proposed by the International League Against Epilepsy (ILAE) and the International Bureau for Epilepsy (IBE). *Epilepsia* 2005;**46**:470–472.

2. Hauser WA, Annegers JF, Kurland LT. Incidence of epilepsy and unprovoked seizures in Rochester, Minnesota: 1935–1984. *Epilepsia* 1993;**34**:453–468.

3. Theodore WH, Porter RJ, Albert P, et al. The secondarily generalized tonic-clonic seizure: a videotape analysis. *Neurology* 1994;**44**:1403–1407.

4. Penry JK, Porter RJ, Dreifuss FE. Simultaneous recording of absence seizures with video tape and electroencephalography. *Brain* 1975;**98**:427–440.

5. Lempert T, Bauer M, Schmidt D. Syncope: a videometric analysis of 56 episodes of transient cerebral hypoxia. *Ann Neurol* 1994;**36**:233–237.

6. Zifkin BG, Dravet C. Generalized tonic-clonic seizures. In: Engel J, Pedley TA, eds. *Epilepsy: a Comprehensive Textbook*. Philadelphia: Lippincott Williams & Wilkins; 2008; 553–562.

7. Krumholz A, Wiebe S, Gronseth G, et al. Practice parameter: evaluating an apparent unprovoked first seizure in adults (an evidence-based review). *Neurology* 2007;**69**:1996–2007.

8. Zivin L, Ajmone Marson C. Incidence and prognostic significance of epileptiform activity in the EEG of non-epileptic subjects. *Brain* 1968;**91**:751–778.

9. Marsan CA, Zivin LS. Factors related to the occurrence of typical paroxysmal abnormalities in the EEG records of epileptic patients. *Epilepsia* 1970;**11**:361–381.

10. Risinger MW, Engel J, Van Ness PC, Henry TR, Crandall PH. Ictal localization of temporal lobe seizures with scalp/sphenoidal recordings. *Neurology* 1989;**39**:1288–1293.

11. Raskin NH, Fishman RA. Neurologic disorders in renal failure. *N Engl J Med* 1967;**294**:143–148.

12. Langendorf FG, Pedley TA, Temkin NR. Posttraumatic seizures. In: Engel J, Pedley TA, eds. *Epilepsy: a Comprehensive Textbook*. Philadelphia: Lippincott Williams & Wilkins; 2008; 2537–2542.

13. Annegers JF, Hauser WA, Coan SP, Rocca WA. A population-based study of seizures after traumatic brain injuries. *N Engl J Med* 1998;**338**:20–24.

14. Annegers JF, Grabow JD, Groover RV, et al. Seizures after head trauma: a population study. *Neurology* 1980;**30**:683–689.

15. Victor M, Brausch C. The role of abstinence in the genesis of alcoholic epilepsy. *Epilepsia* 1967;**8**:1–20.

16. Le Blanc F, Rasmussen T. Cerebral seizures and brain tumors. *Handbook Clin Neurol* 1974;**15**:295–301.

17. Glantz MJ, Cole BF, Forsyth PA, et al. Practice parameter: anticonvulsant prophylaxis in patients with newly diagnosed brain tumors. *Neurology* 2000;**54**:1886–1893.

18. Bladin CF, Alexandrov AV, Bellavance A, et al. Seizures after stroke. A prospective multicenter study. *Arch Neurol* 2000;**57**:1617–1622.

19. Aminoff MJ, Parent JM. Comorbidity in adults. In: Engel J, Pedley TA, eds. *Epilepsy: a Comprehensive Textbook*. Philadelphia: Lippincott Williams & Wilkins; 2008; 2007–2019.

20. Duley L, Gulmezoglu AM, Henderson-Smart DJ. Magnesium sulphate and other anticonvulsants for women with pre-eclampsia. *Cochrane Database Syst Rev* 2003;(2):CD000025.

21. Duley L, Henderson-Smart DJ. Magnesium sulphate versus diazepam for eclampsia. *Cochrane Database Syst Rev* 2003;(2):CD000127..

22. Duley L, Henderson-Smart DJ. Magnesium sulphate versus phenytoin for eclampsia. *Cochrane Database Syst Rev* 2003;(2):CD000128.

23. Hopkins A, Garman A, Clarke C. The first seizure in adult life. *Lancet* 1988;**1**:721–726.

24. Hauser WA, Rich SS, Lee JRJ, Annegers JF, Anderson VE. Risk of recurrent seizures after two unprovoked seizures. *N Engl J Med* 1998;**338**:429–434.

25. Karceski S, Morrell M, Carpenter D. The expert consensus guideline series. Treatment of epilepsy. *Epilepsy Behavior* 2001;**2**:A1–A50.

26. Lacerda G, Krummel T, Sabourdy C, Ryvlin P, Hirsch E. Optimizing therapy of seizures in patients with renal or hepatic dysfunction. *Neurology* 2006;**67**:S28–S33.

27. Annegers JF, Hauser WA, Elveback LR. Remission of seizures and relapse in patients with epilepsy. *Epilepsia* 1979;**20**:729–737.

28. Benbadis SR, Hauser WA. An estimate of the prevalence of psychogenic nonepileptic seizures. *Seizure* 2000;**9**:280–281.

29. Chen DK, So YT, Fisher RS. Use of serum prolactin in diagnosing epileptic seizures. Report of the Therapeutics and Technology Assessment Subcommittee of the American Academy of Neurology. *Neurology* 2005;**65**:668–675.

30. Williamson PD, Spencer DD, Spencer SS, Novelly RA, Mattson RH. Complex partial seizures of frontal lobe origin. *Ann Neurol* 1985;**18**:497–504.

31. Benbadis SR, Agrawal V, Tatum WO. How many patients with psychogenic nonepileptic seizures also have epilepsy? *Neurology* 2001;**57**:915–917.

32. Bourgeois B. Long-term therapy with antiepileptic drugs. In: Wyllie E, ed. *The Treatment of Epilepsy Principles & Practice*. Philadelphia: Lippincott Williams & Wilkins; 2001; 769–774.

33. Altafullah I, Talwar D, Loewenson R, Olson K, Lockman LA. Factors influencing serum levels of carbamazepine and carbamazepine 10,11-epoxide in children. *Epilepsy Res* 1989;**4**:72–80.

34. Kwan P, Brodie MJ. Early identification of refractory epilepsy. *N Engl J Med* 2000;**342**:314–319.

35. Tellez-Zenteno JF, Dhar R, Wiebe S. Long-term seizure outcomes following epilepsy surgery: a systematic review and meta-analysis. *Brain* 2005;**128**:1188–1198.

36. Ben-Menachem E. Vagus nerve stimulation for the treatment of epilepsy. *Lancet Neurol* 2002;**1**:477–482.

37. Medical Research Council Antiepileptic Drug Withdrawal Study Group. Randomised study of antiepileptic drug withdrawal in patients in remission. *Lancet* 1991;**337**:1175–1180.

38. Lowenstein DH, Bleck T, Macdonald RL. It's time to revise the definition of status epilepticus. *Epilepsia* 1999;**40**:120–122.

39. Towne AR, DeLorenzo RJ. Use of intramuscular midazolam for status epilepticus. *J Emerg Med* 1999;**17**:323–328.

Chapter

21 Stroke

Common stroke syndromes

Stroke is a sudden-onset neurological syndrome caused by infarction or hemorrhage within the CNS. While there is no substitute for a detailed understanding of neuroanatomy, recognizing the following common stroke syndromes is a powerful bedside tool for localizing and diagnosing stroke.

Anterior circulation ischemic strokes

Middle cerebral artery syndromes

The anatomy of the circle of Willis, including the origin of the middle cerebral artery (MCA), is shown in Figure 21.1. The MCA is one of the two main branches of the internal carotid artery. Infarction of the MCA or its branches is one of the most common causes of stroke. The first important branches of the MCA are the lenticulostrate arteries, which arise from the stem of the artery and supply the caudate nucleus, internal capsule, putamen, and lateral globus pallidus. After giving rise to the lenticulostrate arteries, the MCA most commonly divides into superior and inferior divisions. The superior division supplies the frontal lobe, while the inferior division supplies the superior temporal lobe.[1] The parietal lobe may be supplied by either the superior or inferior division or by both. Depending on the site of occlusion, MCA strokes lead to the following sensorimotor abnormalities:

- Occlusion at the stem of the MCA produces a severe contralateral hemiplegia, contralateral hemisensory loss, and ipsilateral eye deviation. Stem occlusion may lead to "malignant MCA syndrome" in which swelling of the infarcted territory produces increased intracranial pressure and potentially herniation and death (see below and Chapter 2).
- Infarction of the MCA distal to the takeoff of the medial lenticulostrate arteries produces contralateral weakness of the face and arm, and may be associated with ipsilateral eye deviation.

Hemiparesis tends to be milder than when the occlusion takes place at the stem of the artery.
- Superior division infarction typically produces contralateral weakness and numbness that are greatest in the face and hand.
- Inferior division infarction results in mild contralateral face and hand weakness and numbness, and sometimes a contralateral homonymous hemianopia.

In addition to sensorimotor abnormalities, MCA infarction often produces behavioral manifestations that depend on the hemisphere involved:

- Left MCA. The characteristic behavioral manifestation of left MCA infarction is aphasia, the acquired loss of language (see Chapter 3). Complete left MCA infarction in a patient with left hemispheric dominance for language would be expected to produce global aphasia. Broca's aphasia is associated with superior division infarction, whereas Wernicke's aphasia is associated with inferior division infarction.
- Right MCA. The classical behavioral manifestation of a right MCA stroke is left-sided hemineglect (see Chapter 1). Stroke involving the inferior division of the right MCA may produce an acute agitated delirium.[2]

Anterior cerebral artery syndrome

The anterior cerebral artery (ACA) is derived from the internal carotid artery (Figure 21.1). The proximal ACA, or A1 segment, connects the internal carotid artery and the anterior communicating artery (ACOM). The distal ACA (beginning with the A2 segment) arises from the ACOM, and contains most of the branches that supply the medial frontal and parietal lobes. Anterior cerebral artery stroke results in contralateral leg weakness that is greatest in the foot. Sensory deficits in the leg and foot are usually modest. Stroke involving the left anterior cerebral artery may produce transcortical motor aphasia (Chapter 3). In patients with an azygous

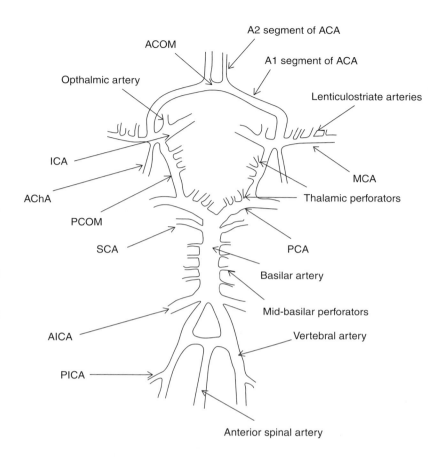

Figure 21.1 The circle of Willis. ACA = anterior cerebral artery, AChA = anterior choroidal artery, ACOM = anterior communicating artery, AICA = anterior inferior cerebellar artery, ICA = internal carotid artery, MCA = middle cerebral artery, PCA = posterior cerebral artery, PCOM = posterior communicating artery, PICA = posterior inferior cerebellar artery, SCA = superior cerebellar artery.

ACA in which both distal segments arise from the same A1, unilateral A1 occlusion leads to infarction of both distal ACA territories, and therefore bilateral leg weakness. Anterior cerebral artery infarction is much less common than MCA infarction.

Internal carotid artery

The common carotid artery bifurcates into the internal carotid artery (ICA) and external carotid artery in the neck at approximately the level of the fourth cervical vertebrae. The ICA enters the skull via the carotid canal and crosses the foramen lacerum before entering the cavernous sinus. After emerging from the cavernous sinus, the carotid artery gives rise to the ophthalmic artery and then trifurcates into the ACA, MCA, and posterior communicating artery (PCOM) (Figure 21.1). The anterior choroidal artery (AChA) usually arises from the ICA just distal to the trifurcation. The following are the common ICA stroke syndromes:

- Internal carotid artery occlusion. Occlusion of the ICA results in the combination of MCA and ACA

syndromes. Deficits are usually severe and may be life-threatening if the occlusion takes place rapidly. Deficits are milder if the occlusion develops slowly, after collateral circulation via the circle of Willis has been established.

- Distal embolization. Distal emboli from the ICA most commonly lodge in the MCA or the ophthalmic artery, but may involve any of its branches. Stroke involving the ophthalmic artery or its branches causes monocular blindness, which, if transient, leads to the clinical syndrome of amaurosis fugax (Chapter 5).
- Watershed infarction. The ischemic watershed or borderzone refers to an area of the brain perfused by the end distributions of two vascular territories. Because these areas have the most tenuous blood supplies, systemic hypotension, often in the context of cardiac arrest, may lead to preferential infarction in a watershed distribution. The most common watershed syndrome involves the territory that is jointly perfused by the ACA

and MCA, leading to weakness with or without sensory disturbance of the proximal arm and leg, the so-called "man in a barrel" syndrome.

- Carotid artery dissection. Headache, ipsilateral eye pain, and Horner's syndrome are the most common symptoms of carotid artery dissection (Chapter 19).
- Anterior choroidal artery infarction. The AChA is usually a branch of the ICA, but it may also arise from the MCA or the PCOM. The AChA variably supplies blood to the motor and sensory fibers within the posterior limb of the internal capsule, the optic tract, the lateral geniculate body, and the optic radiations. Anterior choroidal artery syndrome, uncommon and usually incomplete, includes components of contralateral weakness, sensory loss, and homonymous hemianopia.

Posterior circulation ischemic strokes

The vertebral arteries are derived from the subclavian arteries in the chest and ascend through the foramen transversarium of the C2–6 vertebrae. They then pass through the foramen magnum to enter the skull. The vertebral arteries give rise to the posterior inferior cerebellar arteries at the inferior medullary level and send branches to the anterior spinal artery at the mid-medullary level (Figure 21.1). The vertebral arteries then fuse at the pontomedullary junction to form the basilar artery. The anterior inferior cerebellar arteries are the first branches of the basilar artery. Penetrating branches arise from the basilar artery as it runs along the ventral surface of the pons. The superior cerebellar arteries and the posterior cerebral arteries are the next branches. Finally, the basilar artery gives rise to the paired posterior communicating arteries, which anastomose with the anterior circulation. Posterior circulation infarction is often patchy, producing a variety of deficits such as diplopia, dysarthria, facial and body numbness, vertigo, and nausea and vomiting. Nonetheless, there are several well-defined posterior circulation syndromes, described below.

Wallenberg's syndrome

Occlusion of the vertebral or (less commonly) the posterior inferior cerebellar artery results in infarction of the lateral medulla, leading to Wallenberg's syndrome (Figure 21.2). Common symptoms of Wallenberg's syndrome include vertigo, nausea, vomiting, facial pain, dysarthria, dysphagia, and ipsilateral limb ataxia. Examination findings include nystagmus, loss of pinprick sensation in the ipsilateral face and contralateral body, ipsilateral Horner's syndrome, and ipsilateral limb ataxia.

Mid-basilar artery occlusion

The basilar artery runs along the midline of the ventral pons. Complete occlusion of the basilar artery deprives the descending bilateral corticospinal and corticobulbar tracts of their blood supplies, leading to locked-in syndrome in which the patient is completely paralyzed with the exception of preserved vertical eye

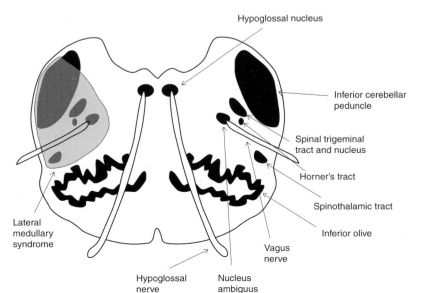

Figure 21.2 Cross section of the medulla showing the structures involved in a lateral medullary infarction (Wallenberg's syndrome). Although there is considerable variety among patients with this syndrome, typical features include vertigo and ipsilateral limb ataxia (inferior cerebellar peduncle), ipsilateral facial sensory loss (spinal trigeminal tract and nucleus), contralateral hemibody sensory loss (spinothalamic tract), ipsilateral Horner's syndrome (Horner's tract), and dysphagia (nucleus ambiguus and vagus nerve).

Hypoglossal nucleus

Inferior cerebellar peduncle

Spinal trigeminal tract and nucleus

Horner's tract

Spinothalamic tract

Inferior olive

Lateral medullary syndrome

Vagus nerve

Hypoglossal nerve

Nucleus ambiguus

Table 21.1 Cerebellar stroke syndromes

Territory	Extracerebellar structures affected	Extracerebellar signs and symptoms
Superior cerebellar artery	Midbrain, thalamus, occipital lobes	Top of the basilar syndrome
Posterior inferior cerebellar artery	Dorsolateral medulla	Wallenberg's syndrome
Anterior inferior cerebellar artery	Lateral pons	Contralateral facial weakness, numbness, and hearing loss

movements and blinking. Although the patient may appear uncommunicative, consciousness is actually preserved because the midbrain and thalamus are spared.

Mid-basilar penetrating branch occlusion

Occlusion of one of the smaller penetrating branches of the mid-basilar artery most commonly produces contralateral hemiparesis. If the abducens or facial nerve fascicles are involved, ipsilateral eye abduction (Chapter 6) and ipsilateral facial movement (Chapter 8) may be impaired.

Rostral basilar (top of the basilar) occlusion

Occlusion of the rostral basilar artery produces a variety of ocular motor and behavioral manifestations, most commonly vertical gaze and convergence impairments.[3] In many cases, the distal basilar branches (the superior cerebellar artery and posterior cerebral artery) are also involved. There is, however, no single unifying clinical feature of rostral basilar occlusion that allows it to be instantly recognized.

Posterior cerebral artery infarction

The posterior cerebral artery (PCA) supplies the visual cortex in the occipital lobes. Visual abnormalities are therefore the most consistent manifestations of PCA infarction (Chapter 5):

- Unilateral PCA infarction leads to macular-sparing contralateral homonymous hemianopia. The patient often does not recognize this problem until their visual fields are tested at the bedside.
- Bilateral PCA infarction results in complete visual loss. In some cases, a patient with bilateral PCA infarction may deny that they are blind and confabulate a detailed visual scene (Anton's syndrome).
- Infarction of the left PCA may produce alexia without agraphia.
- Occasionally, PCA infarction may lead to a state of agitated confusion (Chapter 1).[4]

Thalamic strokes

Thalamic strokes produce a heterogeneous group of clinical deficits. The arteries that supply the thalamus are derived from the posterior cerebral and posterior communicating arteries, and are often quite variable in their origins. The common vascular syndromes of the thalamus involve the following four arteries[5]:

- Thalamogeniculate artery. This artery supplies the lateral thalamus and leads to contralateral hemibody numbness (see "pure sensory lacune", below).
- Paramedian thalamic–subthalamic artery. Medial thalamic infarction leads to problems with consciousness, behavior, and vertical gaze. These patients often present in coma, and when they awaken, appear confused or apathetic (Chapter 2).
- Polar artery. Infarction of the anterior thalamus leads to a variety of behavioral manifestations including amnesia, aphasia, and confusion, in some cases causing "sudden-onset dementia" (Chapter 4).
- Posterior choroidal artery. This artery supplies the lateral geniculate body and leads to contralateral homonymous field deficits, most characteristically the loss of a central wedge of vision (Chapter 5).

Cerebellar strokes

The three arteries that supply blood to the cerebellum are the superior cerebellar artery (SCA), the anterior inferior cerebellar artery (AICA), and the posterior inferior cerebellar artery (PICA). Typical features of cerebellar strokes include occipital–nuchal headache, nausea and vomiting, ataxia, and dysarthria. In some cases, isolated cerebellar infarctions may produce only vertigo and thus resemble a more benign condition such as labyrinthitis (Chapter 9). Unless the adjacent brainstem is involved, it may be difficult to distinguish among infarctions in the three arterial territories (Table 21.1). Although the majority of cerebellar infarcts produce mild, temporary deficits, larger strokes may lead to hydrocephalus or life-threatening brainstem compression if untreated.

Lacunar strokes

Lacunar strokes are small-vessel occlusions that usually occur in the context of hypertension.[6] The following are the most common lacunar syndromes:

- Pure motor lacune. Infarction anywhere in the pyramidal tract may produce contralateral hemiparesis affecting the face, arm, and leg without sensory or behavioral manifestations. Most commonly, the infarction is in the posterior limb of the contralateral internal capsule, although infarction in the contralateral corona radiata, base of the pons, or cerebral peduncle may also result in a pure motor syndrome.
- Pure sensory lacune. Lacunar infarction of the contralateral ventroposterior thalamus (ventroposterolateral and ventroposteromedial nuclei) leads to the sudden onset of contralateral numbness of the face, arm, and leg.
- Ataxic hemiparesis. Small-vessel infarction involving the base of the pons may produce contralateral limb weakness and ataxia. The foot tends to be weaker than the hand, which in turn tends to be weaker than the face.
- Clumsy hand–dysarthria. Lacunes involving the base of the pons or the genu of the internal capsule may produce severe dysarthria with contralateral face and hand weakness.

Intracranial hemorrhage

Intracranial hemorrhage (ICH) accounts for approximately 20% of strokes. It presents in a very similar or identical manner to ischemic stroke, but is more likely to progress over minutes to hours. It is often difficult to distinguish between hemorrhage and infarction by history and physical examination alone. Although headache makes ICH slightly more likely than ischemic stroke, neuroimaging studies are much more reliable in distinguishing between the two stroke types. Evaluation and treatment of ICH is discussed in greater detail below.

Cerebral venous thrombosis

Venous strokes are much less common than arterial ones. Susceptible populations include women in the puerperium, patients with hereditary coagulation defects, and patients with systemic inflammatory diseases. Because headache is the most common presentation of venous sinus thrombosis, it is discussed in more detail in Chapter 19.

Stroke mimics

The rapidity of symptom onset that characterizes stroke is not unique, and in approximately one-third of cases, sudden-onset neurological deficits are produced by other medical, neurological, or psychiatric conditions.[7]

Acute confusional state

While acute confusional states may occasionally be secondary to stroke in the distribution of the left posterior cerebral or right middle cerebral arteries, they are more commonly secondary to toxic or metabolic disturbances.[4,8] Evaluation of confusion is discussed further in Chapter 1.

Focal neuropathies

Deep sleep, usually secondary to heavy intoxication or surgery, may lead to a sudden-onset, painless focal neuropathy that mimics stroke. The best-known focal neuropathy of this type is "Saturday night palsy," which occurs when a patient awakens with a radial neuropathy after sleeping with their arm draped over a chair or bed. Other nerves that are susceptible to focal injuries mimicking stroke include the ulnar, sciatic, and common peroneal nerves. The techniques to distinguish between stroke and focal neuropathy are discussed in further detail in Chapter 11. Although physical examination may help to differentiate focal neuropathies from stroke in most cases, neuroimaging studies or electromyography are often required to solidify the diagnosis. Exercise caution in diagnosing a focal neuropathy rather than a stroke, as infarction of the "hand knob" area of the cerebral cortex may resemble a radial or ulnar neuropathy quite closely.[9]

Metabolic insult causing re-expression of old stroke

The frequently observed, although not formally studied, phenomenon of metabolic insult causing re-expression of old stroke (MICROS) is characterized by the apparent return of prior stroke deficits when patients are subjected to metabolic insults, most commonly urinary tract infections, pneumonia, or medication toxicity. The pathophysiology of MICROS is not well understood, but it is likely that compensatory synaptogenesis, which occurs in the process of stroke recovery, is susceptible to relatively small metabolic perturbations that do not affect otherwise healthy brain tissue. The phenomenon of MICROS should be considered only after thorough evaluation excludes the presence of an actual stroke. Treat MICROS by correcting the responsible medical condition: deficits will improve, sometimes in a few hours but more often over the course of several days.

Migraine aura

Migraine aura may resemble stroke when it is not followed by headache (Chapter 19). Usually, however, the tempo and progression of deficits help to distinguish between migraine aura and stroke. Focal deficits in migraine aura are typically followed by symptoms that develop over several minutes when adjacent cortical areas become involved by a wave of spreading depression. Stroke deficits, in contrast, are maximal at onset and progress very little, if at all. Younger patients with a history of migraine do not require further evaluation for stroke. Older patients and those without any prior history of aura, however, require neuroimaging studies before the diagnosis may be made comfortably.

Todd's paralysis

A combination of neuronal exhaustion and inhibition following a seizure may produce a variety of clinical deficits including focal numbness, visual field cuts, and aphasia (Chapter 20). The most well-known postictal deficit is Todd's paralysis, characterized by focal weakness following a motor seizure. Todd's paralysis and related postictal phenomena are most likely to be misdiagnosed as stroke when the preceding seizure is not witnessed.

Transient global amnesia

Transient global amnesia (TGA) is an acute-onset amnestic state in which a patient loses the ability to encode new memories (Chapter 1).[10] The patient with TGA characteristically repeats the same questions every 2–5 minutes, but is otherwise capable of performing cognitive tasks at a very high level. An episode typically lasts for several hours and resolves spontaneously. The exact pathophysiology of TGA is unclear: it may be related to migraine, seizure, or stroke.

Subdural hematoma

The protean manifestations of subdural hematoma (SDH) include hemiparesis, seizures, and confusion,

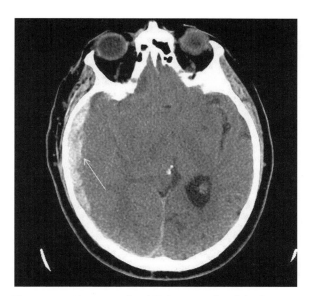

Figure 21.3 Noncontrast head CT showing right subdural hematoma (arrow). Note the presence of a midline shift.

and even the best neurologist may miss the diagnosis by failing to consider it. In the presence of a typical history of head trauma with headache and focal neurological signs, the diagnosis of SDH is fairly straightforward. Head trauma, however, is often occult or not remembered, and the diagnosis may thus be delayed by several days or weeks. Noncontrast head CT is the diagnostic study of choice (Figure 21.3). The first step in treating SDH is to prevent further hematoma expansion by reversing anticoagulation (see below). Indications for neurosurgical intervention include significant midline shift, progression of neurological deficits, and expansion of hematoma size on serial CT scans.

Hypoglycemia and hyperglycemia

Both high and low blood sugar levels may result in focal neurological deficits that closely resemble acute ischemic stroke. Restoring normoglycemia usually resolves any deficits in a few hours, but improvement may sometimes take several days.

Psychogenic disorders

Psychogenic disorders, especially malingering and conversion disorders, may mimic stroke. While these conditions are often quite transparent, mimicry of true neurological deficits may be precise enough to require detailed neuroimaging to secure the diagnosis.

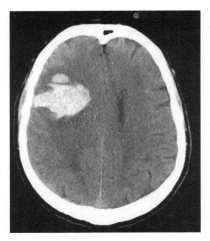

Figure 21.4 Noncontrast head CT showing an intracranial hemorrhage.

Table 21.2 CT changes in early ischemic stroke

Cortical sulcal effacement
CT dot sign
Hyperdense MCA sign
Loss of gray–white differentiation in basal ganglia
Loss of insular ribbon
Obscuration of the lentiform nucleus

Peripheral vestibulopathy

Peripheral vestibulopathy is often difficult to separate from central causes of vertigo such as brainstem or cerebellar infarction (Chapter 9).

Bell's palsy

Bell's palsy is acute facial weakness caused by a peripheral lesion of the facial nerve, and is discussed further in Chapter 8.

Physical examination

Obviously, every patient with a suspected stroke requires comprehensive neurological examination to define the clinical effects of the stroke. Cardiovascular and funduscopic examinations are the most important components of the general physical examination. Auscultation of a heart murmur or atrial fibrillation points to a potential cardioembolic source of stroke. A carotid bruit is often a nonspecific finding of systemic atherosclerosis. A long, high-pitched bruit located high within the neck at the carotid bifurcation, however, suggests the possibility of carotid artery stenosis.[11] Funduscopic examination may disclose Hollenhorst plaques, which are bright white particles that appear at retinal vascular bifurcations and usually suggest an embolic stroke source from the ipsilateral carotid artery or heart. In patients with central retinal artery occlusion, funduscopy shows macular pallor and a cherry-red spot in the fovea (Chapter 5).

Laboratory studies

All patients evaluated for suspected acute stroke require a routine set of laboratory tests, including a complete blood count, basic metabolic profile, coagulation studies, urinalysis, toxicology screen, and chest X-ray. While these tests may have only limited utility in defining the etiology of stroke, they help to diagnose stroke mimics, screen for conditions that may worsen stroke outcome, and determine whether patients are eligible for intravenous thrombolysis.

Neuroimaging

Neuroimaging studies are essential in differentiating between ischemic and hemorrhagic strokes, help to establish the diagnosis when the history or physical examination are unreliable, point to alternative diagnoses such as brain tumor or subdural hematoma, and help to define stroke pathophysiology. Remember that neuroimaging studies are complementary to the history and examination, and that all radiographic abnormalities must be placed in the appropriate clinical context.

Noncontrast head CT

Noncontrast head CT is usually the first and often the only neuroimaging study performed because it is widely available and can be obtained rapidly. In many cases, patients with suspected stroke have already had a head CT before neurological consultation is requested. The main use of a CT scan is to detect intracranial hemorrhage (Figure 21.4). The changes suggestive of acute stroke have only modest sensitivity and interobserver reliability (Table 21.2).[12,13]

Diffusion-weighted MRI

Diffusion-weighted MRI (DWI) is the imaging study of choice for acute ischemic stroke. A bright DWI signal reflecting cytotoxic edema appears within 15–30 minutes of ischemic stroke onset, and its high sensitivity for

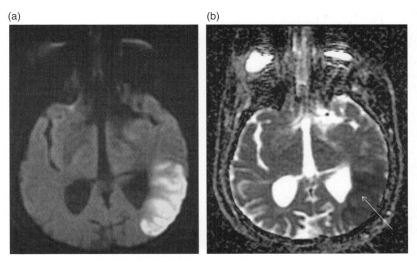

Figure 21.5 An acute occipital–temporal infarction (arrow) as captured by (A) diffusion-weighted imaging and (B) the apparent diffusion coefficient map.

acute stroke makes it ideal for evaluating patients with confusing or atypical presentations (Figure 21.5A).[14] There are two minor limitations of DWI. First, it may be insensitive to very small strokes, particularly those involving the brainstem. Secondly, old T2 lesions may "shine through" and appear bright on DWI, falsely suggesting an acute infarction. The way to differentiate between newly infarcted tissue and an old T2 lesion is by looking at the apparent diffusion coefficient (ADC) map. Acute infarction is bright on DWI, dark on the ADC map, and remains dark on the ADC map for fewer than 10 days (Figure 21.5B).[15] Older T2 hyperintensities are bright on both DWI and the ADC map.

Susceptibility images

Although the sensitivity of DWI for acute ischemia makes MRI the modality of choice for evaluating patients with suspected stroke, compared with CT, routine MRI sequences are less sensitive in detecting hemorrhage. Some patients undergo CT scanning first before they proceed to MRI. Patients who do not have a CT scan before MRI should undergo gradient echo susceptibility-weighted MR imaging (also referred to as T2*) to firmly exclude the possibility of hemorrhage (Figure 21.6). Susceptibility images are as sensitive as noncontrast head CT scan in detecting acute blood.[16]

Perfusion-weighted imaging

Perfusion-weighted imaging (PWI) provides information about relative cerebral blood flow. Areas that

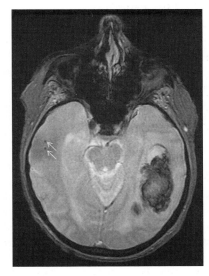

Figure 21.6 Susceptibility imaging showing left temporal–parietal hemorrhage. Note the presence of two cerebral microbleeds in the right temporal lobe (arrows), likely reflective of amyloid angiopathy.

are infarcted or are acutely vulnerable to infarction (the "ischemic penumbra") show decreased perfusion. Mismatch between the infarcted tissue on DWI and the infarcted-plus-vulnerable tissue on PWI therefore theoretically indicates the area that is potentially salvageable by reperfusion therapy.[17] The value of this diffusion–perfusion mismatch, however, is not clear in clinical practice, and PWI remains largely a research tool.

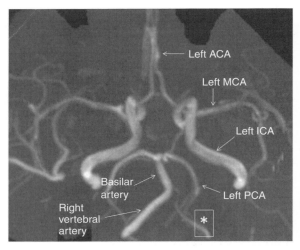

Figure 21.7 Magnetic resonance angiography of the cerebral vasculature. Note the dominance of the right vertebral artery over the left vertebral artery (*) in this patient (normal variant). ACA = anterior cerebral artery, ICA = internal carotid artery, MCA = middle cerebral artery, PCA = posterior cerebral artery.

Vascular imaging studies

Vascular imaging studies such as magnetic resonance angiography (MRA, Figure 21.7) and computed tomographic angiography (CTA) are useful in defining the specific vessel responsible for a stroke. Such information is not essential, however, in the hyperacute stage of stroke management when rapid determination of eligibility for intravenous thrombolysis is essential. Vascular imaging is useful, however, when planning intra-arterial thrombolysis. Other vascular imaging studies that may help in the acute setting include CT or MR angiogram of the neck vessels, which helps to establish the presence of carotid or vertebral artery dissection, and magnetic resonance venography (MRV), which is useful when evaluating possible cerebral venous sinus thrombosis.[18]

Selecting imaging studies

Each stroke center has specific protocols for neuroimaging, which are based largely on the preferences of the stroke specialists and the availability of interventional techniques. If rapid results to exclude hemorrhage are required to determine whether a patient is eligible for intravenous thrombolysis, then treatment should not be delayed, and a noncontrast head CT to exclude hemorrhage is necessary and sufficient. However, if a high-sensitivity study is required to establish the diagnosis of stroke, MRI including DWI, ADC map, and

susceptibility images may be required. Vascular imaging studies help to define the pathophysiology of stroke, and may be necessary if an intervention is planned, but in most cases should not delay acute therapy.

Hyperacute ischemic stroke treatment

Intravenous recombinant tissue plasminogen activator

Intravenous recombinant tissue plasminogen activator (IV rt-PA) is a thrombolytic agent used to treat acute ischemic stroke.[19] Details on the administration of IV rt-PA are found in the protocol in Box 21.1. The randomized, double-blind, placebo-controlled study sponsored by the National Institute of Neurological Disorders and Stroke provides the following data on its safety and efficacy[20]:

- Although IV rt-PA is a "clot-busting" agent, it provides no benefit compared with placebo within minutes or even 24 hours after administration.
- Patients who receive IV rt-PA have a probability of a good neurological outcome (as defined by the modified Rankin scale) of 39% at 3 months compared with 26% for those who do not receive it.
- The most important side effect of IV rt-PA is symptomatic brain hemorrhage, which occurs in approximately 6% of patients.

Intravenous rt-PA is effective when it is given within 3 hours of ischemic stroke onset. Although this may seem like a generous amount of time, few patients undergo thrombolysis because of delays in recognizing stroke, in getting to the emergency room in a timely fashion, in undergoing a directed history and noncontrast head CT, and in excluding contraindications to IV rt-PA. Thus, each minute spent in patient evaluation is critical, and it becomes essential to focus on the four "big picture" questions in order to maximize the chance that a patient receives treatment:

1. When did the problem begin? Intravenous rt-PA is only approved for stroke treatment within 3 hours of symptom onset. It is, therefore, imperative to establish the exact time at which deficits developed. Although initial investigations into IV rt-PA for patients who awaken with stroke seem promising, awakening with stroke is currently an exclusion from undergoing thrombolysis.[21]

2. Is the deficit disabling? It is also necessary to establish that the deficit from the suspected ischemic stroke is disabling. Mild dysarthria or subtle nondominant hand weakness probably does not warrant treatment with IV rtPA, but hemiparesis, aphasia, or neglect do.

3. Is there an explanation for the neurological deficit other than acute ischemic stroke? Hemorrhagic stroke is the most important condition that must be differentiated from acute ischemic stroke. All patients should therefore undergo a noncontrast head CT prior to intravenous thrombolysis. This test will also help to exclude mass lesions, which may mimic an ischemic stroke. Other important stroke mimics, including hypoglycemia, hyperglycemia, and postictal paralysis, are discussed in greater detail above and summarized in Box 21.1.

4. Are there any factors that would exclude the patient from receiving rt-PA? Contraindications to rt-PA administration are listed in Box 21.1.

Intra-arterial tPA and clot retrieval devices

Despite public education campaigns and community outreach programs, most patients with acute ischemic stroke will not reach a stroke center within the approved 3-hour window to receive IV rt-PA. Intra-arterial (IA) tPA is an option for ischemic stroke patients who are not otherwise candidates for IV rt-PA, and may be given up to 6 hours after stroke onset.[22] Risks of IA rt-PA include intracranial hemorrhage and the possibility of stroke or other complications from the angiography itself.[23] Investigational techniques such as mechanical clot retrieval devices may also be considered for patients who are not IV rt-PA candidates.[24]

Acute anticoagulation

The rationale for acutely anticoagulating a patient with acute ischemic stroke is that it may reduce the chance of early stroke recurrence, limit the extent of an existing stroke, and improve neurological outcome. There is no clear evidence, however, that heparin or

---

Box 21.1 Intravenous recombinant tissue plasminogen activator protocol

Intravenous rt-PA is indicated for patients with suspected ischemic stroke within 3 hours of stroke onset. The dose of IV rt-PA is 0.9 mg/kg, with 10% given as a bolus and the remaining 90% infused over 1 hour.

For IV rt-PA candidates with systolic blood pressure >185 or diastolic blood pressure >110 mmHg, use anti-hypertensive medications such as labetalol (10–20 mg IV prn) to lower the blood pressure. Patients who receive rt-PA should be admitted to an intensive care unit for close vital sign monitoring and serial neurological examinations for at least 24 hours. Anticoagulants and invasive procedures such as intravenous catheter and nasogastric tube placement should be avoided for 24 hours. Should the patient develop any change in neurological status, perform a CT scan immediately to exclude the possibility of hemorrhage and treat as discussed in the text.

Absolute exclusion criteria	Relative exclusion criteria
Mild or minimal stroke deficits	Improving stroke symptoms
Prior history of intracranial hemorrhage	Seizure at stroke onset
History of stroke or serious head trauma within prior 3 months	Severe stroke deficits
Major surgery within 14 days	Genitourinary or gastrointestinal bleeding within the previous 21 days
Pregnancy	Arterial puncture or lumbar puncture within prior 7 days
Persistent systolic blood pressure >185 mmHg or persistent diastolic blood pressure >110 mmHg	Serum glucose <50 or >400 mg/l
Intracranial hemorrhage on CT or MRI	
Platelets <100 000	
International normalized ratio (INR) >1.7	
Elevated partial thromboplastin time (PTT) if patient is taking heparin	

low-molecular-weight heparin is effective in doing any of these things. In addition, these anticoagulants increase the risk for hemorrhagic stroke transformation or bleeding in other parts of the body. Until clear evidence is available that anticoagulation provides more benefit than risk, it is best to avoid heparin in patients with acute ischemic stroke. Exceptions to this general statement including arterial dissection, intracardiac thrombi, and venous sinus thrombosis are discussed below.[22]

Blood pressure management

Blood pressure is almost always elevated in patients with acute ischemic stroke. Based on their experience with cardiac patients, emergency room physicians often administer antihypertensive agents to stroke patients prior to neurological consultation. This approach is often deleterious, as rapid blood pressure lowering may lead to hypoperfusion of the vulnerable ischemic penumbra and worsen both acute clinical signs and long-term outcome.[25] The indications for treating elevated blood pressure include:[22]

- intravenous thrombolysis
- excessive hypertension, arbitrarily defined as systolic blood pressure >220 mmHg or diastolic blood pressure >120 mmHg
- signs of malignant hypertension such as retinal hemorrhages and exudates, acute renal failure, and hypertensive encephalopathy
- evidence of compromise of other organ systems including cardiac ischemia or pulmonary edema

Labetalol (10–20 mg IV) is the most commonly employed antihypertensive agent for patients with acute ischemic stroke. In most cases, patients actually benefit from a slightly elevated cerebral perfusion pressure, which may be achieved by lowering the head of the bed. Hold outpatient antihypertensive medications for 24 hours unless there is a compelling reason to continue them in the acute phase.

Surgical treatment of ischemic stroke

Ischemic stroke is rarely treated surgically. The two exceptions are malignant MCA syndrome and cerebellar infarction.

Malignant middle cerebral artery syndrome

Large MCA infarctions, defined as those that involve >50% of the territory of the MCA, are associated with massive edema 24–48 hours after stroke onset

and a high likelihood of death or poor neurological outcome.[26] Medical interventions targeted towards reducing swelling and lowering intracranial pressure are generally ineffective in changing the course of malignant MCA syndrome (Chapter 2). Hemicraniectomy and duraplasty, however, allow room for the swollen brain to expand, thereby reducing the probability of herniation and death. Although surgical intervention reduces the likelihood of poor outcomes, most surviving patients still need assistance with all their activities of daily living and will be unable to walk.[27] Decisions about surgical intervention should therefore be made carefully in conjunction with the patient's family.

Cerebellar infarction

Many patients with isolated cerebellar infarctions recover spontaneously and have no lasting stroke deficits. Other patients, particularly those with large PICA infarctions, develop massive edema 24–48 hours after stroke onset, leading to brainstem compression and obstructive hydrocephalus. A patient with a cerebellar infarction should be monitored frequently, and any change in their level of consciousness should prompt neurosurgical consultation. Suboccipital decompressive craniectomy may reduce the likelihood of death and poor neurological outcome, and many patients who undergo surgery survive with only modest deficits. Because surgical intervention is widely considered the standard of care in rapidly progressing cerebellar infarction, a randomized controlled trial to better define the benefit of surgery is unlikely.

Inpatient evaluation

Cardiac evaluation

Atrial fibrillation (AF) and intracardiac thrombi are important sources of embolic strokes. Evaluation for AF and thrombi begins with careful cardiac examination to screen for irregular rhythms or murmurs. While inpatient cardiac telemetry is routinely ordered in an attempt to capture paroxysmal AF, it is generally of low yield, leading to a change in management in fewer than 2% of patients.[28] The best tool to evaluate structural abnormalities of the heart and intracardiac thrombi is transesophageal echocardiography (TEE). Although it is somewhat more invasive and less readily available than transthoracic echocardiography (TTE), TEE is superior to TTE for detecting abnormalities such as left atrial appendage thrombi, aortic atheromatous disease, patent foramen ovale (PFO), and atrial septal aneurysms.[29]

Vascular evaluation

Assessment of the intracranial circulation using MRA or CTA is typically performed at initial presentation. With the exception of patients who are being evaluated for cervical carotid or vertebral artery dissections, evaluation of the extracranial circulation usually begins when stroke deficits are stable, generally 24 hours or more into the patient's hospital course. Imaging of the extracranial carotid arteries is generally of greatest interest:

- Conventional angiography. While conventional angiography is the gold standard for the assessment of carotid artery stenosis, it is an invasive procedure associated with a 1% risk for serious side effects including death and disabling stroke.[30] Many surgeons, however, still prefer to perform conventional angiography to accurately define vascular anatomy in the planning stages of carotid endarterectomy.
- Carotid duplex ultrasound. This study is noninvasive and readily available, and is generally the first test performed to evaluate carotid artery stenosis.
- CTA and MRA. Because ultrasound may overestimate the degree of carotid artery stenosis, MRA or CTA of the neck vessels often plays a confirmatory role. For patients with posterior circulation strokes, MRA with fat suppression or CTA of the cervical portion of the vertebral arteries is used to evaluate suspected vertebral artery dissection.

Blood tests

Because hyperlipidemia and diabetes are common modifiable risk factors for stroke recurrence, measure lipid levels and hemoglobin A_{1c} percentages in all patients with ischemic stroke. Blood tests for hypercoagulable states are ordered excessively and often incorrectly in stroke patients. The "hypercoagulable panel" includes tests for deficiencies of protein C, protein S, antithrombin III, plasminogen, activated protein C resistance/factor V Leiden mutation, anticardiolipin antibodies, and lupus anticoagulant, and is generally of low yield.[31] Factors that may increase the probability of an abnormal test result include age <50, prior venous thrombosis, multiple family members with venous thrombosis, and personal history of miscarriages .

Secondary prevention

Blood pressure control

In the acute setting, lowering blood pressure is often deleterious to a patient with an ischemic stroke as it may decrease perfusion to vulnerable areas of the brain. For the purposes of secondary prevention, however, hypertension is the most commonly identified treatable stroke risk factor, and must be treated aggressively. Although specific target blood pressure levels are not defined, a common goal is 120/80, with blood pressure reductions by even as little as 10/5 decreasing the likelihood of stroke recurrence.[32] There is no set time after a stroke at which antihypertensive therapy should be initiated or restored, but 1 week poststroke is a reasonable target.

Hyperlipidemia

Statins (3-hydroxy-3-methylglutaryl coenzyme A reductase inhibitors) reduce the risk for stroke recurrence by approximately 20%.[33] Even patients with normal low-density lipoprotein (LDL) and total cholesterol levels benefit from statin therapy.[34] Although the majority of risk reduction is likely secondary to lowering of LDL levels, other important effects of statins include plaque stabilization and anti-inflammatory actions. Diet and other agents capable of lowering cholesterol are not as effective as statins in secondary stroke prevention.[35] Thus, all patients with ischemic stroke should be treated with atorvastatin 80 mg qd, lovastatin 40 mg qd, pravastatin 40 mg qd, or simvastatin 40 mg qd. Side effects of these medications include myotoxicity (Chapter 10), diarrhea, and transaminitis.

Diabetes mellitus

Diabetes mellitus is an independent risk factor for ischemic stroke. Strict glucose control (hemoglobin A_{1c} percentage <7%), whether achieved by diet, oral hypoglycemic medications, or aggressive insulin therapy, decreases the risk for stroke recurrence.[32]

General lifestyle recommendations

While official target weights for stroke patients are not available, it is important to recommend weight loss, as overweight patients (BMI >25 kg/m^2) are at increased risk of stroke recurrence. It is also important to encourage smoking cessation and regular exercise.

Table 21.3 Antiplatelet agents used in stroke prevention

Medication	Dose	Secondary stroke prevention benefits	Important side effects or other considerations
Aspirin	50–325 mg qd	More effective than placebo[38], as effective as clopidogrel[39], less effective than aspirin/extended release dipyridamole[38] or ticlopidine[40]	Gastrointestinal hemorrhage
Aspirin/extended-release dipyridamole	25/200 mg bid	More effective than aspirin[38], as effective as clopidogrel[41]	Headache, expense
Clopidogrel	75 mg qd	As effective as aspirin[39] or aspirin/extended release dipyridamole[41]	Often the best-tolerated antiplatelet agent
Clopidogrel plus aspirin	75 mg of each qd	More effective than clopidogrel alone[42]	Not recommended due to increased risk for brain hemorrhage[32,42]
Ticlopidine	250 mg bid	More effective than aspirin[40]	Infrequently prescribed due to risk of neutropenia, which requires biweekly complete blood counts

Anticoagulation

A small number of stroke etiologies require oral anti-coagulation for secondary stroke prophylaxis:

- Unless there is a clear contraindication (e.g. a bleeding diathesis or high risk of falls), treat all patients with stroke secondary to atrial fibrillation with warfarin, aiming for a goal INR of 2.0–3.0.[32]
- In general, consider treating patients with hypercoagulable states, carotid artery or vertebral dissection, or cerebral venous sinus thrombosis with warfarin for 3–6 months.
- There is no clear evidence supporting anticoagulation for patients with PFO, atrial septal aneurysm (ASA), or the combination of PFO and ASA.[36]
- Anticoagulation is not recommended for patients with ischemic stroke of undefined etiology (cryptogenic strokes).[37]

Antiplatelet therapy

Most ischemic stroke patients are not candidates for anticoagulants and are treated instead with antiplatelet agents. The four most commonly used antiplatelet agents are aspirin, aspirin plus extended-release dipyridamole, clopidogrel, and ticlopidine. Selecting the appropriate agent depends largely on the individual patient and is often the most time-consuming and passionately debated decision in secondary stroke prevention. Table 21.3 provides guidance in choosing an antiplatelet agent. For most patients, aspirin plus extended-release dipyridamole is the agent of first choice. The most common side effect of this medication is headache, which usually resolves on its own without treatment. If the headache is particularly severe and does not improve, clopidogrel is usually the preferred agent. Clopidogrel is also the first-choice medication in patients who do not tolerate aspirin.

Carotid endarterectomy and stenting

As discussed above, carotid artery stenosis is an important cause of stroke and transient ischemic attacks. Carotid endarterectomy (CEA) is the standard surgical approach to prevent ipsilateral stroke or transient ischemic attack from this process, but, because of the risks of surgery, must be considered carefully. The most important variable in determining who should undergo CEA is the degree of carotid stenosis (see also Box 21.2):

- Patients with stenosis between 70 and 99% derive the greatest benefit from CEA, and should undergo surgery, preferably within 2 weeks of their stroke or transient ischemic attack.[43–45]
- Patients with 50–69% stenosis may or may not benefit from surgery. Men with this degree of stenosis tend to benefit more than women.[46] To improve the chances of a good outcome, CEA for 50–69% stenosis should only be performed by surgeons with low complication rates.
- Patients with stenosis <50% or complete occlusion of the carotid artery should be managed with antiplatelet agents and statins.

Carotid artery stenting is a less invasive interventional approach to carotid artery stenosis, which may be used for patients with stenosis between 70 and 99% who have multiple medical comorbidities, extensive or poorly accessible lesions, radiation-induced carotid stenosis, and restenosis after previous CEA.[47]

Box 21.2 Asymptomatic carotid artery stenosis

Carotid bruits are detected frequently on routine physical examination. Primary care physicians often refer these patients to neurologists, or do so after an ultrasound discloses carotid artery stenosis. In some cases, vascular surgeons seek guidance in managing these patients. Because asymptomatic carotid artery stenosis is such a common problem, it is important to understand the data in order to recommend the appropriate course of treatment. Meta-analysis of the three major studies that addressed surgical treatment showed that carotid endarterectomy for patients with moderate-to-severe stenosis (defined as 60–99% in two of the studies and 50–99% in the third) reduced the absolute risk of stroke by approximately 1% for each year of subsequent survival.[48] The benefit of carotid endarterectomy was counterbalanced by a perioperative risk for stroke or death of approximately 3%. Benefits of intervention appeared to be greater for men than for women. Thus, in centers with low complication rates, it seems prudent to consider (although it is not absolutely indicated) carotid endarterectomy for asymptomatic carotid stenosis, especially for men.

Other interventions

Stenting of the vertebral or basilar arteries may be an option for patients with continued symptomatic posterior circulation ischemia despite maximal medical treatment.[32] Surgical or percutaneous closure of a PFO may be employed on a research basis, but should not be used as part of routine clinical care.[32]

Supportive care

Although they often take a back seat to decisions about thrombolysis and antiplatelet agent selection, supportive measures are critical in reducing disability and death from stroke. The pillars of supportive care for stroke patients are:

Treating hyperthermia and infection

Hyperthermia worsens stroke outcome, independent of the presence of underlying infection.[49] Evaluate for sources of fever by performing a complete blood count, blood cultures, chest X-ray, urinalysis, and urine cultures, and treat with antibiotics as appropriate. For patients with unexplained fevers, consider lower-extremity duplex ultrasound studies to investigate for deep venous thrombosis (DVT), echocardiography to evaluate for endocarditis, and infectious disease consultation. Treat mild hyperthermia with antipyretics such as acetaminophen and more severe hyperthermia with antipyretics and cooling blankets.

Correcting hyperglycemia

Because hyperglycemia, like fever, worsens stroke outcome, it is important to maintain strict glucose control.[50]

Maintaining adequate nutrition

Dysphagia, weakness, and cognitive impairments all lead to inadequate nutrition and impede recovery from stroke. If necessary, prescribe parenteral nutrition or tube feedings. Do not use hypotonic fluids, as they may worsen brain edema.

Assessing aspiration risk and preventing aspiration

Patients with strokes involving large hemispheric territories or the brainstem are at increased risk of aspiration, which may lead to both acute airway compromise and aspiration pneumonia. Assess aspiration risk at the bedside by asking the patient to swallow three ounces of water and then observing for coughing or a wet, hoarse voice.[51] A patient who fails this simple swallow test is at risk for aspiration, and should be placed on precautions, which may include monitored eating or restrictions on oral intake. Because difficulties may be subtle (e.g. silent aspiration), patients often require a formal swallowing study to determine whether dysphagia is present.

Deep venous thrombosis prophylaxis

Because patients with severe stroke deficits are generally bed bound for at least several days, DVT prophylaxis is essential to prevent life-threatening pulmonary emboli. Options for DVT prophylaxis include compression stockings, sequential compression devices, unfractionated heparin, and low-molecular-weight heparin. Unless there is a clear contraindication (such as heparin-induced thrombocytopenia or a bleeding diathesis), DVT prophylaxis should consist of unfractionated heparin (5000 units sc tid) or a low-molecular-weight heparin.[22] Treat patients who cannot receive heparin with a sequential compression device.

Preventing falls

Weakness, ataxia, sensory impairments, and cognitive dysfunction are all factors that increase the risk of falls following stroke. Activating bed alarms, employing patient sitters, and even using physical restraints may be necessary to prevent falls and additional injuries.

Initiating a rehabilitation program

Recovery from stroke is a complex process that results from a combination of brain adaptation to injury by new synapse formation and by patient-driven efforts to compensate for irreparable deficits. Improvement is usually maximal 6 weeks after a stroke, and is almost always complete within 3–6 months.[52] Early rehabilitation tends to be more effective than delayed rehabilitation, and for this reason, it is important to involve physical therapists, occupational therapists, speech and swallowing specialists, and cognitive rehabilitation experts as soon as possible.[53]

Evaluation and treatment of intracranial hemorrhage

Intracranial hemorrhage (ICH) is a life-threatening emergency associated with high morbidity and mortality. It may be difficult to differentiate ICH from ischemic stroke on clinical grounds alone. As noted above, possible clues to ICH include headache and the presence of deficits that progress over minutes to hours. Emergency room physicians or other doctors usually make the diagnosis of ICH by noncontrast head CT, well before a neurologist is involved.

Acute life support

Because a patient with ICH may present *in extremis*, the first priority is to assure that they have a patent airway, adequate cardiopulmonary function, and intravenous access for medication administration. A patient with ICH may initially be conscious and then deteriorate rapidly. Thus, it is essential to monitor the patient carefully and transfer them to an intensive care unit should their clinical condition decline.

Reversing anticoagulation

After ensuring basic life support measures, the next step in managing ICH is to discontinue any anticoagulants and reverse their effects if applicable. Review the patient's medication list and check their prothrombin time, PTT, and platelet count.

Warfarin

The three options available for reversing anticoagulation secondary to warfarin are:

- Prothrombin complex concentrate (factor IX complex) 25–50 IU/kg. Factor IX complex reverses the blood-thinning effects of warfarin within several hours, but because of its short half-life, it must be administered with vitamin K. Unfortunately, factor IX complex is quite expensive and may not be available at all medical centers.
- Fresh frozen plasma (FFP) 15–20 ml/kg. This is readily available, but administration may be delayed by thawing and preparation times. In addition, FFP takes several hours to administer and represents a substantial volume load.
- Vitamin K 10 mg IV. Treat all patients with ICH who are taking warfarin with vitamin K. Because vitamin K requires at least 24 hours to work, it is not appropriate monotherapy for reversing ICH in the hyperacute setting.

Heparin

Reverse heparin using protamine sulfate. In general, the dose of protamine is 1 mg per 100 units of heparin if the heparin is being actively infused and between 0.25–0.5 mg per 100 units if the heparin was discontinued >30 minutes prior to beginning protamine infusion. It is good practice to review each case with the pharmacy in order to optimize treatment.

Blood pressure treatment

Blood pressure management in acute ICH is an area of great controversy. Lowering blood pressure reduces the likelihood of hemorrhagic expansion but may also lower perfusion pressure and increase the risk of perilesional ischemia. Similar to ischemic stroke, there is no clearly defined ideal blood pressure, although guidelines suggest a goal blood pressure of no greater than 160/90 for ICH patients.[54] The agents used most commonly to lower blood pressure in ICH are labetalol (10–20 mg IV) or hydralazine (5–10 mg IV) by intravenous push.

Managing increased intracranial pressure

Intraparenchymal hemorrhage may result in increased intracranial pressure, a potentially life-threatening emergency, which is discussed in further detail in Chapter 2.

Surgical hematoma evacuation

Surgical hematoma evacuation has the theoretical potential to rescue vulnerable adjacent brain tissue from ischemia and to reduce the likelihood that ICH will increase intracranial pressure and lead to herniation. Despite these possible benefits, decompressive craniectomy does not appear to improve neurological outcomes or reduce the chance of death in most patients with ICH.[54] Large cerebellar hemorrhages (>3 cm), however, may lead to brainstem compression and obstructive hydrocephalus, and should be evacuated as soon as possible to prevent further neurological deterioration.[55]

Defining the etiology

Defining the etiology of ICH helps to prevent hemorrhage recurrence and points to underlying disease processes that may need specific therapies. Common causes of ICH include:

- Hypertension. This is the most common cause of ICH. Typical locations of hypertensive hemorrhages include the caudate nucleus, thalamus, pons, and cerebellum.
- Amyloid angiopathy. Hemorrhages secondary to amyloid angiopathy tend to involve the parietal and occipital lobes. Other than location, finding cerebral microbleeds with susceptibility imaging studies may help to identify amyloid angiopathy as the source of ICH (Figure 21.6).
- Anticoagulant and thrombolytic agents.
- Bleeding diatheses such as hemophilia and von Willebrand disease. In most cases, these conditions are identified long before ICH occurs.
- Metastatic tumors. Tumors that have a propensity to bleed include renal cell carcinoma, melanoma, thyroid carcinoma, and choriocarcinoma. In patients with a known primary cancer, defining metastasis as the etiology is often straightforward. In patients with no known primary tumor, a careful screening examination must be conducted, as discussed in Chapter 23.
- Arteriovenous malformations. These should be considered as an etiology of ICH in younger patients. Although these masses have a fairly characteristic appearance, they may be masked by the overlying hemorrhage. Arteriovenous malformations are discussed further in Chapter 23.

Table 21.4 Glasgow Coma Scale scores[58]

Parameter	Best response	Points
Eye movements	Opens eyes spontaneously	4
	Opens eyes in response to voice	3
	Opens eyes in response to painful stimuli	2
	Does not open eyes	1
Verbal response	Appropriate conversation	5
	Disoriented	4
	Utters inappropriate words	3
	Groans incomprehensibly	2
	No verbal response	1
Motor response	Obeys commands	6
	Localizes painful stimuli	5
	Withdrawal to painful stimuli	4
	Decorticate posturing	3
	Decerebrate posturing	2
	No movement	1

The GCS score is derived by adding the best eye movement, verbal response, and motor response.

Prognosis of intracranial hemorrhage

Approximately half of patients with ICH will die within 30 days.[56,57] Among the most important prognostic factors are the initial level of consciousness (as summarized by the Glasgow Coma Scale (GCS) score; Table 21.4) and volume of the hemorrhage, which can be estimated from the CT scan using the formula[57]:

$$Volume = (A \times B \times C)/2,$$

where A is the largest diameter of the bleed, B is the diameter perpendicular to the bleed, and C is the number of slices on the CT scan multiplied by the slice thickness. Patients with ICH volumes >60 cm^3 and GCS scores ≤8 had a 30-day mortality of 91%, while those with a volume <30 cm^3 and GCS scores >8 had a 30-day mortality of 19% in one study.[57] Other risk factors for poor prognosis from ICH include older age, intraventricular blood, and early clinical deterioration.[59]

References

1. Neau J-P, Bogousslavsky J. Superficial middle cerebral artery syndromes. In: Bogousslavsky J, Caplan L, eds. *Stroke Syndromes*, 2nd edn. Cambridge: Cambridge University Press; 2001; 405–427.

2. Caplan LR, Kelly M, Kase CS, et al. Infarcts of the inferior division of the right middle cerebral artery: mirror image of Wernicke's aphasia. *Neurology* 1986;**36**:1015–1020.

3. Caplan LR. "Top of the basilar" syndrome. *Neurology* 1980;**30**:72–79.

4. Devinsky O, Bear D, Volpe BT. Confusional states following posterior cerebral artery infarction. *Arch Neurol* 1988;**45**:160–163.

5. Barth A, Bogousslavsky J, Caplan LR. Thalamic infarcts and hemorrhages. In: Bogousslavsky J, Caplan L, eds. *Stroke Syndromes*, 2nd edn. Cambridge: Cambridge University Press; 2001; 461–468.

6. Fisher CM. Lacunar strokes and infarcts: a review. *Neurology* 1982;**32**:871–876.

7. Hand PJ, Kwan J, Lindley RI, Dennis MS, Wardlaw JM. Distinguishing between stroke and mimic at the bedside. The Brain Attack Study. *Stroke* 2006;**37**: 769–775.

8. Mesulam M, Waxman SG, Geschwind N, Sabin TD. Acute confusional states with right middle cerebral artery infarctions. *J Neurol Neurosurg Psychiatry* 1976;**39**:84–89.

9. Gass A, Szabo K, Behrens S, Rossmanith C, Hennerici M. A diffusion-weighted MRI study of acute ischemic distal arm paresis. *Neurology* 2001;**57**:1589–1594.

10. Quinette P, Berengere G, Dayan J, et al. What does transient global amnesia really mean? Review of the literature and thorough study of 142 cases. *Brain* 2006;**129**:1640–1658.

11. Caplan LR. *Caplan's Stroke: a Clinical Approach.* Boston: Butterworth Heineman; 2000.

12. Grotta JC, Chiu D, Lu M, et al. Agreement and variability in the interpretation of early CT changes in stroke patients qualifying for intravenous rtPA therapy. *Stroke* 1999;**30**:1528–1533.

13. Wardlaw JM, Mielke O. Early signs of brain infarction at CT: observer reliability and outcome after thrombolytic treatment – systematic review. *Radiology* 2005;**235**:444–453.

14. Warach S, Gaa J, Siewert B, Wielopolski P, Edelman RR. Acute human stroke studied by whole brain echo planar diffusion-weighted magnetic resonance imaging. *Ann Neurol* 1995;**37**:231–241.

15. Lansberg MG, Thijs VN, O'Brien MW, et al. Evolution of apparent diffusion coefficient, diffusion-weighted, and T2-weighted signal intensity of acute stroke. *AJNR Am J Neuroradiol* 2001;**22**:637–644.

16. Kidwell CS, Chalela JA, Saver JL, et al. Comparison of MRI and CT for detection of acute intracerebral hemorrhage. *JAMA* 2004;**292**:1823–1830.

17. Schlaug G, Benfield A, Baird AE, et al. The ischemic penumbra: operationally defined by diffusion and perfusion MRI. *Neurology* 1999;**53**: 1528–1555.

18. Vertinsky AT, Schwartz NE, Fischbein NJ, et al. Comparison of multidetector CT angiography and MR imaging of cervical artery dissection. *AJNR Am J Neuroradiol* 2008;**29**:1753–1760.

19. Hacke W, Donnan G, Fieschi C, et al . Association of outcome with early stroke treatment: pooled analysis of ATLANTIS, ECASS, and NINDS rt-PA stroke trials. *Lancet* 2004;**363**:768–774.

20. The National Institute of Neurological Disorders and Stroke rt-PA Stroke Study Group. Tissue plasminogen activator for acute ischemic stroke. *N Engl J Med* 1995;**333**:1581–1587.

21. Barreto AD, Martin-Schild S, Hallevi H, et al. Thrombolytic therapy for patients who wake-up with stroke. *Stroke* 2009;**40**:827–832.

22. Adams HP, del Zoppo G, Alberts MJ, et al. Guidelines for the early management of adults with ischemic stroke. *Stroke* 2007;**38**:1655–1711.

23. Kase CS, Furlan AJ, Wechsler LR, et al. Cerebral hemorrhage after intra-arterial thrombolysis for ischemic stroke: the PROACT II trial. *Neurology* 2001;**57**:1603–1610.

24. Stead LG, Gilmore RM, Bellolio MF, Rabinstein AA, Decker WW. Percutaneous clot removal devices in acute ischemic stroke. *Arch Neurol* 2008;**65**: 1024–1030.

25. Oliveira-Filho J, Silva SCS, Trabuco CC, et al. Detrimental effect of blood pressure reduction in the first 24 hours of acute stroke onset. *Neurology* 2003;**61**:1047–1051.

26. Kasner SE, Demchuk AM, Berrouschot J, et al. Predictors of fatal brain edema in massive hemispheric stroke. *Stroke* 2001;**32**:2117–2123.

27. Vahedi K, Hofmeijer J, Juettler E, et al. Early decompressive surgery in malignant infarction of the middle cerebral artery: a pooled analysis of three randomised controlled trials. *Lancet Neurol* 2007;**6**:215–222.

28. Schaer BA, Zellweger MJ, Cron TA, Kaiser CA, Osswald S. Value of routine Holter monitoring for the detection of paroxysmal atrial fibrillation in patients with cerebral ischemic events. *Stroke* 2004;**35**: e68-e70.

29. Pearson AC, Labovitz AJ, Tatineni S, Gomez CR. Superiority of transesophageal echocardiography in detecting cardiac source of embolism in patients with cerebral ischemia of uncertain etiology. *J Am Coll Cardiol* 1991;**17**:66–72.

30. Hankey GJ, Warlow CP, Sellar RJ. Cerebral angiographic risk in mild cerebrovascular disease. *Stroke* 1990;**21**:209–222.

31. Bushnell CD, Goldstein LB. Diagnostic testing for coagulopathies in patients with ischemic stroke. *Stroke* 2000;**31**:3067–3078.

32. Sacco RL, Adams R, Albers G, et al. Guidelines for prevention of stroke in patients with ischemic stroke or transient ischemic attack. *Stroke* 2006;**37**:577–617.

33. Amarenco P, Labreuche J, Lavallee P, Touboul PJ. Statins in stroke prevention and carotid atherosclerosis: systematic review and up-to-date meta-analysis. *Stroke* 2004;**35**:2902–2909.

34. The Stroke Prevention by Aggressive Reduction in Cholesterol Levels (SPARCL) Investigators. High-dose atorvastatin after stroke or transient ischemic attack. *N Engl J Med* 2006;**355**:549–559.

35. Corvol J-C, Bouzamondo A, Sirol M, et al. Differential effects of lipid-lowering therapies on stroke prevention. A meta-analysis of randomized trials. *Arch Intern Med* 2003;**163**:669–676.

36. Messé SR, Silverman IE, Kizer JR, et al. Practice parameter: recurrent stroke with patent foramen ovale and atrial septal aneurysm: report of the Quality Standards Subcommittee of the American Academy of Neurology. *Neurology* 2004;**62**:1042–1050.

37. Mohr JP, Thompson JLP, Lazar RM, et al. A comparison of warfarin and aspirin for the prevention of recurrent ischemic stroke. *N Engl J Med* 2001;**345**:1444–1451.

38. Diener HC, Cunha L, Forbes C, et al. European Stroke Prevention Study 2. Dipyridamole and acetylsalicylic acid in the secondary prevention of stroke. *J Neurol Sci* 1996;**143**:1–13.

39. CAPRIE Steering Committee. A randomised, blinded, trial of clopidogrel versus aspirin in patients at risk of ischaemic events (CAPRIE). *Lancet* 1996;**348**: 1329–1339.

40. Hass WK, Easton JD, Adams HP, et al. A randomized trial comparing ticlopidine hydrochloride with aspirin for the prevention of stroke in high-risk patients. *N Engl J Med* 1989;**321**:501–507.

41. Sacco RL, Diener HC, Yusuf S, et al. Aspirin and extended-release dipyridamole versus clopidogrel for recurrent stroke. *N Engl J Med* 2008;**359**:1238–1251.

42. Diener HC, Bogousslavsky J, Brass LM, et al. Aspirin and clopidogrel compared with clopidogrel alone after recent ischaemic stroke or transient ischaemic attack in high-risk patients (MATCH): randomised, double-blind, placebo-controlled trial. *Lancet* 2004;**364**:331–337.

43. Mayberg MR, Wilson SE, Yatsu F, et al. Carotid endarterectomy and prevention of cerebral ischemia in symptomatic carotid stenosis: Veterans Affairs Cooperative Studies Program 309 Trialist Group. *JAMA* 1991;**266**:3289–3294.

44. North American Symptomatic Carotid Endarterectomy Trial Collaborators. Beneficial effect of carotid endarterectomy in symptomatic patients with high-grade carotid stenosis. *N Engl J Med* 1991;**325**:445–453.

45. Rothwell PM, Ellasziw M, Gutnikov SA, et al. Endarterectomy for symptomatic carotid stenosis in relation to clinical subgroups and timing of surgery. *Lancet* 2004;**363**:915–924.

46. Barnett HJM, Taylor DW, Ellasziw M, et al. Benefit of carotid endarterectomy in patients with symptomatic moderate or severe stenosis. *N Engl J Med* 1998;**339**:1415–1425.

47. Yadav JS, Wholey MH, Kuntz RE, et al. Protected carotid-artery stenting versus endarterectomy in high-risk patients. *N Engl J Med* 2004;**351**:1493–1501.

48. Chambers BR, Donnan G. Carotid endarterectomy for asymptomatic carotid stenosis. *Cochrane Database Syst Rev* 2005:(4):CD001923

49. Azzimondi G, Bassein L, Nonino F, et al. Fever in acute stroke worsens prognosis: a prospective study. *Stroke* 1995;**26**:2040–2043.

50. Baird TA, Parsons MW, Phanh T, et al. Persistent poststroke hyperglycemia is independently associated with infarct expansion and worse clinical outcome. *Stroke* 2003;**34**:2208–2214.

51. DePippo KL, Holas MA, Reding MJ. Validation of the 3-oz water swallow test for aspiration following stroke. *Arch Neurol* 1992;**49**:1259–1261.

52. Jorgensen HS, Nakayma H, Raaschou HO, et al. Outcome and time course of recovery in stroke. Part II: time course of recovery. The Copenhagen Stroke Study. *Arch Phys Med Rehabil* 1995;**76**:406–412.

53. Paolucci S, Antonucci G, Grasso M, et al. Early versus delayed inpatient stroke rehabilitation: a matched comparison conducted in Italy. *Arch Phys Med Rehabil* 2000;**81**:695–700.

54. Broderick J, Connolly S, Feldmann E, et al. Guidelines for the management of spontaneous intracerebral hemorrhage in adults. *Stroke* 2007;**38**:2001–2023.

55. Mendelow AD, Gregson BA, Fernandes HM, et al. Early surgery versus initial conservative treatment in patients with spontaneous supratentorial intracerebral haematomas in the International Surgical Trial in Intracerebral Haemorrhage (STICH): a randomised trial. *Lancet* 2005;**365**:387–397.

56. Flaherty ML, Haverbusch M, Sekar P, et al. Long-term mortality after intracerebral hemorrhage. *Neurology* 2006;**66**:1182–1186.

57. Broderick JP, Brott T, Duldner J, Tomsick T, Huster G. Volume of intracerebral hemorrhage. A powerful and easy-to-use predictor of 30-day mortality. *Stroke* 1993;**24**:987–993.

58. Teasdale G, Jennett B. Assessment of coma and impaired consciousness: a practical scale. *Lancet* 1974;**304**:81–84.

59. Hemphill JC, Bonovich DC, Besmertis L, Manley GT, Johnston SC. A simple, reliable grading scale for intracerebral hemorrhage. *Stroke* 2001;**32**:891–897.

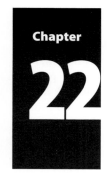
22 Multiple sclerosis

Introduction

Successful treatment of multiple sclerosis (MS), the most common demyelinating disorder of the CNS, requires mastery of four distinct disease stages:

- A clinically isolated syndrome (CIS) suggestive of MS due to a single nervous system lesion often poses a substantial diagnostic challenge, as there is no single definitive diagnostic test for MS, and there are numerous MS imitators.
- Relapsing–remitting MS (RRMS) leads to frequent hospital admissions during MS flares, and requires great familiarity with disease-modifying agents and their potential side effects.
- Progressive MS is characterized by the accumulation of disability. Management of this stage is dominated not only by understanding disease-modifying agents, but also by knowing how to manage the long-term complications of MS.
- Fulminant MS is a rapidly progressive but fortunately uncommon variant of the disease that requires strong immunosuppression for which supporting high-quality evidence is frequently unavailable.

Clinically isolated syndromes suggestive of multiple sclerosis

Visual loss

Optic neuritis is one of the most common presentations of MS (see also Chapter 5). Typically, this condition is characterized by unilateral visual loss and a tugging retrobulbar pain that develops over several days. Eye movements and bright lights may exacerbate the eye pain. Visual acuity may be decreased to any degree (but usually does not lead to an absence of light perception) and color vision is often affected out of proportion to other elements of vision. A relative afferent pupillary defect is present in the affected eye. Ophthalmoscopic examination is usually normal or may show mild swelling at presentation.

Myelopathy

Transverse myelitis is an inflammatory disorder of the white matter of the spinal cord that produces acute or subacute weakness, sensory loss, gait impairment, and urinary incontinence. In patients with MS, transverse myelitis is characteristically incomplete and results in a partial myelopathy rather than dense paraplegia (Chapter 17).

Sensory syndromes

A variety of different sensory syndromes may herald the onset of MS. Typical symptoms include numbness and a perception of abnormal vibration or of pins and needles. Although constant, sharp, burning pains are less consistent with MS, many patients with MS do describe lancinating pains. Common sensory symptom locations include a single limb, both legs simultaneously, a band around the thorax, and in the distribution of the trigeminal nerve. Trigeminal neuralgia in a young person, especially when associated with trigeminal sensory loss, suggests MS. L'hermitte's symptom is a symptom of both MS and other disorders of the upper spinal cord, and occurs when forward flexion of the neck leads to an abnormal electrical sensation shooting down the back.

Motor syndromes

Focal weakness is another common initial MS presentation. A lesion in the subcortical white matter or brainstem may produce weakness of the contralateral face, arm, or leg. Pontine lesions may lead to ipsilateral facial weakness that mimics Bell's palsy. Patchy spinal cord lesions may result in ipsilateral monoparesis. Transverse myelitis, as noted above, may cause bilateral leg weakness.

Diplopia

The best-known pattern of diplopia in MS is internuclear ophthalmoplegia (INO) in which a lesion of the medial longitudinal fasciculus disconnects the contralateral abducens nucleus in the pons from the ipsilateral oculomotor nucleus in the midbrain (Chapter 6). Abduction of the contralateral eye is normal while adduction of the ipsilateral eye is impaired. When INO occurs in MS, it is typically bilateral. Other brainstem lesions may produce a number of different patterns of horizontal, vertical, or oblique diplopia. Diplopia in MS is often complex and difficult to pinpoint to a single site within the brainstem.

Incoordination

Demyelination involving the cerebellar white matter and its brainstem connections, particularly the middle cerebellar peduncle, may lead to incoordination and ataxia. This is usually accompanied by severe action or intention tremor.

Multifocal and progressive presentations

Approximately 20% of the time, MS presents with dysfunction at more than one level of the nervous system.[1] Patients with multifocal presentations may be dismissed as having psychogenic disease because of the great variety of their symptoms. Multiple sclerosis is progressive from onset rather than relapsing in approximately 15% of patients.[1]

Abnormal MRI

The use of MRI to evaluate headaches and other vague neurological complaints is widespread and growing. T2-weighted hyperintensities are common findings on MRI, and many asymptomatic patients with nonspecific lesions are referred to neurologists for MS evaluation. Some patients, however, have radiographically typical MS lesions (see below) without clinical correlation and may be labeled as having "radiologically isolated syndromes." Because these patients have up to a 25% chance of developing a CIS or MS, they should be monitored closely.[2]

Atypical symptoms

A number of signs and symptoms suggest diagnoses other than MS. From an epidemiologic perspective, new MS is unlikely in patients older than 65, and uncommon even in those older than 50. Obvious peripheral nervous system dysfunction including dense distal sensory loss, sensory ataxia, areflexia, and bilateral

hearing loss strongly suggests that MS is not the diagnosis. Symptoms including dry eyes, dry mouth, rash, persistent fevers, and joint aches point to primary rheumatological processes rather than to MS. Mental retardation or psychiatric dysfunction should prompt consideration of mitochondrial disorders, spinocerebellar ataxias, and the leukodystrophies. Strong family histories are uncommon in MS, and suggest spinocerebellar ataxias, the leukodystrophies, hereditary spastic paraplegia, or Leber's hereditary optic neuropathy.

Making the diagnosis

Unfortunately, there is no single symptom, sign, imaging finding, or laboratory test that is 100% reliable in diagnosing MS. The diagnosis is established only by examining the clinical and laboratory data for evidence of demyelination separated in space and time (or progressive demyelination), and then excluding conditions that imitate MS. In some cases, the diagnosis is established by history and physical examination. More often than not, adjunctive tests are necessary to make the diagnosis. Although uncertainty is frequent, early diagnosis is valuable because it allows disease-modifying therapy to be initiated earlier.

Past history

Inquire about prior symptoms typical of MS such as visual loss, weakness, numbness, double vision, vertigo, and clumsiness. Deficits that last longer than 24 hours support the diagnosis while those that last only for several minutes or hours are less suggestive of MS. When reviewing the past history, ask about the evaluation that was performed at the time of each prior symptom and review these results if available.

Physical examination

Physical examination often discloses evidence of prior episodes of demyelination. Most useful among these are findings that suggest prior optic neuritis such as red desaturation, optic atrophy, and relative afferent pupillary defects (Chapter 5), or those that reflect demyelination of the spinal cord such as hyperreflexia and upgoing toes.

MRI

MRI of the brain and spinal cord are the most useful diagnostic studies for patients with suspected MS. As noted above, the diagnosis of MS hinges upon

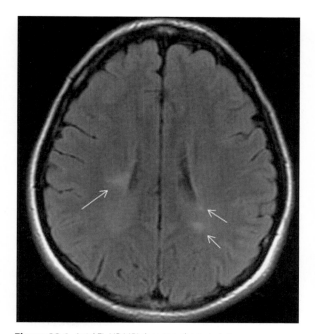

Figure 22.1 Axial FLAIR MRI showing characteristic T2-hyperintense plaques (arrows) in a patient with MS.

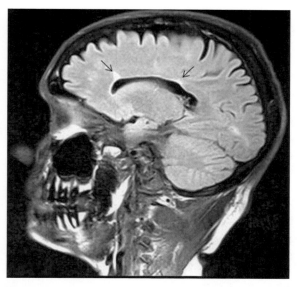

Figure 22.2 Sagittal FLAIR MRI showing Dawson's fingers (arrows): two periventricular plaques oriented perpendicularly to the lateral ventricles, a finding highly characteristic of MS.

demonstrating CNS demyelination separated in both space and time, and MRI is capable of offering important information in both dimensions. Standard MS protocols should include T1, T2, fluid attenuation inversion recovery (FLAIR; in both the axial and sagittal planes), and contrast-enhanced T1 images of the brain. Patients with spinal presentations require T1, T2, and contrast-enhanced T1 images of the spine. A diagnosis of MS is highly unusual when multiple imaging studies are normal.

T2 and fluid attenuation inversion recovery imaging

The T2 hyperintense plaque is the characteristic MRI finding of demyelination secondary to MS (Figure 22.1). Plaques are generally easier to visualize by FLAIR, a sequence in which the bright CSF signal is removed. Common plaque locations are in the periventricular white matter, corpus callosum, centrum semiovale, and middle cerebellar peduncle. Although plaques may have a variety of appearances, those that are ovoid in shape are most suggestive of MS. Lesions in the corpus callosum that are oriented perpendicularly to the lateral ventricles are known as Dawson's fingers (Figure 22.2) and are particularly characteristic of MS. These lesions are best visualized using FLAIR sequences in the sagittal plane. Plaques may accompany both new and old (presumably inactive) MS symptoms.

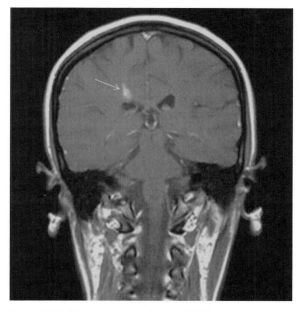

Figure 22.3 Contrast-enhanced coronal MRI showing a contrast-enhancing lesion (arrow) in a patient with relapsing–remitting MS.

Contrast-enhanced T1-weighted imaging

Gadolinium enhancement is used to detect active foci of blood–brain barrier disruption, and therefore active MS (Figure 22.3). Almost 75% of MS lesions will enhance for <1 month, and almost 95% will enhance

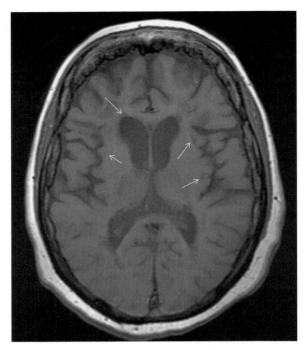

Figure 22.4 T1 black holes (arrows) in a patient with advanced MS. Note also the presence of cerebral atrophy.

for <2 months.[3] It is important to understand, however, that new symptoms may not necessarily correlate with enhancing lesions and that enhancing lesions may not be accompanied by new symptoms.

T1 black holes

The meaning of these hypointense (dark) signals on T1-weighted images is not entirely clear. Although many T1 black holes revert to an isointense signal over time, it is likely that those that persist reflect severe demyelination and irreversible axon loss (Figure 22.4).[4]

Lumbar puncture

Basic studies

CSF abnormalities may support the diagnosis of MS and help to exclude imitators. The typical CSF profile in MS includes a mild elevation in lymphocytes (never exceeding 50 cells/mm³) and a mildly elevated protein (<100 mg/dl). Neutrophilic predominance, very low glucose, and very high protein levels should prompt consideration of other diagnoses.

Oligoclonal banding and antimyelin antibodies

Patients with MS synthesize abnormal IgG intrathecally. These antibodies can be separated using gel electrophoresis into oligoclonal bands (OCBs), preferably by using isoelectric focusing on agarose gels with immunoblotting. Using this technique, 95% of patients with MS will have positive OCBs.[5] When evaluating for OCBs, also perform serum protein electrophoresis to look for distinct bands that are not present in the serum, thus verifying that the IgG is being synthesized intrathecally. Testing for antibodies to myelin basic protein and myelin oligodendrocyte glycoprotein was once popular, but these antibodies are not associated with an increased risk for developing MS.[6]

Visual evoked potentials

Visual evoked potentials (VEPs) are the electrical potentials recorded from the scalp over the occipital lobes in response to visual stimuli. The most commonly used protocol involves presenting an alternating checkerboard pattern to each eye in sequence and measuring the latency of the response recorded in the occipital cortex. Normally, this response has a positive deflection and a latency of approximately 100 ms, and is thus called the P100 response. Patients with prior optic neuritis have prolonged or absent P100 responses recorded from the affected eye. In practice, an abnormal P100 is usually used to establish the presence of an old optic nerve lesion in a patient with an otherwise normal examination.[7]

Patience

In most cases, MS is diagnosed by demonstrating clinical and radiographic white matter lesions separated in both space and time. This is often not possible at the initial encounter despite the most thorough history, examination, and set of investigations. When the diagnosis remains in doubt, a comprehensive re-evaluation in 3–6 months or at a time when further symptoms develop is usually the most appropriate approach.

Differential diagnosis

Other primary demyelinating disorders

Devic's disease (neuromyelitis optica)

The clinical features of Devic's disease are optic neuritis and transverse myelitis. There is a wide range of time intervals between the development of the two symptoms: they are separated by 24 hours in approximately 10%, but the second symptom develops more than a year after the first in a small minority.[8] The disorder usually has a relapsing course similar to MS, but may also be monophasic.[8] Whether Devic's disease is a variant of MS or a distinct syndrome is a subject of controversy. Several features help to differentiate between the two conditions. Optic neuritis in Devic's disease is usually bilateral, which is unusual for MS. The myelopathy of Devic's disease is much more severe and is characterized by involvement of three or more consecutive segments with enlargement and cavitation of the spinal cord, features that are all distinctly unusual in MS.[9] Sparing of the brain both clinically and radiographically also favors a diagnosis of Devic's disease rather than MS. CSF findings that are more consistent with Devic's disease include a neutrophilic pleocytosis during an attack and an absence of OCBs.[8] The diagnosis of Devic's disease is best confirmed by finding antibodies to the aquaporin-4 water channel (also referred to as NMO-IgG) in the serum.[10] Unfortunately, patients with Devic's disease have a worse long-term prognosis than those with MS. Treatment with intravenous steroids and plasmapheresis may be helpful during acute attacks, but once cavitation develops in the cord, treatment is of limited benefit.

Acute disseminated encephalomyelitis

Acute disseminated encephalomyelitis (ADEM) is a multifocal demyelinating disorder of the CNS that usually develops several days or weeks after an infection or vaccination. Symptoms of ADEM are usually more severe and more numerous than those of MS. Cognitive changes, seizures, and even coma may occur in ADEM, but are distinctly unusual presenting symptoms for MS. Imaging features that suggest ADEM rather than MS include white matter changes that extend from the subcortical region to the cerebral cortex, thalamic involvement, and extension of demyelination over multiple contiguous spinal cord levels. Spinal fluid usually shows a mild-to-moderate lymphocytosis. Oligoclonal bands are less common in ADEM than in MS. Despite the apparent abundance of clinical and laboratory clues that help to distinguish between ADEM and MS, the two diagnoses may resemble each other at presentation, and the only definitive way to separate them is by observing the patient over time: the monophasic, nonrelapsing course of ADEM distinguishes it from the relapsing or progressive course of MS. An attack of ADEM is usually treated with methylprednisolone (1 g IV × 5 days). Intravenous immunoglobulin and plasmapheresis are options in patients with severe disease or an incomplete response to steroids.

Secondary demyelinating disorders: reasonable exclusion of multiple sclerosis mimics

A wide variety of medical conditions may mimic MS, but surprisingly little guidance exists as to what constitutes a reasonable exclusion of alternative diagnoses. This is problematic, as many of the other causes of multifocal demyelination are at least partially reversible and do not produce long-term disability if treated properly. In a patient with a CIS, MRI findings highly suggestive of MS, and no other systemic signs of an alternative condition, additional diagnostic testing is seldom worthwhile. Tables 22.1–22.4 contain brief descriptions of the possible alternative diagnoses that should be considered when evaluating a patient with suspected CNS demyelination.

Treatment of clinically isolated syndromes and relapsing–remitting multiple sclerosis

Optic neuritis

Patients with optic neuritis are among the most heavily studied and carefully followed cohorts of patients with neurological disease. Patients in the treatment arm of the Optic Neuritis Treatment Trial (ONTT) received methylprednisolone 250 mg IV qid × 3 days followed by oral prednisone 1 mg/kg/day PO for 14 days. Because this regimen may be impractical in many cases, a methylprednisolone dose of 1 g IV qd × 3 days is often employed without a prednisone taper in clinical practice. Sequential follow-up of patients in the ONTT offers several important pieces of information:

- Treatment with methylprednisolone hastens recovery but does not change the typically excellent long-term visual prognosis of optic neuritis.[11]
- Patients with optic neuritis who receive intravenous methylprednisolone have a decreased probability of developing MS in the short-term (2 years).[12]
- Methylprednisolone does not reduce the lifetime chance that a patient with optic neuritis will develop MS.[13]
- At 15 years, the overall probability that a patient with optic neuritis will develop MS is 50%. The

Table 22.1 Differential diagnosis of multiple sclerosis mimics that may affect the brain, optic nerve, or spine, in combination or in isolation

Disorder	Suggestive features	Evaluation
Adrenoleukodystrophy	X-linked inheritance, adrenal dysfunction, peripheral neuropathy	Elevated very-long-chain fatty acids
Behçet's disease	Oral and genital ulcers	Clinical diagnosis
Lyme disease	Rash, cardiac and rheumatological manifestations	Lyme antibodies, history of exposure and rash
Metachromatic leukodystrophy	Autosomal recessive inheritance, prominent psychiatric dysfunction, peripheral neuropathy	Decreased leukocyte arylsulfatase A levels
Mitochondrial encephalomyelopathy	Mental retardation, short stature, bilateral hearing loss	Elevated serum and CSF lactate, imaging abnormalities may involve the basal ganglia
Neurosarcoidosis	Pulmonary and cardiac symptoms	Biopsy showing noncaseating granulomas
Sjogren's syndrome	Dry mouth, dry eyes	Sjogren's antibodies
Systemic lupus erythematosus	Rash, kidney dysfunction	Anti-dsDNA and anti-Smith antibodies

Table 22.2 Differential diagnosis of predominantly cerebral presentations of multiple sclerosis

Disorder	Suggestive features	Evaluation
CADASIL (cerebral autosomal dominant arteriopathy with subcortical infarcts and leukoencephalopathy)	Dementia, headache, multiple brain infarctions	NOTCH-3 mutation
CNS lymphoma	History of immunosuppression	Brain biopsy
CNS vasculitis	Development of multiple symptoms in short time frame	Brain biopsy
Progressive multifocal leukoencephalopathy	History of immunosuppression	JC virus PCR in CSF

PCR = polymerase chain reaction

Table 22.3 Differential diagnosis of predominantly spinal presentations of multiple sclerosis (see also Chapter 17)

Disorder	Suggestive features	Evaluation
Cervical spondylosis	Neck pain, signs and symptoms of osteoarthritis elsewhere	Imaging of cervical spine
Copper-deficiency myelopathy	Progressive, painless myelopathy	Low serum copper levels
Hereditary spastic paraplegia	Inherited in mostly autosomal dominant fashion, may be associated with other neurological signs and symptoms	Genetic testing available for more common mutations
Spinal cord dural arteriovenous malformation	Sudden-onset waxing and waning symptoms	Spinal angiography
Spinocerebellar ataxia	Ataxia and dysarthria are prominent	Genetic testing available for more common mutations
Tropical spastic paraparesis	Patient from Caribbean, Japan, or Africa	Human T-cell lymphotropic virus PCR testing
Vitamin B_{12} deficiency	Anemia, large-fiber polyneuropathy	Low vitamin B_{12}, high methylmalonic acid, high homocysteine levels
Vitamin E deficiency	Prominent sensory ataxia and diarrhea	Low vitamin E levels

Table 22.4 Differential diagnosis of optic neuropathy

Disorder	Suggestive features	Evaluation
Leber's hereditary optic neuropathy	Subacute bilateral progressive visual loss	Genetic testing available for more common mutations
Nutritional optic neuropathies	Other signs of vitamin B_1 (beriberi) or B_{12} deficiency	Low vitamin B_1 or B_{12} levels
Retinal artery occlusion	Sudden-onset symptoms	Funduscopic examination

long-term risk of developing MS is best stratified with brain MRI at the time of presentation[13]:

- 25% for patients with no lesions
- 60% for patients with one lesion
- 68% for patients with two lesions
- 78% for patients with three lesions

Based on these data, it is important to strongly consider treating a patient with optic neuritis and one or more MRI lesions with disease-modifying therapy as discussed below.

Other clinically isolated syndromes suggestive of multiple sclerosis

The data to support treatment of CIS other than optic neuritis are less robust. Management decisions for patients with CIS depend on the severity of their deficits and the likelihood of developing MS. Patients with mild deficits do not necessarily require any acute treatment. Use methylprednisolone for patients with more severe deficits, as it hastens symptom resolution. Although there is no dosing regimen that is clearly more effective than any others, methylprednisolone 1000 mg IV × 3 days is used most commonly.

Disease-modifying treatment

In addition to managing acute symptoms with corticosteroids, patients with CIS at high risk of developing MS should be treated with a disease-modifying therapy such as beta interferon (IFN-β) or glatiramer acetate, as these agents delay the development of clinically definite MS.[14]

Beta interferon

The exact mechanism of action of IFN-β in MS is unclear, although multiple studies show that it is an effective treatment option for RRMS.[14] The three available IFNs are:

- IFN-β-1a (Avonex) 30 μg IM injection weekly
- IFN-β-1a (Rebif) 22 or 44 μg SC three times a week
- IFN-β-1b (Betaseron) 250 μg SC every other day

Common side effects of IFN therapy include flu-like reactions, joint aches, injection site reactions, headaches, and depression. More serious side effects include lymphopenia, thrombocytopenia, asymptomatic transaminitis, and, rarely, hepatitis. Patients should therefore undergo complete blood counts and liver function tests upon initiation, at 1 month, 3 months, 6 months, and periodically thereafter. Studies suggest that IFN formulations with higher doses reduce the subsequent number of flares compared with lower-dose formulations.[15,16] These benefits are counterbalanced by the need for less frequent dosing and a lower incidence of developing neutralizing antibodies (see Box 22.1) with the lower dose formulations.

Box 22.1 Interferon-neutralizing antibodies

Patients who are treated with IFN-β may develop neutralizing antibodies (NAbs). These antibodies are associated with more frequent clinical relapses and larger numbers of radiographic lesions. The exact incidence with which NAbs develop is difficult to establish due to a variety of study methodologies. What is known is that patients who receive IFN-β more than once per week are more likely to develop antibodies than those who receive only a single weekly injection.[17] Whether this information should merit any consideration in choosing a first IFN is uncertain. The exact role of testing for NAbs is also unclear. Many patients who develop the antibodies show no evidence of clinical worsening. Others may develop the antibodies and later revert to an antibody-negative status. For patients with stable disease, screening for NAbs is not indicated. For those with more frequent flares or evidence of disease progression, the decision to discontinue an IFN in favor of a different disease-modifying therapy should be made on clinical grounds, and little weight should be assigned to the presence or absence of NAbs.

Glatiramer acetate

This semirandom amino acid mixture reduces the number of relapses and possibly slows disease progression in patients with RRMS.[18] Glatiramer acetate is administered subcutaneously at a dose of 20 mg qd. Side effects include injection site reactions, chest pain, flushing, and tachycardia. Patients who take glatiramer acetate do not require any blood tests for monitoring purposes.

Multiple sclerosis flares

New neurological deficits account for the majority of hospitalizations in patients with known MS. The three possible explanations for new symptoms are new demyelinating lesions, unmasking of old deficits by superimposed infectious or metabolic insults, and unrelated neurological disease. Screen all patients with new deficits for possible infectious and metabolic exacerbants including complete blood count, electrolytes, glucose levels, urinalysis, and chest X-rays. Contrast-enhanced MRI is often necessary to distinguish active MS lesions from other causes of neurological symptoms. In general, patients with MS flares should be treated with a 3-day course of 1000 mg IV methylprednisolone. Oral prednisone (1250 mg qd × 3 days) may be used as a substitute if methylprednisolone is unavailable or if outpatient treatment is absolutely required.[19]

Relapsing–remitting multiple sclerosis

This refers to a milder or early stage of the disease characterized by episodic flares separated by remissions in which there is little or no evidence of disease activity. Most trials of disease-modifying therapy in MS are directed at this relapsing–remitting form. Patients with RRMS are generally treated with IFN-β or glatiramer acetate as described above. Relapsing–remitting MS with frequent flares or with evidence of progression usually requires a more aggressive strategy than IFNs or glatiramer acetate. Treatment options in this clinical scenario include:

- Switching from IFN-β to glatiramer acetate or vice versa.
- Natalizumab. This is an α_4-integrin antagonist that theoretically prevents leukocyte migration across the blood–brain barrier, thereby reducing CNS inflammation. It decreases the number of flares, reduces radiological evidence of active disease, and slows disease progression.[20] While it is possible that natalizumab is the most effective single agent available to treat MS, it is associated with an estimated 1 in 1500 annual risk for developing progressive multifocal leukoencephalopathy (PML).[21] Because PML is

difficult to treat and often fatal, this side effect must be discussed seriously with any natalizumab candidate.[22] All physicians who prescribe natalizumab must be enrolled in the TOUCH Prescribing Program to ensure patient safety.

- Mitoxantrone. Mitoxantrone is an immunomodulatory agent that reduces MS flares and slows disease progression.[23] It is prescribed as an infusion of 12 mg/m² every 3 months, with a maximum lifetime dose of 140 mg/m². The two most serious potential side effects of mitoxantrone are cardiotoxicity and bone marrow suppression. All patients must therefore undergo echocardiography prior to each dose, and cannot receive the medication if their ejection fraction is <50% or if it is declining.

Progressive multiple sclerosis and symptomatic treatment

Disease-modifying therapy

Unfortunately, approximately 80% of patients with MS have progressive disease. While flares are less frequent in this stage, disability accumulates and many patients become house bound or lose their ability to live independently. Progressive deterioration from disease onset is known as primary progressive MS, whereas deterioration that develops after several relapses and remissions is known as secondary progressive MS. While there is evidence that IFNs and glatiramer acetate may help to slow disease progression, they tend to be less effective in patients with more severe disability. Natalizumab and mitoxantrone are commonly employed options for patients with advanced MS. Cyclophosphamide is an alkylating agent that may help patients with rapidly progressive disease, although its use is controversial due to conflicting study results.[24,25] Alternative treatment options for patients who continue to progress include monthly steroids, methotrexate, azathioprine, plasmapheresis, and intravenous immunoglobulin.

Symptomatic treatment

Spasticity

Spasticity secondary to MS may lead to intense pain and impaired mobility. Physical therapy emphasizing range-of-motion exercises is only modestly helpful, but in some cases may prevent contractures. Baclofen (initiated at 10 mg tid and titrated upward to a maximum daily dose of 80 mg) is usually the first line of treatment for spasticity secondary to MS. In patients who do not respond to baclofen, alternative treatment options include tizanidine (2–8 mg tid), dantrolene (25–100 mg tid) and diazepam (5–20 mg tid). Consider placing an intrathecal baclofen pump in patients with refractory symptoms. Although botulinum toxin injections are theoretically helpful, most patients require injections in a large number of muscles, which makes them somewhat impractical.

Urinary dysfunction

The majority of patients with MS will develop bladder dysfunction.[26] After excluding urinary tract infection by performing urinalysis and treating any relevant infection, the next step in evaluating bladder complaints is to try to localize the problem:

- Cervical and upper thoracic level lesions produce a spastic bladder and urge incontinence. The patient has a sudden urge to urinate and cannot make it to the bathroom in time.
- Mid-to-lower thoracic level lesions result in detrusor–sphincter dyssynergia in which the urinary detrusor contracts against a closed urethral sphincter. The patient has difficulty voiding and feels an excessive strain in an attempt to produce a weak urinary stream.
- Lumbosacral level lesions lead to bladder hypotonia and overflow incontinence. The patient feels that they are emptying their bladder incompletely and note intermittent urinary leakage.

Patients often describe their urinary symptoms inaccurately, and, as a first step, it is usually best to measure the postvoid urine residual volume in order to better classify the problem. Incontinence in a patient with a postvoid residual of <100 cm^3 is most likely due to a spastic bladder with urge incontinence, and should be treated with an anticholinergic agent such as oxybutinin (5 mg bid–qid) or tolteridone (1 mg qd–2 mg bid). Incontinence in a patient with a postvoid residual of >100 cm^3 is most likely due to a flaccid bladder with overflow incontinence, and should be treated with intermittent straight catheterization. It is often best to refer patients with bladder dysfunction with MS for formal urological evaluation. Refractory symptoms may require a chronic suprapubic catheter, botulinum toxin injections, or sacral stimulator placement.

Fatigue

Although the exact mechanisms by which MS leads to fatigue are not entirely clear, it is often the most prominent and disabling MS symptom. Patients with MS describe exhaustion, myalgias, and impaired concentration, although they usually do not report a specific urge to sleep. The most commonly used agent for fatigue is amantidine 100 mg bid. Other medications that may be effective include selective serotonin reuptake inhibitors (SSRIs), aspirin, and methylphenidate. While modafinil (200 mg qam) helps many patients with daytime sleepiness, it is often ineffective for patients with fatigue related to MS.

Depression and anxiety

Depression and anxiety affect approximately 50% of patients with MS, and are due to a combination of the neurodegenerative process and psychological maladjustment to the disease.[27] Although patients treated with IFN-β were once thought to be at higher risk of depression, the evidence that this is true is unclear. Patients with MS and depression or anxiety usually benefit from a combination of cognitive–behavioral therapy and SSRIs. Short-acting anxiolytics should be used cautiously for patients with anxiety. Social workers and psychologists often play an important role in dealing with adjustment issues related to MS.

Cognitive dysfunction

Cognitive dysfunction develops in about half of patients with MS, and is usually a manifestation of the later stages of the disease.[28] The classic pattern of impairment in MS is "subcortical dementia" in which processing speed and attentional problems outweigh cortical defects such as aphasia and apraxia. Whether disease-modifying agents reduce the probability or slow the onset of dementia is unclear. Patients with dementia secondary to MS are treated in much the same fashion as those with other forms of dementia (Chapter 4). Donepezil is used most frequently, although the evidence for its effectiveness in MS is somewhat limited.

Pain and paresthesias

Sensory symptoms affect almost all patients with MS. Agents such as gabapentin, nortriptyline, and pregabalin are employed in much the same fashion as for other patients with neuropathic pain (Chapter 15). Trigeminal neuralgia is particularly common in patients with MS. Conventional treatments for this condition include carbamazepine, phenytoin, and gabapentin (Chapter 19). The prostaglandin E1 analog misoprostol (600 μg qd) is an additional treatment option specifically for trigeminal neuralgia in the setting of MS.[29] Gamma knife radiosurgery may be useful for patients with refractory symptoms.[30]

Tremor

Tremor is one of the most difficult MS symptoms to treat. The tremor is usually an action tremor (Chapter 14), and in some patients may be of large amplitude and quite disabling. First-line agents used for essential tremor including propranolol and primidone are only marginally effective. Other options include benzodiazepines, carbamazepine, and isoniazid. If tremor fails to respond to medical treatment, thalamotomy or deep brain stimulation of the nucleus ventralis intermedius may help.[31]

Motor impairments

Motor decline is usually the symptom that is of greatest concern to patients with newly diagnosed MS. While the course of each individual MS patient is different and somewhat difficult to predict, most patients will require a walking aid and some will need a wheelchair.

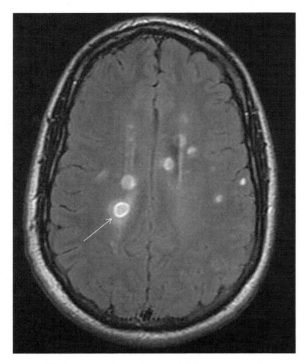

Figure 22.5 Axial FLAIR MRI showing Balo's concentric sclerosis (arrow), a severe variant of MS characterized by alternating concentric rings of demyelination and remyelination.

Early and frequent involvement of physical therapists is often helpful to teach effective compensatory strategies and to determine the need for assistive devices.

Fulminant MS

Rare fulminant variants of MS cause rapidly progressive disability and sometimes death. The two best-known examples are Balo's concentric sclerosis and Marburg variant MS. Balo's concentric sclerosis is pathologically and radiologically characterized by alternating rings of demyelination alternating with rings of preserved myelin (Figure 22.5). The Marburg variant of MS is characterized by progression of deficits to severe disability or death within a few weeks to months.[32] Obviously, immunomodulatory therapy must be initiated quickly and aggressively for patients with rapidly progressive variants. In most cases, patients should undergo plasmapheresis in addition to corticosteroid treatment. Other chemotherapeutic agents including cyclophosphamide may be helpful if prescribed at an early enough stage of the disease.

References

1. Confavreux C, Vukusic S, Moreau T, Adeleine P. Relapses and progression of disability in multiple sclerosis. *N Engl J Med* 2000;**343**:1430–1438.

2. Okuda DT, Mowry EM, Beheshtian A, et al. Incidental MRI anomalies suggestive of multiple sclerosis: the radiologically isolated syndrome. *Neurology* 2009;**72**:800–805.

3. Harris JO, Frank JA, Patronas N, McFarlin DE, McFarland HF. Serial gadolinium-enhanced magnetic resonance imaging scans in patients with early, relapsing–remitting multiple sclerosis: implications for clinical trials and natural history. *Ann Neurol* 1991;**29**:548–555.

4. van Walderveen MAA, Kamphorst W, Scheltens P, et al. Histopathologic correlate of hypointense lesions on T1-weighted spin-echo MRI in multiple sclerosis. *Neurology* 1998;**50**:1282–1288.

5. Freedman MS, Thompson EJ, Deisenhammer F, et al. Recommended standard of cerebrospinal fluid analysis in the diagnosis of multiple sclerosis. A consensus statement. *Arch Neurol* 2005;**62**:865–870.

6. Kuhle J, Pohl C, Mehling M, et al. Lack of association between antimyelin antibodies and progression to multiple sclerosis. *N Engl J Med* 2007;**356**:371–378.

7. Hume AL, Waxman SG. Evoked potentials in suspected multiple sclerosis: diagnostic value and prediction of clinical course. *J Neurol Sci* 1988;**83**:191–210.

8. Wingerchuk DM, Hogancamp WF, O'Brien PC, Weinshenker BG. The clinical course of neuromyelitis optica (Devic's syndrome). *Neurology* 1999;**53**: 1107–1114.

9. Mandler RN, Davis LE, Jeffery DR, Kornfeld M. Devic's neuromyelitis optica: a clinicopathological study of 8 patients. *Ann Neurol* 1993;**34**:162–168.

10. Lennon VA, Wingerchuk DM, Kryzer TJ, et al. A serum autoantibody marker of neuromyelitis optica: distinction from multiple sclerosis. *Lancet* 2004;**364**:2106–2112.

11. Beck RW, Cleary PA, Anderson MM, et al. A randomized controlled trial of corticosteroids in the treatment of acute optic neuritis. *N Engl J Med* 1992;**326**:581–588.

12. Beck RW, Cleary PA, Trobe JD, et al. The effect of corticosteroids for acute optic neuritis on the subsequent development of multiple sclerosis. *N Engl J Med* 1993;**329**:1764–1769.

13. The Optic Neuritis Study Group. Multiple sclerosis risk after optic neuritis. Final Optic Neuritis Treatment Trial follow-up. *Arch Neurol* 2008;**65**:727–732.

14. Goodin DS, Frohman EM, Garmany GP, et al. Disease modifying therapies in multiple sclerosis: Subcommittee of the American Academy of Neurology and the MS Council for Clinical Practice Guidelines. *Neurology* 2002;**58**:169–178.

15. Panitch H, Goodin DS, Francis G, et al. Randomized, comparative study of interferon-β-1a treatment regimens in MS: the EVIDENCE trial. *Neurology* 2002;**59**:1496–1506.

16. Durelli L, Verdun E, Barbero P, et al. Every-other-day interferon β-1b versus once-weekly interferon β-1a for multiple sclerosis: results of a 2-year prospective randomised multicentre study. *Lancet* 2002;**359**:1453–1460.

17. Goodin DS, Frohman EM, Hurwitz B, et al. Neutralizing antibodies to interferon beta: assessment of their clinical and radiographic impact: an evidence report. *Neurology* 2007;**68**:977–984.

18. Johnson KP, Brooks BR, Cohen JA, et al. Copolymer 1 reduces relapse rate and improves disability in relapsing–remitting multiple sclerosis: results of phase III multicenter, double-blind placebo-controlled trial. *Neurology* 1995;**45**:1268–1276.

19. Morrow SA, Stoian CA, Dmitrovic J, Chan SC, Metz LM. The bioavailability of IV methylprednisolone and oral prednisone in multiple sclerosis. *Neurology* 2004;**63**:1079–1080.

20. Polman CH, O'Connor PW, Havrdova E, et al. A randomized, placebo-controlled trial of natalizumab for relapsing multiple sclerosis. *N Engl J Med* 2006;**354**:899–910.

21. Goodin DS, Cohen BA, O'Connor P, et al. Assessment: the use of natalizumab for the treatment of multiple sclerosis (an evidence-based review). *Neurology* 2008;**71**:766–773.

22. Wenning W, Haghikia A, Laubenberger J, et al. Treatment of progressive multifocal leukoencephalopathy associated with natalizumab. *N Engl J Med* 2009;**361**:1075–1080.

23. Goodin DS, Arnason BG, Coyle PK, et al. The use of mitoxantrone (Novantrone) for the treatment of multiple sclerosis. *Neurology* 2003;**61**:1332–1338.

24. Weiner HL, Mackin GA, Orav EJ, et al. Intermittent cyclophosphamide pulse therapy in progressive multiple sclerosis: final report of the Northeast Cooperative Multiple Sclerosis Treatment Group. *Neurology* 1993;**43**:910–918.

25. The Canadian Cooperative Multiple Sclerosis Study Group. The Canadian cooperative trial of cyclophosphamide and plasma exchange in progressive multiple sclerosis. *Lancet* 1991;**337**:441–446.

26. Fowler CJ, Panicker JN, Drake M, et al. A UK consensus on the management of the bladder in multiple sclerosis. *J Neurol Neurosurg Psychiatry* 2009;**80**:470–477.

27. Siegert RJ, Abernethy DA. Depression in multiple sclerosis: a review. *J Neurol Neurosurg Psychiatry* 2005;**76**:469–475.

28. Chiaravalloti ND, DeLuca J. Cognitive impairment in multiple sclerosis. *Lancet Neurol* 2008;**7**:1139–1151.

29. Evers S. Misoprostol in the treatment of trigeminal neuralgia associated with multiple sclerosis. *J Neurol* 2003;**250**:542–545.

30. Zorro O, Lobato-Polo J, Kano H, et al. Gamma knife radiosurgery for multiple sclerosis-related trigeminal neuralgia. *Neurology* 2009;**73**:1149–1154.

31. Koch M, Mostert J, Heersema D, De Keyser J. Tremor in multiple sclerosis. *J Neurol* 2007;**254**:133–145.

32. Mendez MF, Pogacar S. Malignant monophasic multiple sclerosis or "Marburg's disease". *Neurology* 1988;**38**:1153–1155.

Introduction

Intracranial mass lesions may come to clinical attention by producing headaches, seizures, or other focal neurological findings. Some mass lesions are life-threatening, placing the patient at risk for increased intracranial pressure or recurrent seizures. Others are "incidental-omas," which grow slowly and bear watching, but have a more benign prognosis. The important factors in diagnosing a mass lesion are its location, the patient's immune status, and their geographic background. This chapter reviews common intracranial mass lesions in adults. Many pediatric tumors or less common masses are not discussed, and the reader is instead referred to a more comprehensive neuro-oncology text.[1]

Supratentorial, brainstem, and cerebellar masses

Metastatic tumors

Metastatic tumors are the most common intracranial tumors in adults. Their diagnosis is usually fairly straightforward in patients with a known primary tumor, but metastatic lesions may also be the first presentation of cancer. Three radiological features help to differentiate metastatic lesions from other intracranial masses: they tend to be multiple, they are located at the gray–white junction, and they are associated with large amounts of surrounding vasogenic edema (Figure 23.1).[2]

The first steps in evaluating a patient with cerebral metastasis are to control the surrounding edema and address or prevent increased intracranial pressure (Chapter 2). Treat patients with vasogenic edema with a 10 mg loading dose of dexamethasone followed by 4 mg qid. When prescribing dexamethasone, be sure to provide ulcer prophylaxis with an agent such as ranitidine (150 mg bid).

Cerebral metastases also pose an increased risk for seizures (Chapter 20). Unless the patient presents with a seizure, however, anticonvulsant prophylaxis is not indicated, as it does not prevent seizures and has the potential to interact with chemotherapy.[3]

The next step in managing a patient with cerebral metastasis is to define the origin of the tumor. Common tumors that metastasize to the brain include carcinomas of the lung, breast, kidney, and colorectal region, and melanoma. Evaluation for a primary tumor should therefore include a CT scan of the torso with and without contrast and careful dermatological assessment. Women should undergo mammography. Although tumors of the prostate and testicular region are less frequent sources of metastases, men require directed testicular examination, scrotal ultrasound, and prostate-specific antigen measurement if no other primary source is found. In some patients, a thorough medical evaluation does not disclose the source of the metastasis, and the primary tumor is defined only after brain biopsy.

Definitive management of newly discovered cerebral metastasis depends on patient age and the status of the primary cancer. As might be expected, younger patients and those with a lower burden of systemic disease have better prognoses and are better candidates for more aggressive management. Patients with surgically accessible lesions and otherwise favorable prognosis should undergo tumor resection followed by whole-brain radiation therapy. Those with inaccessible lesions but otherwise good prognosis should undergo stereotactic radiosurgery. Patients with poor prognosis should receive palliative whole brain radiotherapy. Unfortunately, most patients with cerebral metastasis have a poor overall prognosis, with most surviving for just a few months.

Primary brain tumors

Glial tumors

Glial tumors are the most common primary intracranial neoplasms. High-grade gliomas, including glioblastoma multiforme and high-grade oligodendrogliomas,

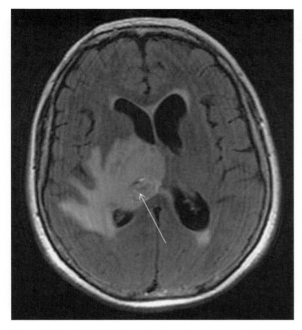

Figure 23.1 Axial fluid attenuation inversion recovery (FLAIR) MRI showing metastasis (arrow) with large amounts of surrounding cerebral edema.

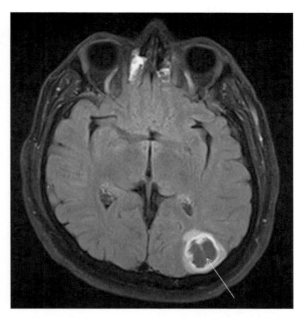

Figure 23.2 Contrast-enhanced T1-weighted MRI of a high-grade glial tumor showing a hypodense occipital lesion with a ring of surrounding enhancement and scant edema (arrow).

are typically hypodense on T1-weighted images and enhance heterogeneously (Figure 23.2). Common presentations include headache and seizures. The diagnosis must be made by examining tissue, either by stereotactic biopsy or at the time of resection. Unfortunately, high-grade gliomas have a poor prognosis. Patients who choose aggressive therapy should be treated with a combination of maximal resection, adjuvant radiation therapy, and temozolomide.

Low-grade gliomas are unlike many other brain tumors in that they often exert minimal mass effect. They have a propensity to produce refractory seizures, which often brings them to clinical attention (Chapter 20). Optimal management of low-grade gliomas is not entirely clear. Because they may transform into higher-grade tumors, aggressive treatment including surgical resection and radiotherapy would seem to be the most reasonable approach. However, some low-grade gliomas follow a fairly benign course and may be followed with serial MRI every 3 months, with surgery being reserved for patients with tumor growth or transformation.

Meningiomas

Meningiomas are the second most common primary intracranial tumors. They are often asymptomatic, but some come to clinical attention by producing headaches, seizures, or focal neurological findings. Radiologically, meningiomas are typically dural-based masses that enhance homogeneously with contrast (Figure 23.3). Asymptomatic meningiomas may be followed with serial MRI, initially every 6–12 months. When possible, symptomatic meningiomas and those that show evidence of expansion should be removed surgically. Patients with surgically accessible higher-grade lesions should undergo postoperative radiation therapy, while those with inaccessible lesions should be treated with radiotherapy.

Primary CNS lymphoma

Primary CNS lymphoma (PCNSL) usually presents with headaches or focal neurological findings. They are most commonly solitary, invasive, periventricular lesions. A classic but uncommon radiographic finding is crossing of the corpus callosum. Lymphomas are extremely sensitive to steroids, and for this reason, steroids may obscure the diagnosis and should not be administered until PCNSL is confirmed histologically. The mainstay of treatment of PCNSL is chemotherapy with systemic methotrexate. Although adding radiation therapy to methotrexate may improve survival, this combination may be quite toxic and should be considered with extreme caution, especially in older patients.

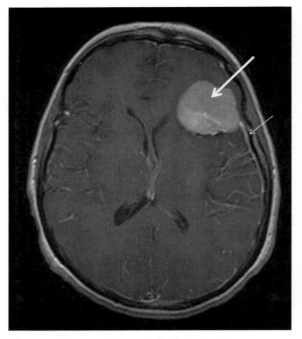

Figure 23.3 Contrast-enhanced T1-weighted MRI of a meningioma showing a homogeneously enhancing mass (thick arrow). Note the dural tail (thin arrow), a helpful sign in diagnosing meningioma.

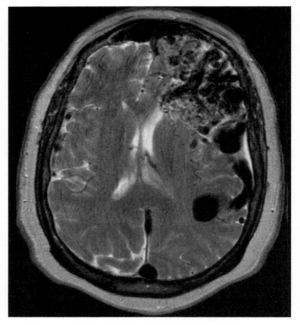

Figure 23.4 T2-weighted axial MRI showing large frontoparietal arteriovenous malformation. The flow voids seen on T2 resemble a "ball of worms."

Arteriovenous malformations

Arteriovenous malformations (AVMs) produce a variety of symptoms including hemorrhages, seizures, headaches, and focal neurological signs such as hemiparesis or visual field cuts. They often present for the first time in childhood or young adulthood. The annual risk for hemorrhage from AVMs is approximately 2–3%, and 20% of these hemorrhages will be fatal.[4] Beyond imaging studies, little is generally needed to make a diagnosis of an AVM: the vascular flow voids, which resemble a ball of worms on MRI, are pathognomonic (Figure 23.4). Decisions concerning management of AVMs depend on their size, location, and the presence of deep venous drainage (Table 23.1). In general, lesions with a Spetzler–Martin grade of I, II, or III should undergo microvascular surgery, endovascular surgery, or radiosurgery.[4] Procedures for grade IV and V AVMs are associated with high morbidities, and decisions about intervention should be made very carefully based on the experience and comfort level of the neurosurgeon.

Abscesses

Intracranial abscesses are life-threatening infections, which are usually acquired via direct spread (e.g.

head trauma, neurosurgery, or sinus infection) or as a result of hematogenous dissemination of an infection elsewhere. Headache is the most common sign of abscess. Because fever is present inconsistently, the diagnosis is often missed because it is not considered. In more severe cases, abscesses may produce seizures or encephalopathy. The preferred neuroimaging study for evaluating abscesses is MRI with contrast, which characteristically shows a ring-enhancing lesion. The diagnosis is established via brain biopsy, with blood cultures playing a potentially important role prior to tissue confirmation. Common causes of abscesses in immunocompetent patients include Gram-positive cocci, Gram-negative rods, and anaerobic bacteria. Empiric therapy should be designed with the assistance of an infectious disease specialist, and usually includes a combination of vancomycin, ceftriaxone or cefotaxime, and metronidazole. Surgical drainage of the abscess is definitive.

Tumefactive multiple sclerosis

Multiple sclerosis (MS) may produce demyelinating lesions that resemble gliomas both clinically and radiographically. This so-called tumefactive MS leads to symptoms that are otherwise unusual in MS, including

Table 23.1 Spetzler–Martin arteriovenous malformation grading scale[5]

Size	
0–3.0 cm	1
3.1–6.0 cm	2
>6.0 cm	3
Location	
Noneloquent	0
Eloquent	1
Deep venous drainage	
Absent	0
Present	1

The Spetzler–Martin grade is obtained by adding the numbers in the second column.

seizures and headache. Although there are no radiological features that reliably distinguish between glioma and tumefactive MS, findings that are more consistent with MS include young age of onset, the presence of multiple lesions, and minimal perilesional edema.[6] In patients with known MS, it may be appropriate to perform magnetic resonance spectroscopy to differentiate between tumefactive MS and glioma.[7] Unfortunately, brain biopsy is the only definitive way to make the diagnosis.

Sellar region masses

Masses in the sellar region are often noted as incidental findings in patients with nonspecific headache. In other patients, sellar masses are first detected when ocular motor abnormalities, visual field cuts, or hypothalamic–pituitary dysfunction develop. Approximately 90% of pituitary masses in adults are adenomas.[8] Less common masses include craniopharyngioma, meningioma, metastases, abscesses, and cysts. Unfortunately, it is often difficult to distinguish among these masses radiographically. Although biopsy is the definitive way to diagnose a sellar region mass, the first step in the evaluation is to classify the mass by size, prolactin level, and whether it is causing any neuro-ophthalmologic abnormalities[9]:

- Masses that secrete prolactin are prolactinomas, and should be treated with dopamine agonists.
- Masses that secrete hormones other than prolactin are functional adenomas, and should undergo excision.
- Masses that produce neuro-ophthalmologic abnormalities should undergo excision.

- Masses that are smaller than 10 mm and that do not produce neuro-ophthalmologic abnormalities should be re-evaluated with MRI at 1 year. If there is no growth, repeat imaging studies only if neuro-ophthalmologic or endocrine symptoms develop.
- Tumors larger than 10 mm that do not produce neuro-ophthalmologic abnormalities should be evaluated with MRI at 6 months and then yearly if no growth is observed.

The assistance of an endocrinologist should be obtained in all but the most straightforward of cases.

Cerebellopontine angle masses

The most common presentation of a cerebellopontine angle (CPA) mass is hearing loss due to compression of the vestibulocochlear nerve. Because most CPA lesions grow slowly, compression of the vestibular portion of this nerve does not usually produce frank vertigo, but patients may complain of a mild sensation of feeling off balance. Other structures in the CPA that may be compressed include the trigeminal nerve, facial nerve, cerebellum, and brainstem.

Vestibular schwannomas (acoustic neuromas) account for the majority of CPA tumors. In patients with neurofibromatosis type 2, these tumors are bilateral. Meningiomas represent a small but important minority, and other masses such as cholesteatomas, gliomas, and metastases are uncommon. Decisions concerning treatment of a CPA tumor depend on the size of the tumor, its histology, and the symptom burden it produces. Surgical resection is the best approach for patients with large, symptomatic tumors. Because vestibular schwannomas and meningiomas grow slowly, patients with smaller, minimally symptomatic tumors may be followed with serial MRI scans every 6–12 months, or sooner if symptoms progress.

Masses in immunocompromised patients

AIDS patients, bone marrow transplant recipients, and other immunocompromised patients are susceptible to intracranial mass lesions that do not affect immunocompetent people. The two most important of these are toxoplasmosis and PCNSL. Fungal abscesses are also relatively specific to immunocompromised patients. Obviously, when evaluating an immunosuppressed patient with an intracranial mass lesion, it is

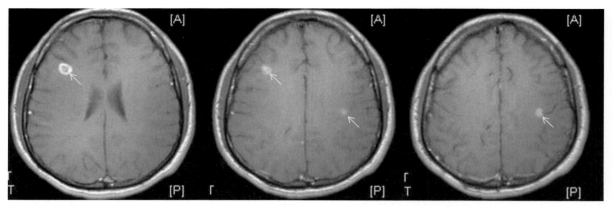

Figure 23.5 Multiple contrast-enhancing T1 lesions, some of which are ring-enhancing, in a patient with HIV infection and a CD4 count of 90 cells/μl, consistent with toxoplasmosis.

important to not neglect the possibility of masses that affect immunocompetent patients including primary and metastatic tumors.

Toxoplasmosis and primary CNS lymphoma

Toxoplasmosis (caused by reactivation of infection with the protozoan parasite *Toxoplasma gondii*) and PCNSL are the two intracranial masses that should be considered first in immunosuppressed patients. Both lesions occur in patients with CD4 counts lower than 100 cells/μl. Radiographic features may help to differentiate between the two, but are not entirely reliable: toxoplasma lesions are more likely to be multiple and to have a ring-enhancing pattern (Figure 23.5), while PCNSL is more likely to be a solitary mass and to involve or cross the corpus callosum. The usual protocols to differentiate between toxoplasmosis and PCNSL are:

- In stable patients, treat toxoplasmosis empirically with pyrimethamine (200 mg loading dose followed by 75 mg/day) and sulfadiazine (1.5–2 mg/kg qid) for 2 weeks. If the lesions decrease in size on repeat MRI, the diagnosis is toxoplasmosis, and appropriate treatment should be continued with the guidance of an infectious disease specialist. If the lesions do not decrease in size, arrange for brain biopsy.
- In patients with severe mass effect and impending herniation, initiate dexamethasone (10 mg × 1 followed by 4 mg qid) and arrange for diagnostic brain biopsy and resection of the mass.

Fungal abscesses

In addition to the typical organisms that form intracranial abscesses in immunocompetent patients, immunocompromised patients are also susceptible to abscess formation by fungi such as *Aspergillus*, *Candida albicans*, *Coccidioides immitis*, and *Cryptococcus neoformans*. Evaluation of a suspected fungal abscess should include fungal blood cultures and spinal fluid analysis, provided that the abscess is not producing substantial mass effect. Treatment should be conducted with the supervision of an infectious disease specialist. Unfortunately, the outcome of fungal abscesses in immunocompromised patients is poor.

Masses in patients from the tropics and developing world

Neurocysticercosis

Infection with the pork tapeworm *Taenia solium* leading to neurocysticercosis is common in Latin America, Africa, and Asia. Although understanding the transmission and entire life cycle of the organism is helpful in managing the disorder, the two stages that are clinically relevant to the neurologist are active cysts and calcified cysts. Active cysts leading to seizures are the best-known neurological manifestation of neurocysticercosis (Chapter 20). Calcified cysts are usually asymptomatic and are noted only incidentally upon neuroimaging for other indications (Figure 23.6). Neurocysticercosis may also lead to ventricular obstruction, which in turn produces headaches and increased intracranial pressure. Both MRI and CT are used to diagnose neurocysticercosis. Active lesions enhance on MRI, and in some of tuberculoma is quite variable: the most common appearance is a mass lesion with a T2-hypointense core and hyperintense rim, with approximately two-thirds of patients having more than one and sometimes numerous lesions.[11] Treatment of tuberculoma includes a four-drug regimen (isoniazid, pyrazinamide, rifampin, and either ethambutol or streptomycin) supervised by an infectious disease specialist. Lesions that produce severe mass effect may require neurosurgical intervention.

References

1. Bernstein M, Berger M. *Neuro-oncology: the Essentials*. New York: Thieme; 2008.

2. Delattre JY, Krol G, Thaler HT, Posner JB. Distribution of brain metastases. *Arch Neurol* 1988;**45**:741–744.

3. Glantz MJ, Cole BF, Forsyth PA, et al. Practice parameter: anticonvulsant prophylaxis in patients with newly diagnosed brain tumors. *Neurology* 2000;**54**:1886–1893.

4. Ogilvy S, Stieg PE, Awad I, et al. Recommendations for the management of intracranial arteriovenous malformations: a statement for healthcare professionals from a special writing group of the Stroke Council, American Stroke Association. *Stroke* 2001;**32**:1458–1471.

5. Spetzler RF, Martin NA. A proposed grading system for arteriovenous malformations. *J Neurosurg* 1986;**65**:476–483.

6. Giang DW, Poduri KR, Eskin TA, et al. Multiple sclerosis masquerading as a mass lesion. *Neuroradiology* 1992;**34**:150–154.

7. Butteriss DJA, Ismail A, Ellison DW, Birchall D. Use of serial proton magnetic resonance spectroscopy to differentiate low grade glioma from tumefactive plaque in a patient with multiple sclerosis. *Br J Radiol* 2003;**76**:662–665.

8. Freda PU, Post KD. Differential diagnosis of sellar masses. *Endocrinol Metabol Clin North Am* 1999;**28**: 81–117.

9. Serhal D, Weil RJ, Hamrahian AH. Evaluation and management of pituitary incidentalomas. *Clev Clin J Med* 2008;**75**:793–801.

10. Carpio A, Kelvin EA, Bagiella E, et al. Effects of albendazole treatment on neurocysticercosis: a randomised controlled trial. *J Neurol Neurosurg Psychiatry* 2008;**79**:1050–1055.

11. Wasay M, Kheleani BA, Moolani MK, et al. Brain CT and MRI findings in 100 consecutive patients with intracranial tuberculoma. *J Neuroimaging* 2003;**13**:240–247.

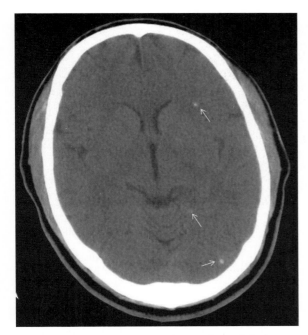

Figure 23.6 Noncontrast head CT showing three calcified cysts (arrows) in a patient with neurocysticercosis.

cases, a scolex of the organism may be visible. CT is better suited for identifying calcified cysts. The diagnosis is confirmed by finding a positive enzyme-linked immunoelectrotransfer blot assay result in the serum. Treat patients with active lesions with albendazole 800 mg for 8 days with close infectious disease consultation; patients with multiple lesions and those that produce ventricular obstruction may require longer courses of treatment.[10] When initiating albendazole, be sure to include a rapid prednisone taper, as antiparasitic agents may produce a life-threatening inflammatory response as the organisms die. Supportive care is an important component of treating neurocysticercosis: patients with seizures should be treated with anticonvulsants and those with ventricular obstruction may require neurosurgical intervention.

Tuberculoma

Hematogenous seeding of *Mycobacterium tuberculosis* may lead to an accumulation of organisms in the brain known as a tuberculoma. This is particularly common in patients from the Indian subcontinent and East Asia. Tuberculomas are often clinically silent, but may also produce a wide variety of serious neurological problems including seizures, headache, stroke, and meningitis (Chapter 1). The radiographic appearance

Index